AF556841

CHEMOTHERAPY

Volume 7
Cancer Chemotherapy I

CHEMOTHERAPY

Volume 1 **Clinical Aspects of Infections**
Prophylaxis; life-threatening infections; infection in leukaemia; surgical infection; anaerobic infection; respiratory and urinary tract infections; amikacin.

Volume 2 **Laboratory Aspects of Infections**
Sensitivity testing; assay methods; animal models of infection; sisomycin; tobramycin.

Volume 3 **Special Problems in Chemotherapy**
Tuberculosis; genital tract infections; antibiotic resistance and mode of action; topical chemotherapy and antisepsis.

Volume 4 **Pharmacology of Antibiotics**
Tissue concentrations; pharmacokinetics; untoward effects of antibiotics.

Volume 5 **Penicillins and Cephalosporins**
Penicillins and cephalosporins; betalactamases; new agents.

Volume 6 **Parasites, Fungi, and Viruses**
Parasitic infections; fungal infections; chemotherapy of viruses; co-trimoxazole.

Volume 7 **Cancer Chemotherapy I**
Symposia – new drugs and approaches; cell and pharmacokinetics; potentiators of radiotherapy; in vitro screening systems; immunological aspects.

Volume 8 **Cancer Chemotherapy II**
Free papers – new drugs and approaches; cell and pharmacokinetics; mechanisms of action; new analogues; cancer chemotherapy of specific organs.

CHEMOTHERAPY

Volume 7
Cancer Chemotherapy I

Edited by
K. Hellmann
Westminster Hospital
and Imperial Cancer Research Fund

and
T. A. Connors
Chester Beatty Research Institute

Plenum Press · New York and London

Library of Congress Cataloging in Publication Data

International Congress of Chemotherapy, 9th, London, 1975.
Cancer chemotherapy I-

(Chemotherapy; v. 7-)
1. Cancer–Chemotherapy–Congresses. I. Hellmann, Kurt. II. Connors, T. A., 1934- III. Title. IV. Series.
RM260.2.C45 vol. 7, etc. [RC271.C5] 615'58s [616.9'94'061] 76-1944
ISBN 0-306-38227-X

Proceedings of the Ninth International Congress of Chemotherapy held in London, July, 1975 will be published in eight volumes, of which this is volume seven.

A Division of Plenum Publishing Corporation
227 West 17th Street, New York, N. Y. 10011

United Kingdom edition published by Plenum Press, London
A Division of Plenum Publishing Company, Ltd.
Davis House (4th Floor), 8 Scrubs Lane, Harlesden, London, NW10 6SE, England

Printed in the United States of America

CHEMOTHERAPY

Proceedings of the
9th International Congress of Chemotherapy
held in London, July, 1975

Editorial Committee

K. Hellmann, *Chairman* (Anticancer)
Imperial Cancer Research Fund, London.

A. M. Geddes (Antimicrobial)
East Birmingham Hospital.

J. D. Williams (Antimicrobial)
The London Hospital Medical College.

Congress Organising Committee

International Society
of Chemotherapy Executive - to July 1975

Preface

The International Society of Chemotherapy meets every two years to review progress in chemotherapy of infections and of malignant disease. Each meeting gets larger to encompass the extension of chemotherapy into new areas. In some instances, expansion has been rapid, for example in cephalosporins, penicillins and combination chemotherapy of cancer - in others slow, as in the field of parasitology. New problems of resistance and untoward effects arise; reduction of host toxicity without loss of antitumour activity by new substances occupies wide attention. The improved results with cancer chemotherapy, especially in leukaemias, are leading to a greater prevalence of severe infection in patients so treated, pharmacokinetics of drugs in normal and diseased subjects is receiving increasing attention along with related problems of bioavailability and interactions between drugs. Meanwhile the attack on some of the major bacterial infections, such as gonorrhoea and tuberculosis, which were among the first infections to feel the impact of chemotherapy, still continue to be major world problems and are now under attack with new agents and new methods.

From this wide field and the 1,000 papers read at the Congress we have produced Proceedings which reflect the variety and vigour of research in this important field of medicine. It was not possible to include all of the papers presented at the Congress but we have attempted to include most aspects of current progress in chemotherapy.

We thank the authors of these communications for their cooperation in enabling the Proceedings to be available at the earliest possible date. The method of preparation does not allow for uniformity of typefaces and presentation of the material and we hope that the blemishes of language and typographical errors do not detract from the understanding of the reader and the importance of the Proceedings.

K. HELLMANN, Imperial Cancer Research Fund
A. M. GEDDES, East Birmingham Hospital
J. D. WILLIAMS, The London Hospital Medical College

Contents

ADVANCES IN CANCER CHEMOTHERAPY

Emil Frei III

Director and Physician-in-Chief

Sidney Farber Cancer Center, Boston, Mass, USA

INTRODUCTION

Like all therapeutics, cancer chemotherapy began as a largely emperical effort with a major emphasis on the interplay between serendipity and screening. The first major point I would like to make in this presentation is that a scientific base for cancer chemotherapy and for the construction of clinical trials has developed rapidly in the past five to 15 years. Basic research on the nature of the neoplastic cell has provided an increasing number of leads with respect to therapeutic targets exploitable by chemotherapy and immunotherapy (Fig. 1). The sciences of pharmacology and its subsets and of cytokinetics and biostatistics, which some refer to as "bridging sciences", now impinge daily and importantly on the development and application of chemotherapeutic programs to man (Fig. 1). I would like to cite one important recent example that relates to structure activity studies.

Drug Development. One of the most important classes of antitumor agents are the anthracyclines (Fig. 2)(1). Adriamycin was introduced into the clinic four years ago and has substantial antitumor activity, not only in the hematologic neoplasms, but also in carcinomas and sarcomas (2). Adriamycin has a substantially superior therapeutic index in experimental systems and in man as compared to daunorubicin. Since the difference between these two compounds relates only to substitution on the 14 carbon further manipulation of this position seemed rational. The amino group of the aminosugar (Fig. 2) has been proposed, on the

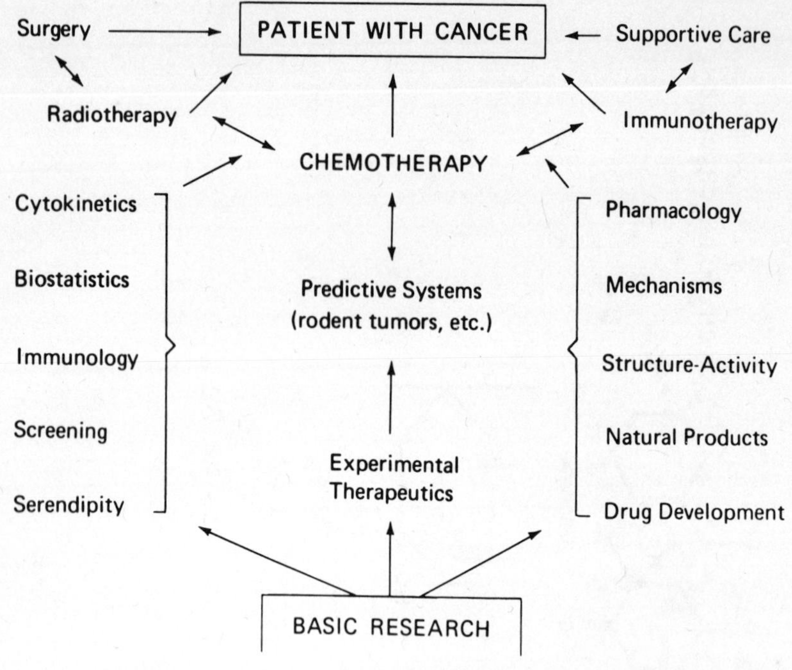

FIGURE 1
Chemotherapy: Relation to Clinical and basic disiplines.

basis of biochemical and by x-ray diffraction studies, to anchor the tetracycline portion of the molecule which intercalates between nucleotide base pairs in DNA to the phosphodiester exoskeleton of the DNA molecule (3). Hence manipulation of the amino group was also studied. Systematic substitutions in both of these positions led to the development of a compound known as AD 32, which has a 5 carbon ester substituted in the 14 position and in which the positive charge of the amino group in the amino sugar is reduced by a trifluoroacetyl substitution. At optimal that is, at equitoxic doses, AD 32 is superior to adriamycin with respect to both increasing the life span and curing the tumor bearing animals (Fig. 3). While these results remain to be confirmed, they provide an example of a rational, semiempirical approach to the development of a new compound.

Multimodality Therapy (Adjuvant Chemotherapy). The second major point I would like to make relates to multimodality treatment of cancer with particular emphasis on

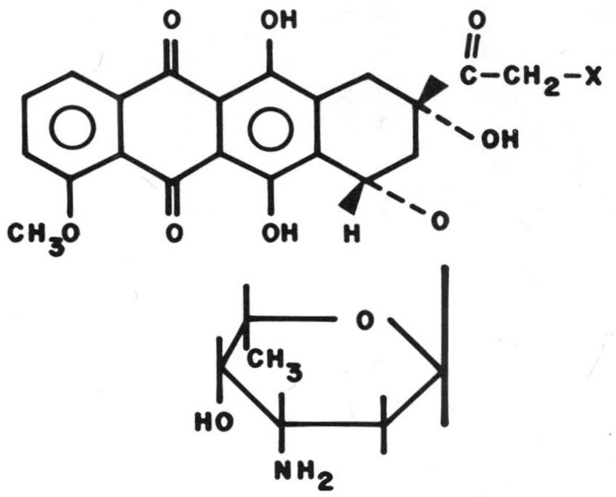

Daunorubicin: $X = H$
Adriamycin: $X = OH$

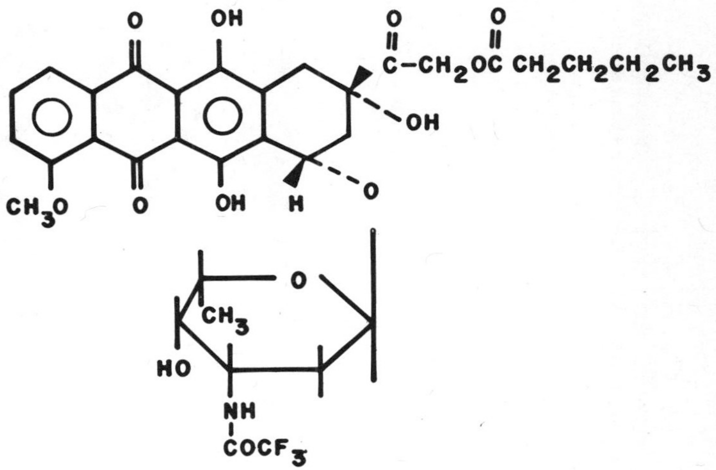

AD 32

FIGURE 2

Structural relationship between daunorubicin, adriamycin and AD 32

Mouse Leukemia	Drug	Optimal Dose mg/kg/day, ip days 1-4	Increase in Median Life Span (%)	"Cure"*
L1210	Adriamycin	4	45	0/5
	AD 32	60	445+	4/5
P388	Adriamycin	4	132	0/6
	AD 32	40	429	4/5'

*"Cure" = 30 day tumor-free survivors, expressed as a fraction of surviving/treated leukemic mice

FIGURE 3
Effect of Adriamycin Analog N-Trifluoroacetyl-14-Valerate (SFCC AD 32) on Experimental Leukemias.

DISEASE	SCHEMA PRIMARY	CONTROL OF PRIMARY ACHIEVED WITH	SYSTEMIC METASTASES (MICROSCOPIC) %	SYSTEMIC METASTASES (MICROSCOPIC) LOCATION	SYSTEMIC (ADJUVANT) CHEMOTHERAPY
Breast Cancer Stage II	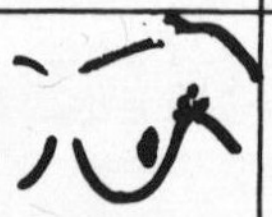	Surg. + XRT	70	Liver, Lung, Bones	Designed to eradicate microscopic disease
Osteosarcoma	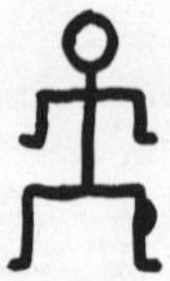	Amputation	90	Lungs	

FIGURE 4
Adjuvant Chemotherapy

the concept of adjuvant chemotherapy, that is, chemotherapy employed immediately following primary treatment with surgery and/or radiotherapy (Fig. 4). For examples of adjuvant chemotherapy I will employ osteogenic sarcoma and Stage II breast cancer. In both of these diseases the primary can usually be totally eradicated by surgery and/ or radiotherapy. Unfortunately, at the time that such treatment is applied approximately 70% of patients with Stage II breast cancer have blood borne microscopic metastases usually in the lungs, liver and/or bones. For patients with osteogenic sarcoma, the respective figure is 90%, and such microscopic metastases are present almost exclusively in the lungs. The classical approach has been to hope that a given patient was in the 10 or 30% of patients who did not have blood borne metastases and, therefore, to wait. The approach that I am about to present involves the use of systemic treatment or adjuvant treatment with chemotherapy, immunotherapy or both in an effort to eradicate microscopic metastases.

There is strong experimental basis for such studies. These are presented in abbreviated form in Fig. 5. First, it has been known since the studies of Goldin and thoroughly quantified in recent years by Schabel that, for any given effective treatment, microscopic tumor in rodents can frequently be cured whereas the same tumor allowed to advance until it is grossly evident, may undergo transient regression only (4). The number of tumor cells in a patient with microscopic disease, is estimated to be less than 10^9 whereas for overt metastases greater than $5x10^9$ cells must be present (5). In homogeneous *in vivo* experimental systems it has been demonstrated that destruction of tumor cells by chemotherapy follows first order kinetics (4). Thus, it is the fractional reduction of tumor cells by a given treatment rather than the absolute reduction that tends to be constant. Because of this, exponential considerations become paramount, and it is evident that a given treatment has a far greater likelihood of destroying, for example, 10^5 as compared to 10^{10} neoplastic cells. Employing sophisticated cytokinetic studies, it has been demonstrated that as tumors increase in size, the growth fraction, that is the proportion of cells in mitotic cycle decreases (4). It has been demonstrated that cells not in cycle are not necessarily end stage cells and may re-enter cycle when transplanted into syngeneic rodent systems. Since almost all of our drugs have varingly greater potency against cycling as compared to noncycling cells, the high growth fraction for microscopic tumor makes such tumor much more vulnerable to chemotherapeutic attack. Recent *in vivo* studies indicate

	Disseminated Metastases	
	Microscopic	Overt (bulk)
Transplanted tumor response to chemo.	Frequency cured	Rarely cured
No. of tumor cells First order Kinetics	$<10^9$ (ca 1 Gm)	$>5 \times 10^9$
Growth Fraction	$>90\%$	$<10\%$
Drug membrane active transport	3-4+	0-1+
pO_2	Normal	↓
Vascular supply	Adequate	Compromised
Competing metabolites	0	?+

FIGURE 5 : Experimental Data Supporting Adjuvant Chemotherapy.

that as a generality, cycling cells have a substantially greater capacity for drug transport than noncycling cells though this may relate simply to the fact that cycling cells are larger and therefore have a larger surface area (5). While the blood supply of microscopic metastases is presumably normal it is frequently comromised in patients with overt metastases and many of the above factors may relate to this compromised blood supply (6). Finally, competing metabolites derived from marginally viable tumor in the center of bulk metastases may prevent antimetabolite effect. In short, experimental models and experimental studies derived from basic and bridging sciences along with well conceived and designed clinical experiments provide a sound basis for the adjuvant approach.

Within the past three years two treatment programs, one involving high dose methotrexate followed by citrovorum rescue and the other, adriamycin, have been shown to be capable of producing tumor regression in 30-50% of patients with advanced metastatic osteosarcoma (7-9). Because of this, starting two to four years ago such treatment was applied in the adjuvant situation, that is immediately following amputation which is usually used to control the primary lesion (10, see references). In the historical control group at the Farber Center and in other

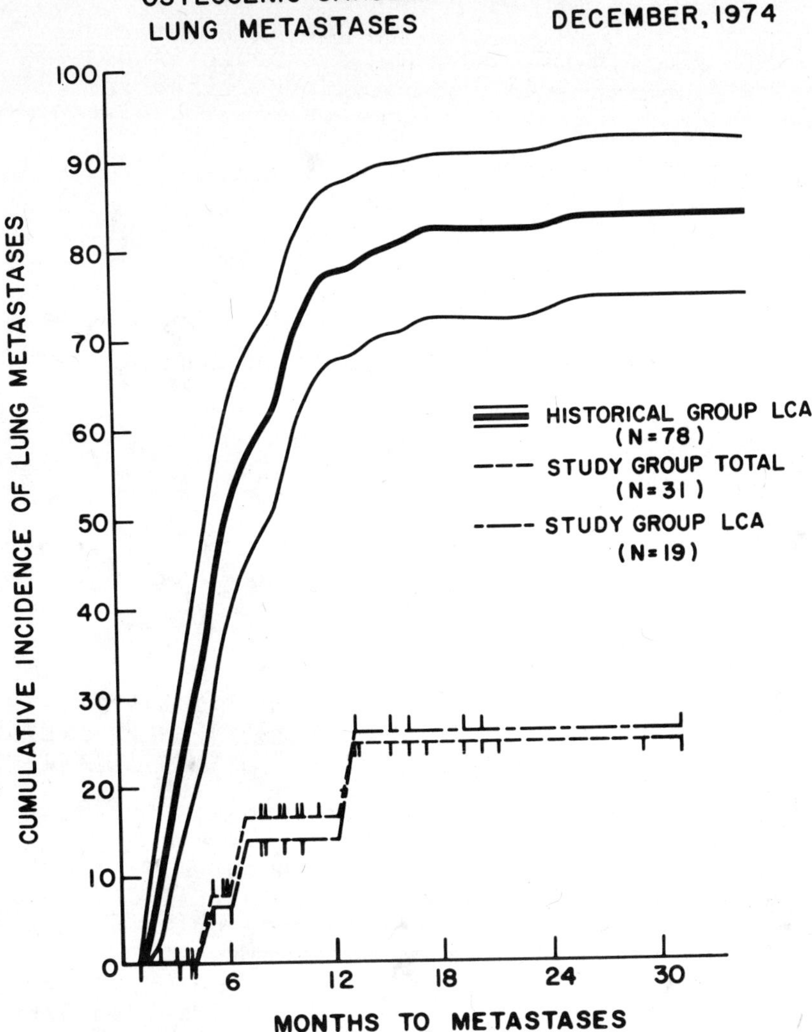

FIGURE 6 : Pulmonary Metastases in Historical and Study Groups (Adapted from Jaffe, et al)

centers such as Memorial-SKI, tumors appear in the lungs after local control has been achieved (Fig. 6). Thus, by six months over 50% have pulmonary metastases and by 12 months 80% of patients have developed pulmonary metastases.

Thus 80 to 90% of patients eventually die of pulmonary metastases. Most of the 10-20% of patients who remain free of metastases at 12 months remain so thereafter and are cured. Our adjuvant treatment program started three years ago. The rate of relapse during the first year was significantly reduced and, as with the controls, relapses did not occur after 12 months though the number of patients was small (Fig 6). In more recent studies employing more advanced principles of combination chemotherapy it has been observed that Mtx-CF rescue combined with adriamycin has reduced the proportion of patients relapsing during the first year in two series to less than 10%. The crucial question in any such study is whether such treatment has simply delayed the development of relapse by suppressing but not eradicating metastases. If such were the case, overt metasteses would continue to appear particularly after cessation of adjuvant treatment. There was evidence from other Centers as well that metastases, if they occurred, tended to occur early and not after 12 months. Patient data from the major Centers employing adjuvant chemotherapy for osteogenic sarcoma was collected and pooled and the relapse after 12 months for those patients who were relapse free 12 months after the initiation of adjuvant treatment was plotted (Fig 7).

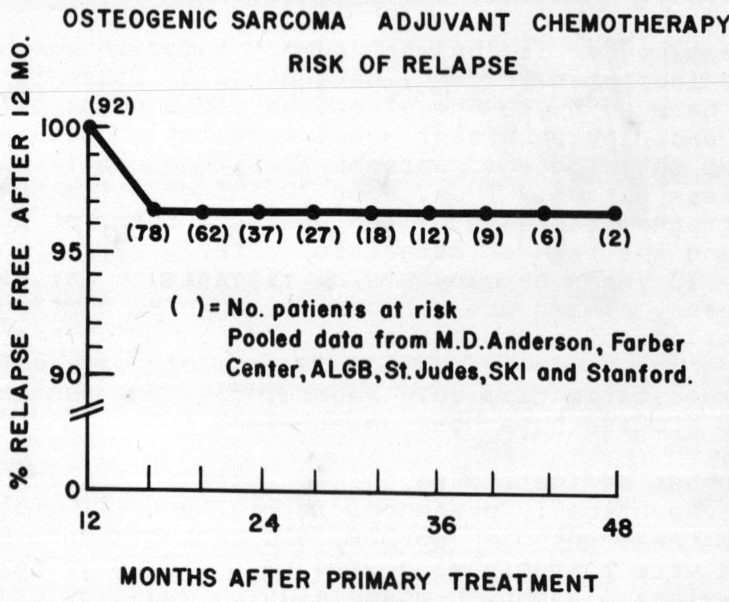

FIGURE 7

From studies at these institutes, 55-95% of patients by life table plot were free of metastases at 12 months and the number at risk falls off progressively up to a total of four years. Two patients relapsed in the 13th month after which there were no further relapse. This curve after 12 months was the same whether the adjuvant treatment was given for a total of only six months following amputation or for as long as 24 months. It thus seems increasingly probable that microscopic metastases in these patients are indeed eradicated and that a substantial increase in cure rate has probably been achieved.

These chemotherapeutic advances in osteogenic sarcoma have lead to preliminary studies involving treatment of the primary. Thus, in selected patients, chemotherapy is initiated prior to operation and depending upon the site of the primary and the degree of reduction in size as the result of chemotherapy, a segment of bone sometimes including a joint is removed and replaced by a titanium prosthesis. The effectiveness of such an approach to controlling the primary and the function of the preserved extremity will require more extended follow-up.

These observations in osteosarcoma have also been demonstrated for Wilm's tumor, Ewing's sarcoma, embryonal rhabdomyosarcoma and Stage IIIB Hodgkin's disease (10, see references). However, these are relatively rare diseases.

Breast cancer is the most common tumor in women and as already indicated (Fig. 4) patients with Stage II breast cancer have a 70% chance of having blood borne metastases as evidenced by recurrent overt metastatic disease. In contrast to osteogenic sarcoma breast cancer is kinetically less active. Thus, some 30-40% of patients will demonstrate metastases by two years, a total of 60% by 5 years and the risk of metastases after 5 years continue so that by 10 years as many at 70% of patients may manifest metastases. There are a number of agents, particularly combinations of chemotherapeutic agents which are capable of producing tumor regression in patients with established overt metastatic disease. Accordingly, adjuvant chemotherapy studies have been undertaken.

A number of institutes collaborated in the comparative study schematically presented in Fig. 8 (11). Following primary treatment with surgery all patients with Stage II disease were randomly allocated to the drug or to placebo. The alkylating agent, L-phenylalanine mustard, or L-PAM was chosen for the initial adjuvant study because it has significant activity against advanced disease and because

ADJUVANT TREATMENT--BREAST CANCER

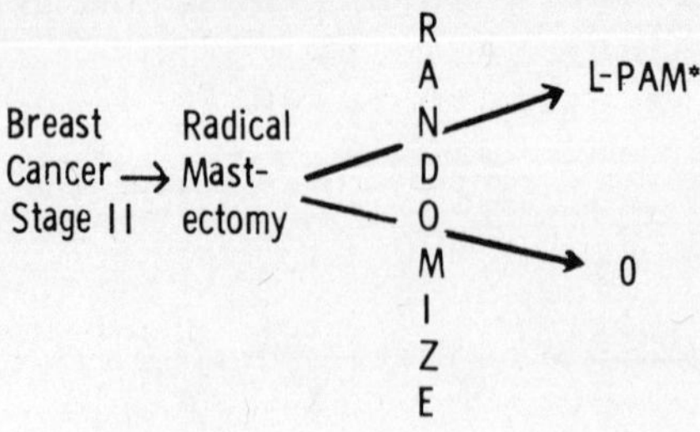

*L-phenylalanine mustard 0.15 mg/kg/day x 5 q 6 wks. for 2 yrs.

FIGURE 8

ADJUVANT TREATMENT--BREAST CANCER

	Relapse by 18 mo.		
	Placebo	L-PAM	
Total patients	24/100	10/96	p=0.01
Premenopausal patients	11/37	1/30	p=0.008
Postmenopausal patients	13/63	7/66	p=>0.05<0.1

Fischer, Carbone et al. Jan '75.

FIGURE 9

it is well tolerated. At the time of this analysis over 269 patients had accrued to the study over a two year period. There were significantly fewer relapses by 18 months for patients receiving adjuvant chemotherapy, a difference which was highly significant for premenopausal patients and suggestively significant for postmenopausal patients (Fig. 9). When this data is presented by life table plot a progressive separation of the curves in favor of L-PAM is apparent and differences calculated using the life table plot are similar.

It is a reasonable assumption that the most effective treatment for patients with advanced metastatic breast cancer will also be more effective when employed in the adjuvant design. Thus while the single drug PAM produces

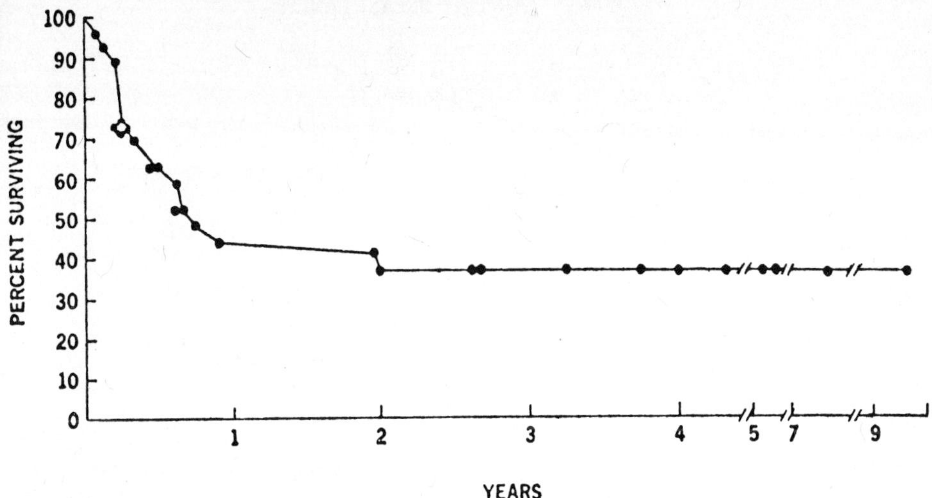

Life-table analysis of survival of entire group of patients with advanced histiocytic lymphoma.

FIGURE 10

an objective response rate in advanced disease of 19% the combination of cytoxan, methotrexate and fluorouracil produces an objective response rate of 53% in such patients (12). An adjuvant study using this combination has been ongoing for almost two years and the risk of relapse is significantly decreased for both pre- and post-menopausal patients (14).

It is predicted that the major advances in definitive treatment other categories of neoplastic disease will result from combined initial therapy with the best local and systemic therapeutic modalities. Thus there are preliminary positive results and major ongoing studies involving surgery and/or radiotherapy plus chemotherapy in such neoplastic disease categories as testicular cancer, ovarian cancer, soft tissue sarcoma and tumors of the gastrointestinal tract.

Combination Chemotherapy. The experimental basis and the clinical extrapolation of the experimental basis for combination chemotherapy has advanced substantially over the past five to 10 years (13,14). The use of agents in combination involves toxicologic, biochemical, pharmacologic, cytokinetic, immunosuppressive and other considerations. The experimental and clinical basis for

RESPONSE ACCORDING TO DIAGNOSIS

IN VA-DIC (SWG 7210) AND CY-VA-DIC (DT 73-02)

DIAGNOSIS	SWG 7210 EVALUABLE	SWG 7210 CR/PR*	SWG 7210 PERCENT RESPONSE+	DT 73-02 EVALUABLE	DT 73-02 CR/PR*	DT 73-02 PERCENT RESPONSE+
Angiosarcoma	7	0/4	57%	5	0/4	80%
Chondrosarcoma	3	0/0	0%	6	0/2	33%
Ewing's Sarcoma	5	1/1	40%	1	0/0	0%
Fibrosarcoma	10	1/5	60%	23	4/9	57%
Leiomyosarcoma	22	0/8	36%	28	2/17	68%
Liposarcoma	15	0/7	47%	10	1/5	60%
Mesothelioma	6	0/0	---	6	0/2	33%
Neurofibrosarcoma	3	1/0	33%	13	3/5	62%
Osteogenic Sarcoma	13	0/3	23%	11	1/2	27%
Rhabdomyosarcoma	9	2/4	67%	15	6/4	67%
Synovial Cell Sarcoma	2	0/1	50%	3	0/2	67%
Undifferentiated Sarcoma	12	4/3	59%	15	2/4	40%
	107	9/36	42%	136	19/56	55%

*CR/PR = Number of complete responders / Number of partial responders

+Percent response = CR + PR / Number of evaluable patients

FIGURE 11

combination chemotherapy have been reviewed. Essentially all of the major effective chemotherapeutic programs involved combinations. There is now convincing evidence in childhood acute leukemia and in patients with disseminated Hodgkin's disease that combination chemotherapy provides definitive treatment. With follow-up studies in excess of 10 years, a substantial and increasing proportion of patients arrived at the flat portion of the relative survival and the disease-free actuarial curves. This has been employed as the definition of cure by Russel and Easson (15) and has been widely accepted. The most common type of non-Hodgkin's lymphoma is diffuse histiocytic lymphoma. This disease, up until the past year, has been considered to be incurable. It has recently been demonstrated and confirmed that those patients who achieve complete remission (40% in Figure 10) and continue in remission two years after the initiation of treatment, remain free of disease with a maximum follow up of 10 years (16). Recent efforts to increase the complete remission rate have been successful and it is hoped that, consistent with the above, this will increase the long-term definitive treatment rate (17).

In summary, combination chemotherapy continues in a state of rapid evolution. In addition to increasing complete remission rates and the duration of complete remission combination chemotherapy may result in curative treatment for some patients with disseminated disease.

An excellent example of the extraordinary rate of progress that can be achieved in a disease with combination chemotherapy is soft tissue sarcoma. Prior to four years ago there was no effective treatment for patients with disseminated soft tissue sarcoma. With the introduction of adriamycin and with experimental and clinical studies indicating synergism between adriamycin and DTIC on the one hand and adriamycin and cyclophosphamide on the other, a series of studies led to a progressive increase in the objective response rate so that now between 40 and 60% of such patients respond (Fig. 11)(18). The median duration of such responses has varied from four to seven months. Perhaps most important is the fact that complete tumor regression is achieved in 5 to 15% of patients and for this group of patients the median duration of response is in excess of two years. Disseminated testicular cancer provides another good example of where combination chemotherapy has resulted in increasing complete remission rate. A substantial proportion of patients in complete remission would appear to remain so indefinitely.

Dose Response Curve. Relatively few clinical trials in responsive tumors have employed dose as a randomized variable. Where this has been done the dose response curve is steep both with respect to host effect and antitumor effect (19). The experimentalists have been emphasizing for years the steepness of the dose response curve for the majority of antitumor agents just as they have been telling us that, for a given treatment program, minimal disease is far more easy to erradicate than bulk disease. One example of the steepness of the dose response curve is that of fluorouracil in the Ridgeway osteogenic sarcoma (Fig. 12). In this study Dr. Schabel employed or adapted clinical criteria. Note that a difference in dose rate of only 20% is enormously important. Thus at 66 mg/kg dose the complete remission rate is

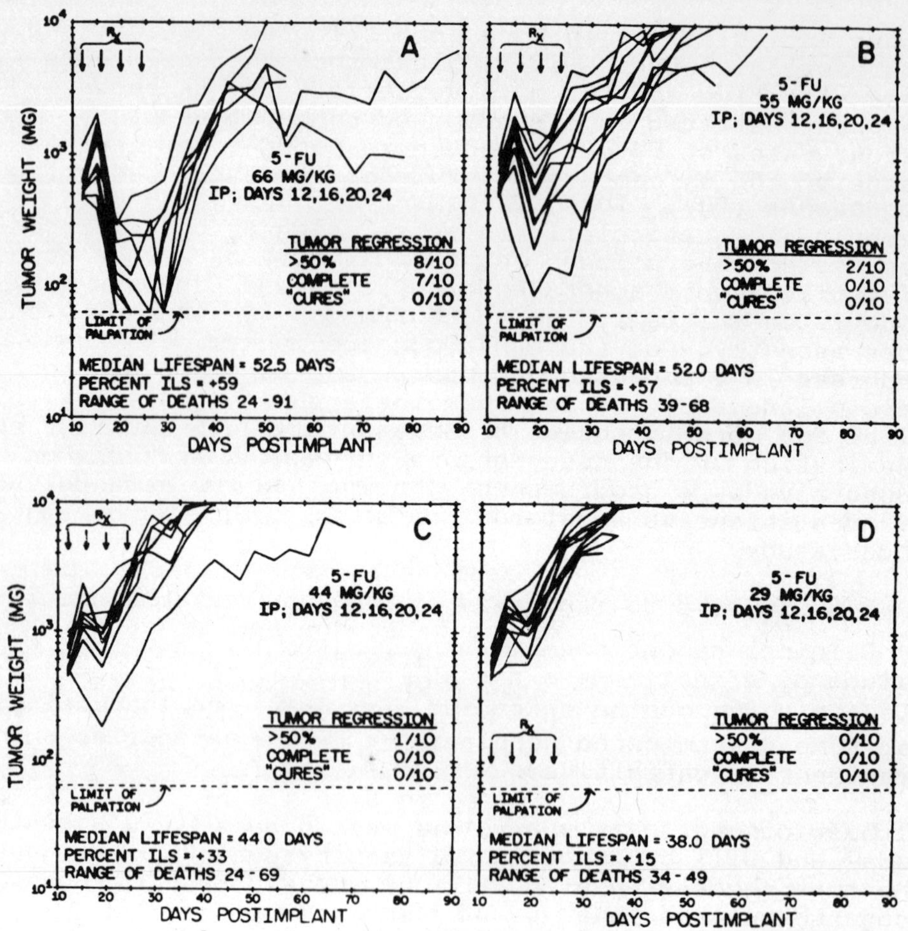

FIGURE 12 Individual tumor response of advanced Ridgway osteogenic sarcoma in a dose-response study with 5-FU. Treatment was begun 12 days post-implant of tumor.

70% whereas at 55 mg/kg it is 0%. Generally similar results are achieved with other classes of antitumor agents and in other experimental tumors (19). Given no loss in therapeutic effect we physicians will gravitate to that program which has the least side effects and is most convenient to the patient. Thus the dose of FU has been progressively reduced, the compound has been given weekly, and it has been administered orally with the general impression that the response rate for colorectal cancer will be in the range of 15-20% regardless of the above variables. With more sophisticated clinical and pharmacologic studies it is clear that the oral route is less effective and far more variable. It has recently been demonstrated in a randomized comparative study that larger doses of FU will produce response rates in the range of 40% as compared to 20% for currently conventional approaches (20). The development of supportive care techniques, particularly those relating to bone marrow depression have allowed for the delivery of larger doses of antileukaemic agents and thus improved complete remission rates initially for acute lymphocytic leukamia, and more recently, for acute myelogenous leukemia. Recent progress in the control of nausea and vomiting of central origin induced by cancer chemotherapeutic agents may allow for more intensive treatment (21). In short, a re-examination of the dose reponse curve with emphasis on supportive care programs which allow for the safe delivery of more intensive treatment for solid tumors is currently under study.

I would like to summarize by re-emphasizing 3 points:

1) Clinical cancer chemotherapy is moving. Both the magnitude of effectiveness and the spectrum of neoplastic disease which can be effectively treated are increasing. For some disseminated neoplastic disease categories such treatment is definitive.

2) Multidisciplinary evaluation and treatment is essential today and will be increasingly so in the future. Perhaps the most compelling example for treatment and therapeutic research relates to adjuvant chemotherapy.

3) Last, but most certainly not least, is the fact that the experimental basis for cancer chemotherapy is provid ing an increasing number of areas for therapeutic research and of hypotheses and leads for application to preclinical systems and to patients.

REFERENCES

1. Di Marco, A., & Lenaz, L. Daunomycin and Adriamycin. In _Cancer Medicine_, Eds. J.F. Holland and E. Frei III, Lea & Febiger, Philadelphia, 1973, pp. 826-835.

2. Blum, R.H. & Carter S.K. A new cancer drug with significant clinical activity. Ann. Internal Med. 80, 249-259, 1974.

3. Pigram, W.J., Fuller, W. & Hamilton, L.D. Stereochemistry of intercalation: interaction of daunomycin with DNA. Nature New Biol. 235: 17-19, 1972.

4. Skipper, H.E., Schabel, F.M. Jr. Quantitative and cytokinetic studies in experimental tumor models. In Cancer Medicine, Eds. J.F. Holland, E. Frei III, Lea & Febiger, Philadelphia, 1973, pp. 629-650.

5. Hakala, M.T. Transport of antineoplastic agents. In Antineoplastic and Immunosuppressive Agents. Chapter 13, pp. 240-269, 1974.

6. Tannock, I.F. The relation between cell proliferation and the vascular system in transplanted mouse mammary tumour. Brit. J. Cancer, 22: 258-273, 1968.

7. Djerassi, I., Rominger, C.J. Kim, J.S. et al. Phase I study of high doses of methotrexate with citrovorum factor in patients with lung cancer. Cancer 30:22-30, 1972.

8. Jaffe, N. Recent advances in the chemotherapy of metastatic osteogenic sarcoma. Cancer 30:1627-1631, 1972.

9. Cortes, E.P., Holland, J.F., Wang, J.J. et al. Doxorubicin in disseminated osteosarcoma. JAMA 221:1132-1138, 1972.

10. Frei, E III, Jaffe, N, Tattersall, M.H.N., Pitman, S. New approaches to cancer chemotherapy with methotrexate New Engl. J. Med. 292: 846-851, April 17, 1975.

11. Fisher, B., Carbone, P., Economou, S.G. et al. l-Phenylalanine mustard (L-PAM) in the management of breast cancer: A report of early findings. New Engl. J. Med. 292:117-122, 1975.

12. Canellos, G.P., Taylor, S.G.III., Band, P. & Pocock, S. Combination chemotherapy for advanced breast cancer: randomized comparison with single drug therapy. Prox. XI Intern. Cancer Congress 3:596, 1974 (abstr.)

13. Frei, E. III. Combination cancer therapy: Presidential address. Cancer Research Vol 32:2593-2607, 1972.

14. Sartorelli, A.C. Combination chemotherapy. Cancer Medicine, Eds. J.F. Holland and E. Frei III, Lea & Febiger, Philadelphia, 1973, pp. 706-716, 1973.

15. Easson, E.C. & Russel, M.H. The cure of Hodgkin's disease. Brit. J. Med. 1:1704-1707, 1963.

16. DeVita, V.T. Jr., Canellos, G.P., Chabner, B. et al. Advanced diffuse histiocytic lymphoma, a potentially curable disease: results with combination chemotherapy Lancet 1:248-250, 1975.

17. Skarin, A., Rosenthal, D., Moloney, W. & Frei, E.III. Treatment of advanced non-Hodgkin's lymphoma (NHL) with bleomycin (B), adriamycin (A), cyclophosphamide (C) and vincristine (O) and prednisone (P)(BACOP), AACR/ASCO Proceedings 15:133, 1974.

18. Gottlieb, J., Baker, L.H., O'Brien, R.M. et al. Adriamycin used alone and in combination in soft tissue and bone sarcomas. Cancer Chemotherapy Reports (In press).

19. Frei, E. III & Freireich, E.J. Progress and perspective in the chemotherapy of acute leukemia. Advances Chemother. 2:269, 1965.

20. Ansfield, F.J. A randomized phase III study of four dosages regimens of 5-fluorouracil - A preliminary report. 11th Annual Meeting of the American Society of Clinical Oncology, Abstract 1014, p. 224, 1975.

21. Sallan, S., Zinberg, N., Frei, E, III. Oral delta-9-tetrahydrocannabinol (THC) in the prevention of vomiting (V) associated with cancer chemotherapy (CC) 66th Annual Meeting of the American Association for Cancer Research, Abstract 575, p. 144, 1975.

EXPERIMENTAL BASIS OF CANCER CHEMOTHERAPY

Norbert Brock

Asta-Werke A.G., Chemische Fabrik

D-4800 Bielefeld 14, Brackwede, West Germany

In the course of its 30 years of development, chemotherapy has acquired a firm place in the treatment of human cancer in addition to the classical methods of surgery and radiation therapy, which have been of considerable benefit in fighting primary tumours. By their very nature, surgery and radiation therapy are local or regional measures. By the time of diagnosis more than two thirds of all malignant tumours have spread beyond their local borders so that therapeutic benefit can only be expected from additional systemic treatment and therefore chemotherapy has its preferential potentialities in such generalized tumour conditions. This conclusion invariably applies irrespective of whether the present drugs are satisfactory or not.

As pharmacologists, we have to restrict ourselves to the field of experimental research, and therefore we can only briefly point out its clinical conclusions, which should eventually be drawn and critically assessed by the clinician. However, close cooperation between pharmacologist and clinician is of utmost importance. Particularly in this intricate field the pharmacologist should supply the clinician with clear-cut data so as to enable him to assess both possibilities of treatment and its limiting risks. Such data can only be obtained under uniform conditions as they are provided by animal experiments.

This paper is to describe the most important pharmacological bases of cancer chemotherapy without going into such details as to discuss all pertinent agents and their actions, especially in view of the great number of agents which are continuously developed, and some of which are rapidly superseded. Therefore, description of fundamental mechanisms, the knowledge of which is indispensable for further efficient and successful development, appears to be most important. At the same time, it opens up new perspectives to future approach.

1.0 Prerequisites of cancer chemotherapy

Cancerous degeneration of body cells is due to irreversible changes in the latter's "genetic information". These changes are defects in organospecific differentiation which are transferred to the daughter cells. Thus the cancer cells represent a mutated, exogenous strain of cells. Therefore any type of treatment such as surgery, irradiation or chemical agents should aim at destroying the cancer cells completely, damaging the body of the host as little as possible. Cancer chemotherapy is hampered by two principal difficulties: The first one, unknown in classical chemotherapy of infectious diseases, is due to the close relationship between cancer cells and normal cells of the host: The biochemical differences between the two cell types are not sufficient to allow a specific chemotherapeutic approach without any risk of toxic lesions to the normal body cells. The second difficulty is that the objects of treatment i.e. the cancer cells, are not at all uniform, but differ greatly from patient to patient: Cancer is a collective term for the most varied types of neoplasms.

Thus it is comprehensible that in spite of numerous advances, the very aim of healing cancer by means of chemical agents has so far only been reached in a few types of tumour.

Malignant tumour growth results from the difference between multiplication and mortality rate of cells. Both processes offer possibilities for a chemotherapeutic approach. Inhibition of cellular multiplication and its underlying biochemical syntheses may be attained by "starvation" of the cells, i.e. by what has been called Ehrlich's atreptic therapy. Damage to, or destruction of, cancer cells - and thus an increased mortality rate of the tumour cells - is aimed at by using oncocidal agents. As early as at the beginning of this century Paul Ehrlich realised that only oncocidal treatment could be expected to produce genuine therapeutic benefit. Since this ideal has so far not yet been reached, a combination of the two possible approaches appears to be useful.

The characteristic feature of the cancer cell is its rapid multiplication, which has been considered an important possibility of cancer chemotherapy, since rapidly growing cells have a high metabolic rate and thus are not only much more susceptible to many cellular poisons than cells at rest, but they are also in particular need of suitable metabolites for the synthesis of essential nucleic acids in nuclei and cytoplasma. The intense search for such cellular poisons and antimetabolites has led to the development of a great number of cytostatic compounds.

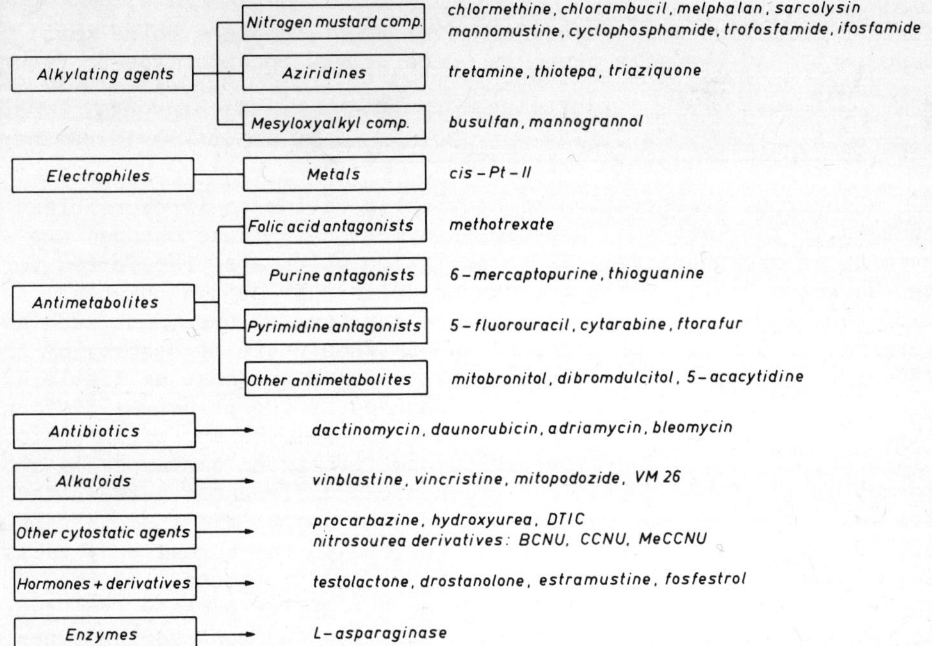

Fig. 1. Pharmacotherapy of cancer

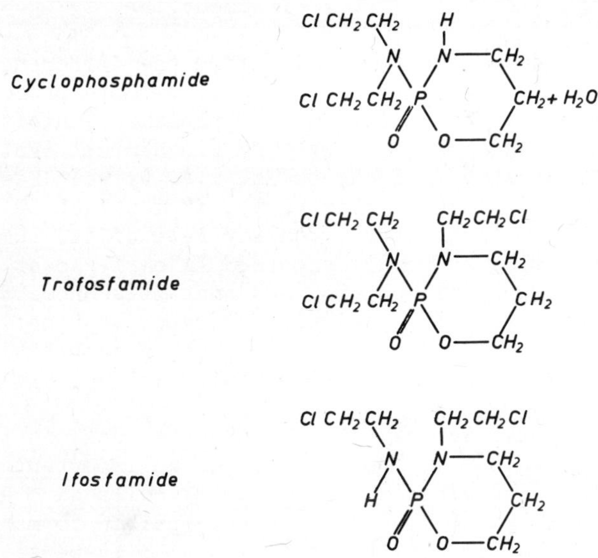

Fig. 2. Structural formulas of cyclophosphamide, trofosfamide, and ifosfamide

2.0 Cytostatic agents as anticancer drugs

Fig. 1. shows the anticancer drugs which are now preferably use and which have been developed by cooperative research groups of many countries. According to their mechanism of action, these drugs can grouped in the following main classes:

Alkylating agents
Antimetabolites
Antibiotics
Alkaloids
Miscellaneous.

The majority of these cytostatics have been tested in animal experiments and in detailed clinical trials. Some recently introduced compounds, which are of major clinical interest or importance for the theoretical conceptual bases of cytostatic treatment, will be described briefly.

From among the group of alkylating agents, the two new oxazaphosphorine derivatives trofosfamide (4) and ifosfamide (3) have acquired definite clinical importance (Fig. 2) (21). Like cyclophosphamide they follow the transport form/active form principle. Trofosfamide has the same pharmacological and clinical spectrum of activity as cyclophosphamide, but it exerts only a relatively slight immunosuppressive effect and is therefore particularly suited for maintenance treatment. Ifosfamide, which shows definitely different antitumour action and metabolic behavious (27), can be given in higher doses because of its reduced toxic cumulation and less pronounced leucotoxicity. Thus clinical remissions were obtained even in cyclophosphamide-resistant tumours.

In the group of anthracycline antibiotics, adriamycin is of particular interest (fig. 3) (14). The only difference between this compound and its parent structure of daunorubicin is in the C14 position, which is hydroxylated in the case of adriamycin. Whereas daunorubicin is only used in haemoblastoses, adriamycin has been proved to be of value also in quite a number of solid tumours, sometimes along with other agents. This difference in clinical action cannot yet be explained on structural grounds.

The nitrosourea derivatives (fig. 4) can pass the blood/brain barrier (29) and thus exert their effect even in primary and especially secondary tumours of the central nervous system. In animal experiments, nitrosourea derivatives have been proved to exert a cytostatic effect on CNS tumours, their significance for the clinical treatment of brain tumours has not yet been definitely confirmed. Some derivatives have gained special important in association with other cytostatics.

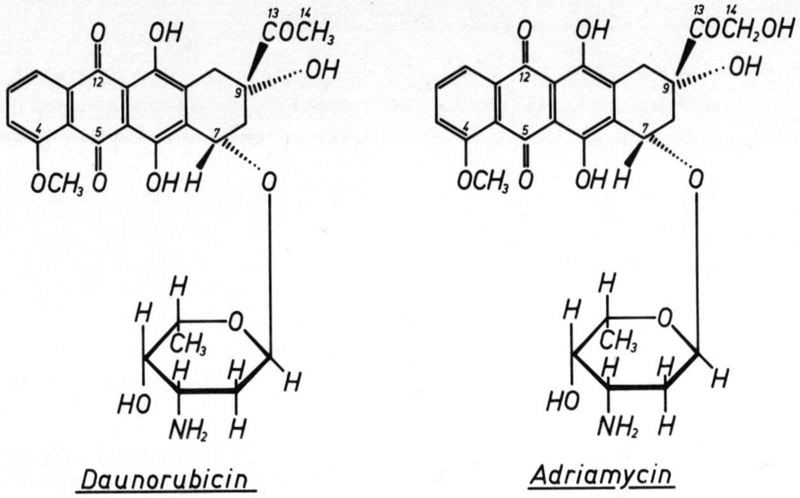

Daunorubicin Adriamycin

Fig. 3. Structural formulas of daunorubin and adriamycin

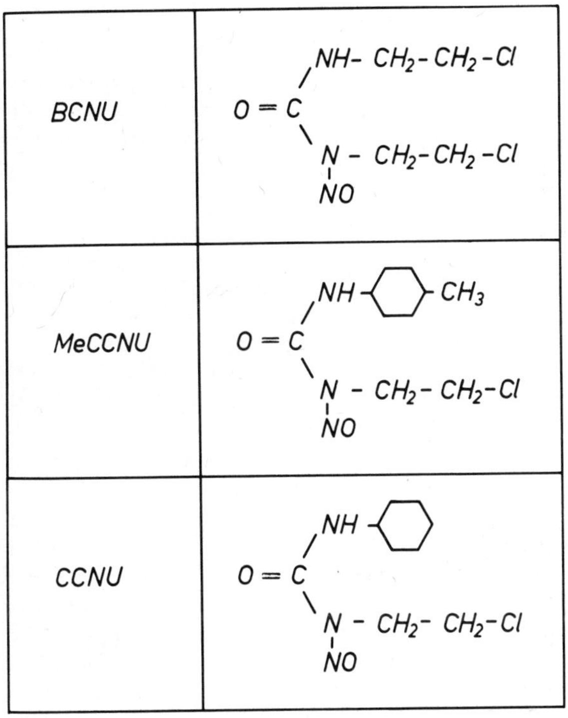

BCNU	$O=C$ (–$NH-CH_2-CH_2-Cl$)(–$N(NO)-CH_2-CH_2-Cl$)
MeCCNU	$O=C$ (–NH–(4-methylcyclohexyl) CH_3)(–$N(NO)-CH_2-CH_2-Cl$)
CCNU	$O=C$ (–NH–cyclohexyl)(–$N(NO)-CH_2-CH_2-Cl$)

Fig. 4. Structural formulas of BCNU, MeCCNU, and CCNU

To increase the selectivity of the cancerotoxic effect, the cytostatics were attached to various carrier molecules such as amino acids, carbohydrates and proteins. However, the increase in selectivity was disappointing. Using DNA as a carrier molecule has also been attempted. e.g. for daunorubicin, adriamycin and actinomycin. The cytostatic/carrier complex is considered to be selectively absorbed by the tumour cell by what has been called pinocytosis, the cytostatic being released under the influence of intracellular lysosomal enzymes. For instance, in Leukaemia L1210 of the mouse, the daunorubicin/DNA complex proved to have a greater therapeutic index than free daunorubicin alone (12). However, these findings have not yet been confirmed clinically.

3.0 Fundamental bases of further development

It is really astonishing that so many different active principle have been discovered without understanding the very nature of cancer and without adequate knowledge of fundamental biochemical differences between cancer cells and the normal host cells. However, most drugs have the drawback of not only damaging the tumour cells, but also the normal proliferation centres of the body such as blood, bone marrow, intestinal epithelium and gonads. Any future development of cancer chemotherapy must therefore aim at increasing the selectivity of the antitumour action. To achieve this it is necessary to base the development of more specific drugs on theoretical concepts and on the results of biophysical and biochemical research. In his paper "Creative ideas and their potentialities in drug research", Wolfgang Heubner, one of the pioneers of modern pharmacology, critically examined this decisive possibility, drawing particular attention to the development of the transport form/active form principle by Druckrey (15). The possibility of organospecific actions has also been proved by inducing cancer by means of nitrosamines and nitrosourea.

In future, pharmacological screening should be conducted with even more systematic consequence so as to "sift the chaff from the wheat" from the very outset. This is not only an essential prerequisite in experimental cancer research, but it is of fundamental importance in any type of pharmacotherapy. If in the past, and occasionally even today, the transfer of results of animal experimentation to man has been queried, it should be emphasized that, like in general pharmacotherapy, all essential advances in cancer chemotherapy have been made by animal experiments. In recent years their possibilities have been considerably increased by widening the tumour spectrum, providing adequate model systems for assessing the drug's antitumour and toxic effects, by elaborating more rigid criteria and using quantitative test methods, especially the dose/action analysis, and by pharmacokinetic studies. Nowadays no new agent should be released for clinical trials unless it has been thoroughly assessed in pharmacotherapeutic tests in animals.

Thorough knowledge of its pharmacological and toxicological properties is even more important in view of the fact that new drugs are nowadays usually administered in the form of polychemotherapy along with other agents, which adds to complicating further action analysis of the individual agent.

4.0 Screening principles and methods of test

The quantitative methods for the assessment of the therapeutic qualities of a new drug are based on experiments in intact animals. In vitro methods - whether biochemical or biological - do not yield any information on the anticancer selectivity of the drug. They may however be useful for the study of specific problems such as that of the mechanism of action.

The quantitative determination of the various therapeutic and toxic actions of a drug in animal experiments should preferably be made by establishing the corresponding dose-action relations. For this purpose it is important to use a clear and simple test for each particular action, which should simulate the physiopathological and clinical conditions as closely as possible. In the pharmacological studies on cytostatics, this has not yet been adequately achieved so far. For instance, a short-term inhibition of tumour growth observed in the experimental animals does not allow an adequately safe assessment of the drug's curative action. Clear-cut and fully reproducible results were only obtained when we used the animals' definite cure as a yardstick, which is considered to be reliable in rats whenever the animals remain free from tumours for a period of 90 days. In more chemoresistant tumours, in which a definite cure cannot be obtained by chemotherapy, the increase in survival time is the essential criterion for assessment of the drug's effect.

For the tests in the intact animals a great number of various tumour types are available as model systems. They were first selected on purely empirical grounds. Nowadays adequate model systems are selected by assessing their effectiveness with regard to certain standard agents. In addition, selection of a model system on the basis of certain biochemical properties or on the type of the affected organ appears to be promising.

The tumours are either grafted onto the experimental animals, or produced by means of carcinogenic agents. For practical reasons, the following types of model systems are distinguished:

(1) Heterologous graft tumours, in which the primary tumours are not grafted in the same, but in a different strain of animals.
(2) Homologous graft tumours, which are invariably regrafted in the same strain.
(3) Autologous tumours, which develop either spontaneously in the experimental animal or which are produced by carcinogenic

agents. The latter method allows to produce highly specific tumours in almost any organ.

Chemosensitivity is most pronounced in heterologous graft tumours in accordance with their great malignancy, whereas it is least pronounce in the less malignant autologous tumours. To obtain comparable conditions and thus ensure reliable results, all studies should be started with graft tumours, and switched over to autologous tumours in a second stage.

Close simulation of clinical conditions is not only an essential requirement for the characterization of the curative action, but also for that of the toxic effects For this purpose, determination of the lethal dose will not be sufficient. The lethal effect is the last of all toxic lesions to occur and it is usually highly complex so that far-reaching conclusions cannot be drawn with regard to clinical conditions. In pharmacotherapeutic analysis the most important toxic actions should be determined separately. The cytostatics are meanwhile known to exert quite a number of organotoxic actions - acute and chronic - which limit their therapeutic use. Of the acute organotoxic actions, leucopenia and immunosuppression should be mentioned, of the chronic ones, the carcinogenic action is of special importance. In future it will be necessary to develop adequate quantitative tests with respect to possible adverse reaction occurring with the heart, lung, kidneys and gonads.

We have developed model systems which allow quantitative determination and comparative assessment of some of these actions. This is of great significance for the pharmacotherapeutic characterization; the more so as therapeutic doses alone are of little value. Reliable comparison, and thus comprehensive assessment of the margin of safety is only possible when the therapeutic doses are related to the toxic doses. The quality of a drug depends on its reliability in producing a definite cure without giving rise to toxic lesions. For the assessment of a drug's chemotherapeutic value we used the therapeutic index, which is the quotient resulting from the LD 5 and CD 95 (fig. 5). However, this index is only valid for a definite type of tumour. The same applies to the D 50 index (LD 50: CD 50). The more the needed therapeutic dose approaches toxic dose levels as they doubtless do in chemotherapy of cancer, the more they must be considered only in relation to the toxic and lethal doses. Therefore Druckrey (17) suggested expressing the administered curative dose as a percentage of the exactly determined medium lethal dose. As non-dimensional quantities, these so-called therapeutic units can be generally applied and allow direct numerical comparison of the potencies of various agents in different types of tumour.

For the quantification of the organo-toxic effects, the danger coefficient has proved of particular value (6). It is determined by the situation of the organotropic regression line in relation to the

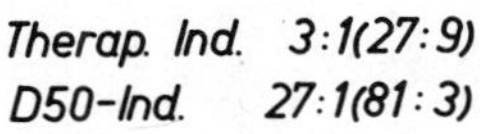

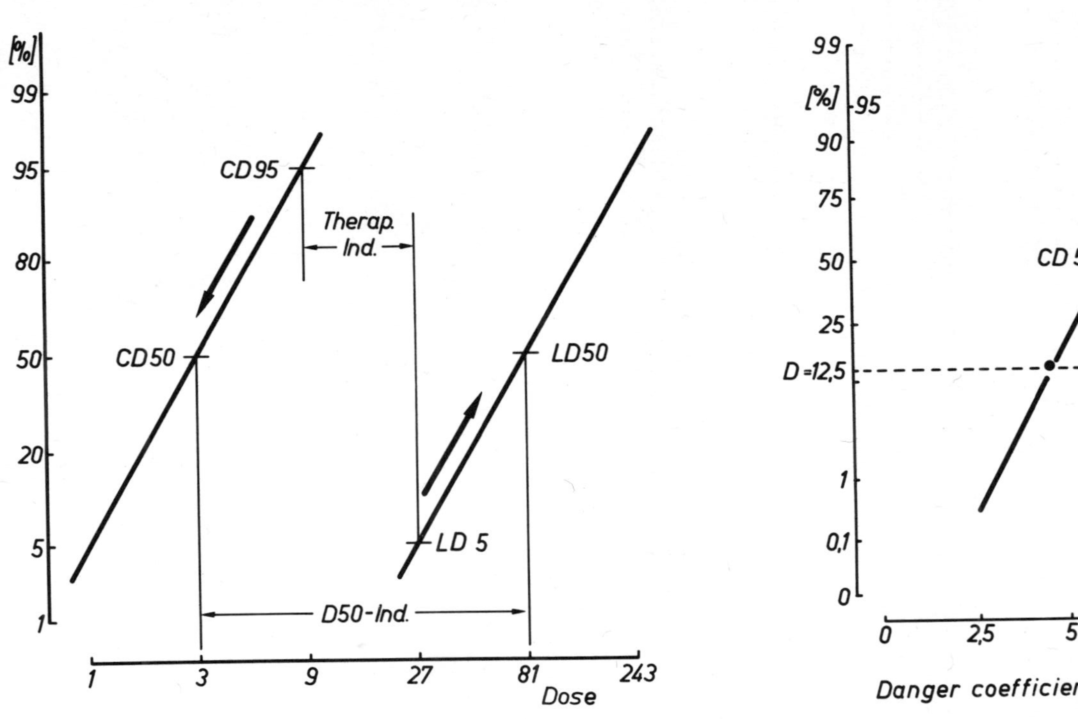

Fig. 5. Determination of the therapeutic index by means of the dose/action regression lines (8)

Fig. 6. Determination of danger coefficient D for the CD95 by means of the curative (CD) and leukotoxic (ED) regression lines (11)

curative regression line and indicates the degree of organotropic risk, e.g. leucotoxicity or immunosuppression of a certain curative dose, for instance the CD 95 (Fig. 6). If the danger coefficient of a newly developed agent is related to that of a well-known standard, the risk of organotropic toxic complications can be easily assessed for any curative effect.

5.0 Pharmacotherapeutic assessment of cancerotoxic agents

Pharmacotherapeutic assessment of antitumour agents, just as of any other drugs, can be divided into 3 stages:

(1) Primary screening
(2) Special pharmacological and toxicological characterization
(3) Preclinical pharmacology

These 3 stages should not be considered apart from each other as independent units, but they should continuously increase the relevant information about the drug's therapeutic and toxic properties with regard to its clinical use. In each stage the drug's properties are quantitatively assessed in special animal test systems which provide definite biometric figures. The predictive value of these indices depends e.g. on the chosen test model (tumour strain, chemoresistance) on the experimental set-up (dose, number of animals, route and sequence of administration) and on the method of evaluation. For the sake of continuity of the test procedure, all stages of the model system, its design and evaluation must be adapted to each other, taking into account the specific requirements and limitations of the individual phases.

5.1 Screening of antitumour agents

5.11 General prerequisites

The development and use of adequate test models for the screening of antitumour agents is of particular importance. Since, in primary screening, investment should be kept as low as possible, only a few generally applicable test models should be used. Such a limitation is a real problem since a uniform tumour system for the investigation of chemically different compounds and different mechanisms of action cannot be developed because of the differences in tumour types. Therefore several tumour systems are needed for such a variety of different agents as alkylators, antimetabolites, antibiotics, alkaloids and hormone-like compounds.

At the suggestion of Goldin (18) and Larionov (26) a WHO-supported international conference on "Screening Methodology for Antitumour Drugs" was held at Geneva in 1974. A great number of experts from all over the world discussed the problems of screening and achieved real progress.

Some points of the agreements will be described briefly:

(1) Even in future all research centers will be free to develop adequate methods for the solution of their own problems.
(2) All pharmacological methods - especially of the quantitative type - should be fully used in primary screening and in pharmacological characterization before an agent can be released for clinical trials.
(3) Interesting drugs developed by the individual cooperative groups, should be tested in a standard tumour system such as Leukaemia L1210 of the mouse. In addition, the effect of newly developed preparations should be related to a standard agent such as cyclophosphamide in some sort of a positive control. All prerequisites associated with these recommendations were clarified.

5.12 Our own procedure

For more than 20 years our cooperative group has concentrated on alkylating agents, and therefore we will present our method of screening and pharmacological characterization by the example of alkylators. With this limitation, some problems of screening are considerably simplified, since the individual screening methods decisively depend on the type and mechanism of action of the respective type of compound. However, in principle all pharmacological screening techniques are so closely related to each other that it appears justified to describe their basic principles by presenting this one example. In view of the strong and general cytotoxic action of the alkylators, it was our goal to apply the "transport form/active form" principle, first recommended by Druckrey (15) for the treatment of prostatic carcinoma (stilboestrol diphosphate), in order to increase the selectivity and reduce the toxicity to the nitrogen mustards. For this purpose it was necessary to transform the highly active nitrogen mustard into an inert "transport" form by suitable substitution, which would allow this transport form to be activated in the body: This principle was successfully utilized in the case of cyclophosphamide (1,2) and later with trofosfamide and ifosfamide. These compounds are practically inert in vitro, but they are converted in the body into the proper active form. Pharmacological screening of alkylators has to take into account both directly acting forms and inert transport forms.

The sensitivity of tumours to alkylating agents shows "individual variations" which is in accordance with the general laws of pharmacology. It is not of principal, but only of quantitative nature. Even in tumours, which appear to be completely resistant, a therapeutic effect can be obtained, if the drug is supplied to the tumour in adequate concentrations. If cell suspensions of various sensitive or resistant rat tumours are incubated in vitro

Table 1. Mean effective concentrations of chlormethine-N-oxide in various tumour systems in vitro (1 h at 37°C) according to Druckrey (1961)

Tumours		Conc. µg/ml
Heterologous tumours	Walker ascites carcinoma	0,15
	Yoshida ascites sarcoma	1,0
	Jensen sarcoma (homogenate)	3,0
Homologous tumours	T-ascites sarcoma	25
	DS-ascites carcino-sarcoma	25
	C-sarcoma (homogenate)	65

Table 2. Comparison of chlormethine, chlormethine-N-oxide, and cyclophosphamide in 7 different tumour strains of the rat according to Druckrey (17)

Test system	Transplantation	Medium curative doses in therapeutic units % LD 50		
		Chlormethine	Chlormethine-N-oxide	Cyclophosphamide
Yoshida ascites sarcoma	heterologous	21	4,7	3,0
Jensen sarcoma		40	4,3	4,5
Walker carcinoma		100	8,2	4,2
DENA carcinoma	homologous	»100	60	21
T-sarcoma		»100	›100	50
DS-carcinoma		»100	»100	~100
C-sarcoma		»100	»100	›100

for 1 hour with chlormethine N-oxide in Ringer's solution, determination of the limit concentrations, which counterbalance the tumour's transplantability, will show (Table 1) that the effective concentrations vary considerably (at a ratio of 1:100), whereas the full cytostatic effect can be obtained in all types of tumour, even in the highly resistant DS-carcinosarcoma (14). Similar results were seen in adequate tests on intact animals, where sublethal or lethal doses abolished the transplantability even of resistant tumours. The use of all effective compounds is limited by their toxicity. The more compounds with a wider margin of safety were developed, the more the number of tumours increased amenable to treatment (Table 2). Thus it can be concluded that quantitative methods, such as they are used for the determination of the margin of safety, allow the transference of the results obtained in a definite type of tumour, to other tumour types and to clinical conditions. For this purpose two prerequisites are essential:

(1) Concurrently with the assay compound a standard agent should be tested, the pharmacological and clinical actions of which are known on various tumour types.
(2) The quantitative results obtained with test agent and the standard should be the same in both animal and clinical trials.

If the above requirements are complied with, the animal experiment can be considered as an adequate model for the clinical conditions, which has meanwhile repeatedly been confirmed in animal experimentation and by clinical experience.

5.13 Primary screening

For primary screening we use the following model systems:

Yoshida ascites sarcoma AH 13 (rat BD II)
Walker 256 carcinosarcoma (rat Sprague-Dawley)

These two relatively chemosensitive tumour types were chosen because under the given test conditions with cyclophosphamide as a standard, they allow complete dose/action regression lines to be established for the curative effect. Our own screening method is characterized by great economy, its criterion is the therapeutic index and it allows the calculation of the probability of acceptance (operation characteristic curve). Our method has been published in all details (9).

5.2 Special pharmacological characterization

The agents accepted in the primary screening are subsequently assessed in detailed pharmacological characterization, nowadays hardly more problematic than that of any other drug. This will be

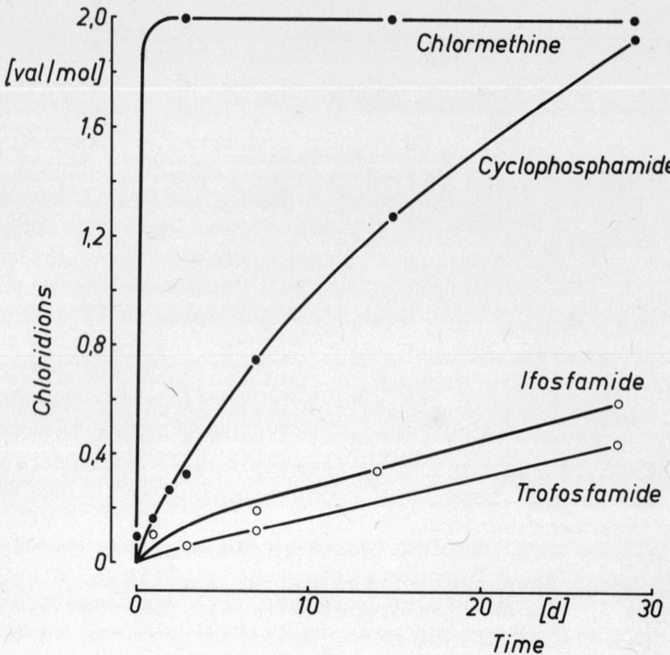

Fig. 7. Chloride ion liberation of chlormethine, cyclophosphamide, ifosfamide, and trofosfamide (bicarbonate buffer solution pH 7.5; 0.026 M; 37°C)

Table 3. Cytotoxic concentration of ifosfamide, cyclophosphamide, Nor-nitrogen mustard, chlormethine-N-oxide, and chlormethine in the incubation test with Yoshide ascites cells in vitro

Compound	Yoshida ascites sarcoma in vitro (37°C, 1h) EC 50 [μg/ml]
Ifosfamide	> 1000
Cyclophosphamide	> 1000
Nor-nitrogen mustard	1,0
Chlormethine-N-oxide	0,5
Chlormethine	0,1

demonstrated by the example of oxazaphosphorines: cyclophosphamide, trofosfamide and ifosfamide, for which I have my own data available.

5.21 Chemical and biological reactivity

With the alkylating cytostatics, the direct reactivity of the individual compound plays an important role, as is particularly seen in the case of nitrogen mustard and some ethylenimine compounds the toxicities of which considerably interfere with their general therapeutic use. Therefore the agents' reactivity should be carefully determined. For such an assessment several methods are available, e.g. the chemical corroborative test with 4-(4'-nitrobenzyl)-pyridine (NBP), or in mustard compounds, the determination of chloride ion liberation in aqueous solution, and the biological incubation test with living tumour cells. In comparison to nitrogen mustard and other directly acting alkylators, the chloride ion liberation from oxazaphosphorine derivatives is considerably reduced (fig. 7). In the NBP test, the 3 oxazaphosphorine compounds practically exert no activity at all. In the incubation test, the cytotoxic concentration of the oxazaphosphorines is four orders of magnitude greater than that of the direct alkylators (Table 3). Determination of the chemical reactivity and the result of the biological tests always show the 3 oxazaphosphorines to be practically inert in vitro, thus being genuine "transport" forms of nitrogen mustard.

5.22 Chemotherapeutic studies for the determination of the margin of safety.

The margin of safety should preferably be determined in various types of tumours on the basis of the toxicological tests. The lethal dose/action regression lines are assessed for various routes of administration (e.g. i.v. and orally), preferably in the type of animal in which the curative and organotropic effects are determined.

In our cooperative group we determine the curative potency in vivo in a number of tumour systems of rats and mice (Table 4). The table shows 4 rat tumours, selected from the point of view of increasing chemoresistance; in addition, a monocytic myeloid leukaemia L5222, which is characterized by a specific biochemical property, i.e. a high nonspecific esterase activity (23); furthermore, 3 mouse tumours, among them Leukaemia L1210. In this spectrum of rat and mouse tumours, as well as leukaemias, we effect a detailed assessment of the dose/action relations.

For the so-called transport forms, the cancerotoxic effectiveness *in vivo* is considered to be proof of their intracorporeal conversion into the active form, and thus as proof of the mechanism of action.

Table 4. Test systems for characterization of new antitumour drugs (Asta Laboratories)

Test systems	Host strain	Tumour inoculum		Treatment route	Treatment schedule	Parameter of response
		Type	Route			
Yoshida ascites sarcoma (Tokyo)	rat Sprague-Dawley heterologous	AF	i.p.	i.v. (i.p.)	Day 0	Cured animals
Walker-256 carcinosarcoma	rat Sprague-Dawley heterologous	TS	i.m.	i.v. (i.p.)	Day 4	TWI Day 14 ILS
Yoshida ascites sarcoma (Asta)	rat Sprague-Dawley heterologous	AF	i.p.	i.v. (i.p.)	Day 0	Cured animals
DS-carcino-sarcoma	rat BD II homologous	TS	i.m.	i.v. (i.p.)	Day 10	Cured animals ILS
Leukemia L5222	rat BD IX homologous	SpS B	i.p.	i.v. (s.c.)	Day 5 qd, Days 5 - 8	Cured animals ILS
Leukemia L1210 early	mouse DBA heterologous	AF	i.p.	i.p.	qd, Day 1 - death	ILS
Ehrlich ascites sarcoma	mouse Swiss heterologous	AF	i.p.	i.v. (i.p.)	qd, Day 0 - 3	ILS
Nemeth-Kellner lymphosarcoma	mouse Swiss heterologous	AF	i.p.	i.v. (i.p.)	qd, Day 0 - 3	ILS

AF = ascites fluid; TS = tumour suspension; SpS = spleen cell suspension; B = blood (heart puncture);

qd = daily; Day 0 $\hat{=}$ 3 hours after tumour inoculation; Cured animals = percentage of 90 days' survivors;

ILS= percentage of increase in life span over controls; TWI = percentage of tumour weight inhibition compared with controls

From among the great number of *in vivo* results, only a few will be described: Table 5 shows the results of comparative studies in Yoshida's ascitic sarcoma AH 13 of the rat on single i.v. administration and on fractionated administration (distribution of the total dose over 4 consecutive days). The data and indices of the table show the oxazaphosphorine compounds to have about the same curative potency as the standard chlormethine N-oxide, whereas they are considerably less toxic than this and other active nitrogen mustards. Thus toxic and therapeutic actions are not necessarily related to each other, so that a higher selectivity can actually be reached.

The assessment of cyclophosphamide in leukaemia L5222 showed an interesting result (fig. 8). In the lower dose range (0.5 to 2.0 mg/kg) the curative rate appears to depend directly on dosage with between 2 and 10 mg/kg of the leukaemic animals are definitely cured. Whenever a dose of 10 mg/kg is exceeded, the results are worse again and the animals die from leukaemia. In this type of tumour, the close relationship between the drug's chemotherapeutic action and the body's readiness for defence can be demonstrated with special clarity. The curative effect of a cancerotoxic compound does not only depend on its cytocidal effect, but also on the body's defensive powers. If these are hampered by immunosuppression, surviving cancer cells may cause a relapse.

5.23 Time/action relation

The lethal doses, by means of which the margin of safety is calculated, are usually determined in what might be called a "timeless" method on single administration. This is however only permissible, if the drug's action is practically a function of its concentration, i.e. if its action is due to a relatively rapidly reversible concentration effect. Since the cumulative toxicity of almost any cancer drug such as antimetabolites, alkaloids and alkylating agents is very high and often additive, the pharmacologist has to study in detail all possible risks of long-term treatment.

Although the cumulation of toxicity of any drug is dangerous, cumulation of its therapeutic action may be desirable and highly useful. Therefore the therapeutic value of an antitumour agent is the greater, the more rapidly its toxic effect is reversible and the more its curative effect is cumulated. According to Druckrey (17), the cumulative properties may be assessed quantitatively by determining that part of the cumulative action which is reversible within a certain period of time, e.g. 24 hours. The cumulation residue C is the complement of the quantity R following the equation R+1-C. The C values are calculated by comparative determination of the D 50 values on single dose administration and on subdividing the total dose into 4 individual doses.

The results of comparative studies on cyclophosphamide and

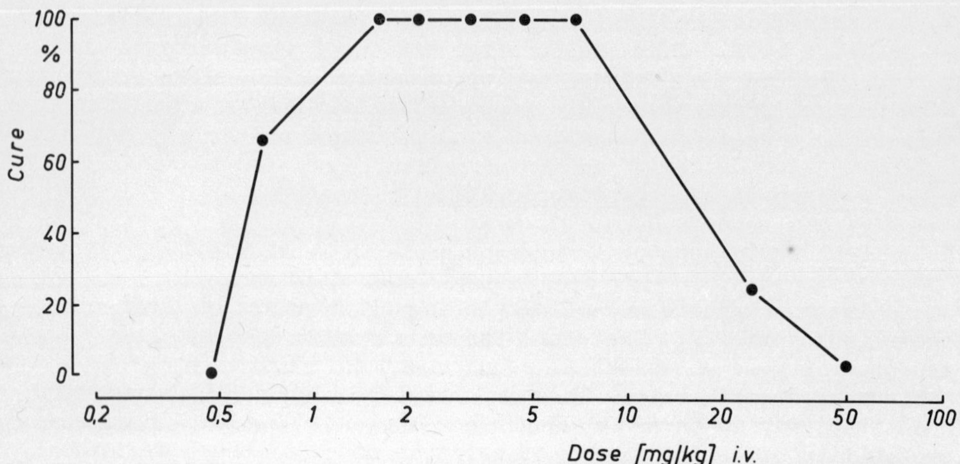

Fig. 8. Dependence of the cure rate on the height of a single iv dose applied 5 days after inoculation with 5 x 10^6 leukemic cells (Leukemia L5222) ip in adult BD IX rats

Table 5. Curative and lethal doses as well as D50 indices of chlormethine-N-oxide, cyclophosphamide, trofosfamide, and ifosfamide with one single dose and 4 separate doses in the Yoshide ascites sarcoma of the rat (AH 13)

Compound	Number of administrations	LD 50 [mg/kg]	CD 50 [mg/kg]	LD 50 / CD 50	Therapeutic units % LD 50
Chlormethine-N-oxide	1	50	5,4	9,3	10,8
	4	90	7,8	11,5	8,7
Cyclophosphamide	1	150	3,9	38	2,6
	4	140	8,0	17,5	5,7
Trofosfamide	1	63	2,1	30	3,3
	4	80	6,5	12,3	8,1
Ifosfamide	1	150	7,7	19,5	5,1
	4	190	6,3	30	3,3

ifosfamide are shown in fig. 9. The toxic cumulation rest of ifosfamide after 24 hours is about 83%, of cyclophosphamide nearly 100%. The curative action behaves just the other way round, for cyclophosphamide the C value is about 45%, whereas for ifosfamide it is about 100%. Thus the curative action of ifosfamide is much more cumulative than that of cyclophosphamide. Therefore on fractionated dosage, ifosfamide would yield definitely better results, whereas on single adminstration, cyclophosphamide would be superior.

5.3 Assessment of organotropic effects

5.31 Leukotoxic action.

The therapeutic use of alkylating cytostatics is limited by their leukotoxicity. Therefore the development of compouns of low leukotoxicity is an essential requirement for further progress in antitumour chemotherapy. This important problem can be elucidated quantitatively in terms of danger coefficient. Table 6 shows the probability of leukotoxicity of curative doses of the 3 oxazaphosphorine derivatives to be considerably smaller than that of the direct alkylator chlormethine N-oxide and in addition they still appear to have certain differences in potency.

5.32 Immunosuppressive effect

In tumour therapy with alkylating agents the inhibition of specific and unspecific defence reactions is known as an "undesirable side effect". Therefore it is important for clinical use to assess the cancerotoxic and immunosuppressive effect in its dependency on dosage and in relation to toxicity. The humoral immunoreaction was produced on rats by administration of Brucella antigens. For this purpose the danger coefficient can be used again (28). D 1 indicates the probability of immunosuppressive action of a curative dose (CD 84), D 2 the probability of toxicity of the immunosuppressive dose. The indices reveal cyclophosphamide and ifosfamide to exert a more pronounced immunosuppressive effect than trofosfamide, which has a relatively slight immunosuppressive effect. That is of practical importance in maintenance therapy (Table 7).

5.33 Assessment of the carcinogenic risk of cytostatic agents in man

Late effects of alkylating agents are due to their nucleotoxic and genotoxic action, which might produce teratogenic, mutagenic and carcinogenic effects just like antimetabolites and antibiotics. These effects can now be assessed both qualitatively and quantitatively in a relatively small number of animals.

An essential prerequisite for all tests is to know the spontaneous tumour rate of the experimental animals. Specifically carcinogenic action should preferably be tested in a strain with a low

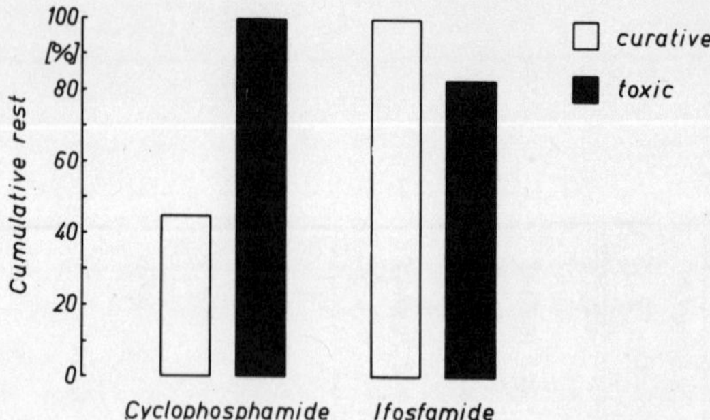

Fig. 9. Cumulative rest C of the curative and toxic activities of cyclophosphamide and ifosfamide. C = the fraction of activity still present after 24 hours and able to cumulate when dividing the total dose into 4 daily doses.

Table 6. Leukotoxic effects of cyclophosphamide, trofosfamide, ifosfamide, and chlormethine-N-oxide. Correlation between curative and leukotoxic effects (Yoshide ascites sarcoma) following 1 single iv injection in rats

Compound	ED 50 [mg/kg]	ED 50 / CD 50	D CD 84 [%]	D CD 95 [%]
Cyclophosphamide	21.3	4,75	1,2	12
Trofosfamide	17	8,1	1,0	5
Ifosfamide	44	6,8	0,6	10
Chlormethine-N-ox.	11	2	44	86

Table 7. Danger coefficient obtained from the curative; immunosuppressive and lethal regression lines for cyclophosphamide, ifosfamide, and trofosfamide

Danger coefficient	Cyclophosphamide	Ifosfamide	Trofosfamide
DI 1)	0,90 %	4,0 %	‹0,02 %
DII 2)	‹0,02 %	0,8 %	4,50 %

1) Probability of immunosuppressive action of the DC 84

2) Probability of toxic (lethal) action of the fully immunosuppressive dose

TABLE 8. Establishing of the pharmacotherapeutic values of three different derivatives of nitrogen mustard.

Drug	7% LD 50	CD 50	CD 95	LD 50	LD 50 / CD 50	LD 5 / CD 95	D (CD 84) [%]	Carcinogenicity		
	[mg/kg]							a. Weis-burger	acc. Schmähl tab. 1	acc. Schmähl tab. 2
Chlormethine	0,11	0,43	–	1,57	3,6	<1	95	++	+	not tested
Chlormethine-N-oxide	4,2	5,4	15,0	50,0	9,3	2,2	44		+	not tested
Cyclophos-phamide	13,0	4,5	13,0	160,0	35,5	8,5	1,2	(+)	?	(+)

CD = curative dose (Yoshida sarcoma)
LD = lethal dose
D = danger coefficient of the leukotoxic effect (related to the CD 84)

Carcinogenicity : ++ = pronounced carcinogenicity
+ = significant carcinogenicity
(+) = slightly significant carcinogenicity compared with controls
∅ = no significant carcinogenicity compared with controls

spontaneous tumour rate; nonspecific tumour development such as increased tumour growth induced by immunosuppression, is preferably tested in a strain with a higher spontaneous tumour rate.

To clarify the relations between chemotherapeutic potency, margin of safety and carcinogenic effect, the most important pharmacotherapeutic indices including the carcinogenic ones are shown in Table 8 (10).

The pharmacotherapeutic development of cyclophosphamide from chlormethine via chlormethine N-oxide does not only reveal the considerable reduction of toxicity (LD 50 value, danger coefficient for the leukotoxic action) and the marked increase of the therapeutic index, but also the pronounced reduction of carcinogenicity. The pharmacotherapeutic advance becomes even more conspicuous if the carcinogenic effect is not only related to the absolute dose (as a percentage of the LD 50), but if the single-dose curative effect is also taken into account. Comparison clearly shows that a drug's carcinogenic action is not necessarily related to its chemotherapeutic potency. Therefore the development of new drugs of a wider margin of safety appears to be basically possible and of urgent necessity.

Since the individual carcinogenic effects are practically irreversible, the decision to institute clinical treatment must be based on rigid principles. On the other hand, the risk should not be overrated, since experience has shown that latency periods of 10 years or even more are to be expected. Cancer is a vital indication which necessarily implies certain risks. Even radiation therapy may eventually induce cancer, and surgery is not at all free from any risk. Therefore the demand for rigid principles of indication equally applies to all three types of treatment. The use of suitable chemotherapeutic agents in inoperable and chemosensitive systemic tumour conditions is not only justified, but urgenly indicated for vital grounds. Even in juvenile patients drug treatment may be vitally indicated, as for instance in Burkitt's tumour, which can be cured in about 60% of the cases with high cyclophosphamide doses without any carcinogenic effect having been observed so far.

The drugs should be selected for the individual conditions from a pharmacotherapeutic point of view, carefully pitting their therapeutic effectiveness in the respective type of tumour against the risks involved.

For post-operative use, chemotherapy is indicated whenever the primary tumour is sensitive to chemotherapy and whenever there is a risk of general spreading. In this connection, important pharmacotherapeutic principles have been elaborated in animal experiments. Fig 10 shows that in DS-carcinoma of the rat, which is known to be relatively resistant to cyclophosphamide, radical surgery alone

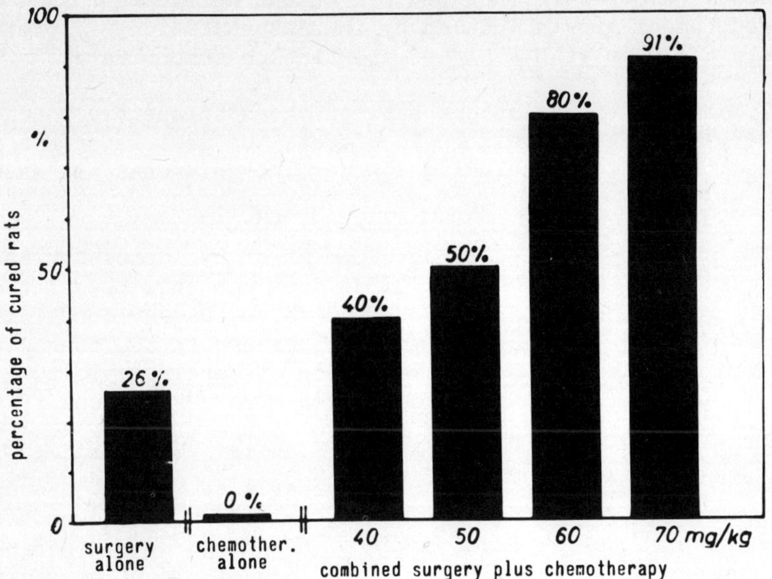

Fig. 10. Surgical removal of DS-carcinosarcomas (30 g) without and combined with chemotherapy (cyclophosphamide, single dose). Test: definite cure (according to Druckrey).

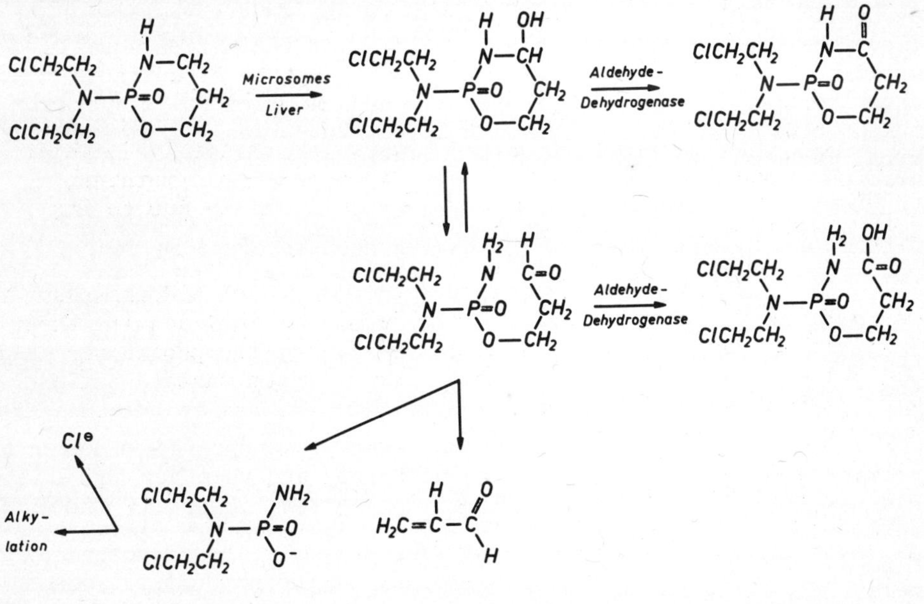

Microsomes Liver

Aldehyde-Dehydrogenase

Aldehyde-Dehydrogenase

$Cl^{\ominus}$

Alkylation

Fig. 11. Activation of cyclophosphamide in the liver

produced cures in a few rats only, whereas concurrent administration of cyclophosphamide allowed a definite cure in up to 90% of the animals in dependence on dosage.

5.4 Mechanism of action

The question of the relative selectivity of cyclophosphamide and other potential slkylators, whose action is based on the transport form/active form principle, has intensely been treated in the last 10 years. At the beginning of July 1975, the Chester Beatty Research Institute held a Symposium on this subject, which was attended by a great number of experts.

Shortly after administration of cyclophosphamide to warm-blooded animals, the serum, various bloodfree extracts, urine and bile contain high concentrations of compounds which differ from cyclophosphamide by their cytotoxic activity on isolated ascitic cancer cells in the incubation test, by the spontaneous alkylation in the NBP test, and which are separately determinable (5). These primarily activated metabolites are preferably formed in the liver by means of a microsomal enzyme system with the consumption of $NADPH_2$ and oxygen (7). The chemistry of the metabolic breakdown in vivo has been elucidated in many individual stages, as can be seen from the following scheme (fig. 11).

Of special importance are the primarily activated metabolites of cyclophosphamide, the tautomers 4-hydroxy-cyclophosphamide and aldophosphamide, which can be considered as transport forms of higher reactivity. These two compounds are not so highly reactive as the direct alkylators, but on the other hand, they are not so stable as cyclophosphamide or 4-keto-cyclophosphamide. Their cytostatic activity in vitro shows an outstanding cytotoxic quotient of 63 (cytostatic units per µmol of N-mustard derivative), which is only exceeeded by chlormethine. In contrast to chlormethine, 4-hydroxycyclophosphamide has a wide margin of safety due to its considerably reduced in vivo toxicity (Table 9).

The tautomers 4-hydroxy-cyclophosphamide and aldophosphamide do not represent direct alkylating compounds, but they acquire their alkylating properties only through cleavage of the phosphoric acid ester bond, which leads to acrolein and nitrogen mustard phosphoric acid diamide which is an intense alkylator and has to be considered as the proper active form of cyclophosphamide.

This assertion appears to be contradictory to the relatively weak cytostatic effect of nitrogen mustard phosphoric acid diamide on isolated cells of Yoshida's ascitic tumour. This discrepancy is probably due to the slight permeability of the anionic nitrogen mustard diamidophosphoric acid. A specific cancerotoxic effect can only be expected if the active form is liberated from 4-hydroxy-

Table 9. Chemical reactivity and biological activity of nitrogen mustard compounds and cyclophosphamide metabolites

Nitrogen mustard derivatives	mol. weight	in vitro			in vivo		
		alkylating activity 1) [%]	Cl^--hydrolysis 2) 1 val/mol in	cytotoxic activity 3) [CU/µmol]	CD 50 4) [mg/kg]	LD 50 [mg/kg]	D50-Index ($\frac{LD\ 50}{CD\ 50}$)
Cyclophosphamide	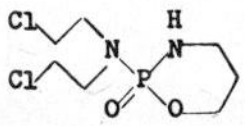 279	1.3	> 7 d	< 0.03	1.25	220	175
4-Keto-cyclophosphamide	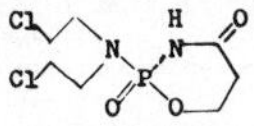 275.1	1.2	> 7 d	< 0.07	> 800	> 800	-
4-Hydroxy-cyclophosphamide	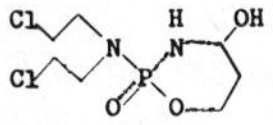 277.1	65	480 min	63	1.25	150	120
4-Hydroperoxy-cyclophosphamide	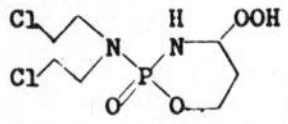 293	40	240 min	21	1.25	97.5	78
Carboxy-phosphamide	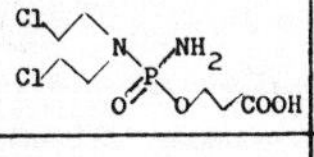 293	85	> 7 d	0.1	~ 200	~ 800	~ 4
N,N-Bis-(2-chloroethyl) phosphorodiamidic acid	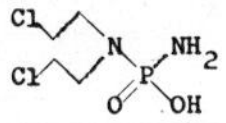 221	90	60 min	2.5	20	61	3.5
Acrolein	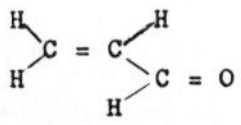 56.06	(1.9)	-	0.4	2.15	7.3	-
Nor-nitrogen mustard	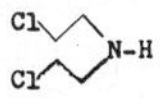 178.5	100	60 min	1.35	40	100	2.5
Chlormethine	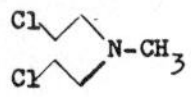 192.5	100	15 min	138	0.25	1.1	4.4
Chlormethine-N-oxide	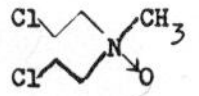 208.6	100	180 min	1.5	5	60	12

1) NBP-test 2) pH 7,5; 37° C 3) Yoshida sarcoma 4) Yoshida sarcoma

cyclophosphamide within the cancer cell. Of special consequence is the observation (13), that the active tautomers are enzymatically transformed into the inactive 4-keto-cyclophosphamide and carboxy-phosphamide. Further to this the degree and site of the hydrolytic cleavage of the oxazaphosphorine ring in the cell may be altered by reactions between the 4-OH group of 4-hydroxy-cyclophosphamide or the oxo function of aldophosphamide and free thiol groups. These complex possibilities, the kinetics of which have to be studied more intensely, are ultimately the underlying principle of the selectivity of the transport forms (22,31).

5.5 Models for preclinical pharmacology

The clinician expects the pharmacologist to supply him with reliable data for the best possible clinical use of the drug. Thus it is understandable that in recent years many pharmacologists have tried to study the drug's basic principles of action and to elucidate its mechanism so as to obtain an even better basis for optimum therapeutic administration.

5.51 Optimum dosage

The question of optimum dosage is of general importance and should be clarified for any drug before its involvement into polychemotherapeutic schemes. With special regard to the oxazaphosphorines, quite a number of experience is available. One has to distinguish between the conventional dosage (2 to 3 mg/kg) and massive-dose treatment (20 to 60 mg/kg). The oncologist has invariably to make the decision on the individual dosage suited for each patient in accordance with the type of tumor condition. In animal experimental studies Druckrey (17) has clearly shown that with rising dosage of cyclophosphamide, not only the curative rates of certain tumour types shows an increase, but also other tumours become amenable to the drug (fig. 12). On the other hand, treatment with fractionated doses or doses which are evidently too low might induce tumour resistance (fig. 13). Massive-dose treatment, e.g. with cyclophosphamide or ifosfamide, facilitates individual dosage, since the physician has enough time to observe the reaction of both patient and tumour, and then to determine the size and time of administration of each of the following doses. If the tumour does not respond to the maximum tolerated dose, the drug should be discontinued, since it would only throw an unnecessary burden on the patient.

5.52 Polychemotherapy

Another possibility of increasing the selectivity of the anti-tumour action and therby improving the therapeutic results, is the institution of polychemotherapy, where various agents are combined in the hope to obtain better therapeutic results with concurrent reduction of toxicity. Combination therapy is expected to lead

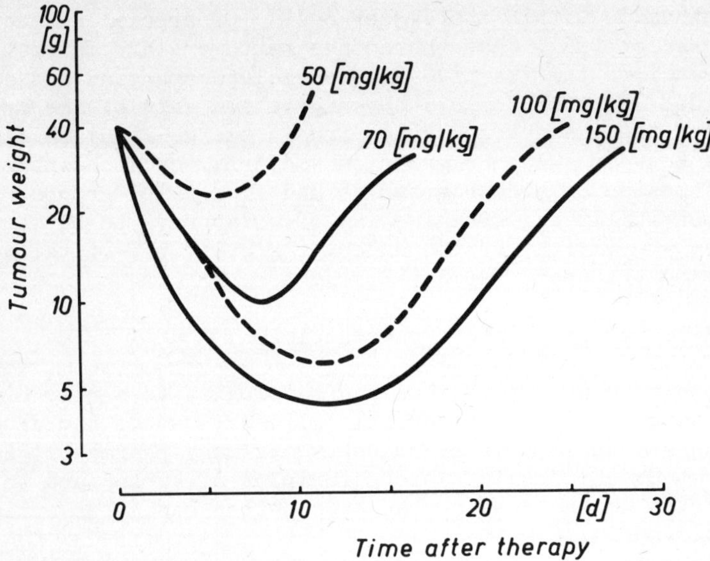

Fig. 12. Degree and duration of regression of DS-carcinoma depending upon the dosage of cyclophosphamide (single iv injection, medium values) (according to Druckrey)

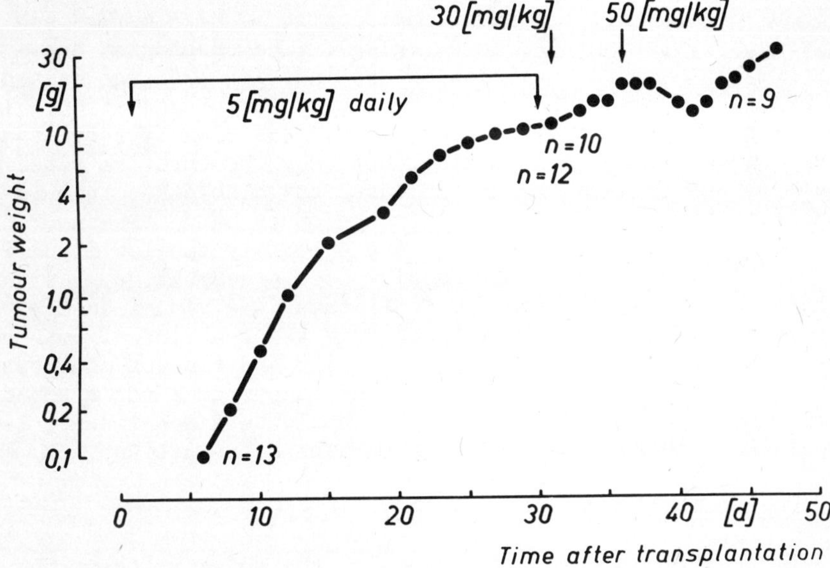

Fig. 13. Therapeutic ineffectiveness of 30 daily doses of 5 mg/kg of cyclophosphamide and increase of resistance in the DS-carcinoma (according to Druckrey)

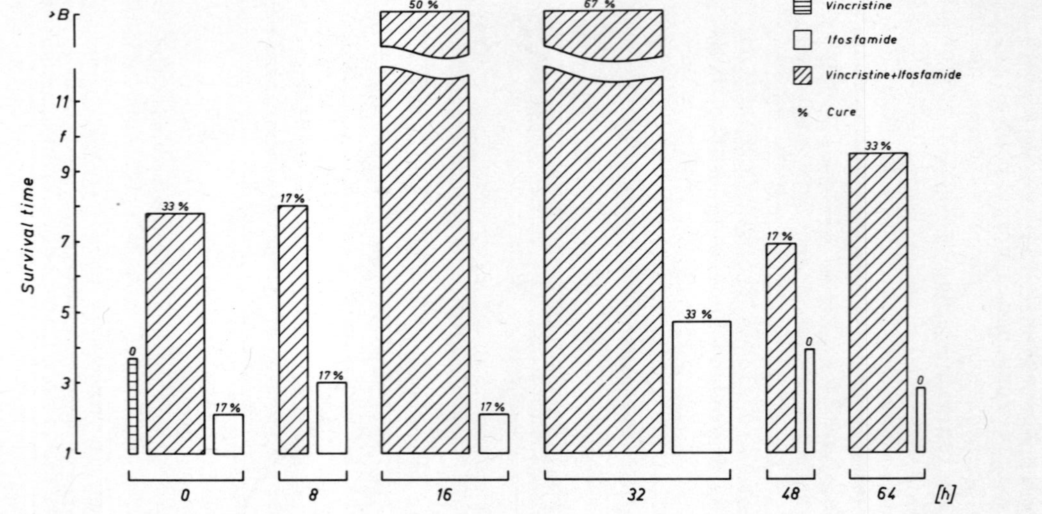

Fig. 14 : Survival time and cure rates obtained in the chemoresistant Yoshica ascites sarcoma (Asta) under treatment with vincristine, ifosfamide and the combination of vincristin and ifosfamide.

Ordinate: Survival time as a multiple of the survival time of untreated tumour animals. If more than 50% of the treated tumour animals survive, the average survival time is called B.

Abscissa: Sequence of the various administrations:

Time 0 = 24 h after tumour grafting — vincristin sulphate (Lilly); ifosfamide (Asta); vincristin + ifosfamide

Time 8,16,32,48,64 = 8,16,32,48,64 h after time 0 — ifosfamide in untreated tumour animals; ifosfamide in animals pretreated with vincristin at time 0

Percentage above the columns: definitely cured animals per group of treatment either to simple summation or even to potentiation of the therapeutic effects of each of the components, whereas the toxic effects are not increased. Such a polychemotherapy requires adequate dosage at appropriate time intervals, and careful choice of the individual drugs. Taking these factors into account, in adequate animal model systems Goldin (19) as well as Schabel and Skipper (30) have elaborated an essential basis for the large-scale use of modern polychemotherapy. By the advent of reasonable polychemotherapy-schemes it became feasible to control human tumour diseases so far out of range. In practice, the individual agents should preferably be chosen from among different classes of compounds with different points of attack. For instance, an alkylator should be combined with an antimetabolite, an alkaloid, an antibiotic or a hormone. Each of the involved compounds should, if given alone, produce a well defined anticancer effect in the respective type of tumour. In spite of greater therapeutic benefit, combination therapy may also lead to an increase in untoward side effects or even to undesirable complications such as increased intensity of the drugs well-known reactions, or new toxic disorders which had remained latent in monotherapy. Therefore polychemotherapy continuously requires particularly careful supervision of the patients.

5.53 Significance of proliferation kinetics and synchronization of human tumour cells for cytostatic treatment.

Since many of the usual cytostatics exert an intense inhibitory effect on definite stages of the cell cycle it is absolutely essential to know not only the cytostatic mechanism of action, but also the proliferative behaviour of the tumour cells if one wants to obtain greater selectivity of action.

Of the cytostatics, for instance, vincristine interferes with mitosis, 5-fluorouracil and methotrexate with the terminal phase of the G_1 stage, cyclophosphamide and other alkylating cytostatics with the S and G_2 stages. For a cell-stage-specific tumour treatment it is important to know the proliferation kinetics of the respective tumour cells so as to find out, in which phase of the cycle the synchronized cells are most probably to be found. The cell kinetic parameters cannot be determined in man by means of labelled DNA precursors because of the risk of radiation lesions. Such studies can however be carried out in vitro with the aid of the double-labelling method in human biopsy material.

The efficacy of synchronization therapy was first demonstrated in animal experiments, e.g. in diploid Ehrlich ascitic cells or in the resistant Yoshida ascitic sarcoma. Thus ifosfamide, administered during the S stage of the previously vincrinstin-synchronized tumour cells, exerts a considerably greater cytostatic effect than after administration to the asynchronously growing tumour (fig. 14).

This proof of greater effectiveness and higher selectivity has repeatedly been produced even in clinical use by Klein, Gross, Lennartz (24), Hartwich (20) and Körner (25). Since vincristin is administered only for a short period of time at relatively low doses, synchronization therapy can in fact be considered as a monotherapy. Its side effects, measured by its leukopenic reaction, are not more pronounced than those of a usual scheme of cytostatic treatment.

6.0 Prospects

I intentionally confined myself to describing the scientific and experimental principles of modern cancer chemotherapy. The approach to pharmacotherapeutic screening described above is characterized by consequently adjusting the individual stages of one test to the others. As early as in primary screening in animals the results are related to the therapeutic index and to standard agents, which provides a basic yardstick for the drug's assessment in view of its later clinical use, and which in principle can be employed until the last stage of test. Thus it is possible to obtain a maximum of information from animal experiments and to speedily identify genuine advances. It is to be hoped that the above principles of screening and assessing antitumour agents will soon become generally accepted. This would allow uniform assessment of the results of diverse cooperative groups.

Any investigator is of course free to go on using his own methods in approaching specific problems. However, the increase in selectivity of the cancerotoxic effect should be aimed at in all future work. In view of the fact that in the field of carcinogenesis we elaborated the principles or organospecific actions and elucidated the interrelation between chemical constitution and specific action (16), it should basically be possible to transfer such an organotropic principle to antitumour agents as well. In analogy to carcinogenesis, one might couple a suitable organotropic compound with alkylators in terms of the transport form/active form principle. The prospect for the development of such a principle has considerably improved, since suitable model systems for nearly all types of tumours have been developed.

A target-aimed improvement of the efficacy of the available anti-cancer drugs requires a precise knowledge of their mechanism of action. Studies of this mechanism again require detailed knowledge of the cellular metabolism onto which the drug acts. Therefore, still increased efforts to clarify the various processes involved in malignant growth are necessary. All the metabolic processes related to cell proliferation are undoubtedly of great practical interest for all possibilities of developing target-aimed chemotherapeutic action on cancer cells. There is no doubt that the oncologist has to consider all available therapeutic possibilities and in particular to include the modern chemotherapy (and immunology) into the well-established methods of surgery and radiation therapy. Chemotherapy of cancer, which usually has to be conducted along the limit of toxicity, requires greater knowledge and experience than most other types of drug treatment and is virtually an art. As experimental experience has shown, the essential potentialities for an effective remission lie in the first dose the patient is given. If it is too low, such an error can never be corrected again. Thus practical chemotherapy is a typical "do it yourself" task for the oncologically experienced specialist. Obsolete illusions, such as assigning the cancer patient to separate wards, are no longer tenable, rather it is urgently necessary to institute special oncological units in all university hospitals and large clinics, and to appoint appropriate specialists to such units.

Whenever possible, the clinicians should enlist the cooperation of qualified oncologists who work in the field of experimental chemotherapy and who would be able to provide them with adequate advice and scientific information. Such cooperation would be of utmost importance for effecting the urgently needed advances in cancer chemotherapy to the benefit of the patient. Even in the future, definite cure of advanced cases of cancer will continue to be possible in a few isolated cases only. Therefore the most effective means of fighting cancer is to prevent it. For this purpose we must know its possible causative agents, their action, when and where they become dangerous, and how people can be protected against them. Even in the control of infectious diseases, prophylaxis through modern hygiene has proved to be the most effective instrument.

The carcinogenic agents are particularly dangerous, because they also exert mutagenic and teratogenic effects, and therefore the most essential task of preventive medicine is to use every possible means for the realization of our scientific knowledge to the benefit of mankind.

REFERENCES

1. Arnold, H., Bourseaux, F., Brock, N. Naturwiss 45, 64 (1958).
2. Arnold, H., Bourseaux, F., Brock, N. Drug Res. 11, 143, (1961).
3. Brock, N. vth Int. Congress of Chemotherapy, Vol 11/1, 1967p.155.
4. Brock, N. Med. Mschr. 27, 390 (1973)
5. Brock, N. Symposium Chester Beatty Research Institute, London July 1975.
6. Brock, N., Geks, F.J. Naturwiss, 38, 351, (1951).
7. Brock, N., Hohorst, H.J. Drug Research 13, 1021 (1963).
8. Brock, N., Schneider, B. Drug. Res. 11, 1, (1961).

9. Brock, N., Schneider, B. Drug Res. 14, 171 (1964).

10. Brock, N., Schneider, B. Drug Res. 21, 435 (1971).

11. Brock, N., Wilmanns, H. Dtsch. med. Wschr. 83, 453 (1958).

12. Calendi, E., DiMarco, A., Reggiani, M. et al. Biochem. Biophys. Acta 103, 25 (1965).

13. Connors, T.A., Cox, P.J., Farmer, P.B., Foster, A.G., Jarman, M. Biochem. Pharmacol. 23, 115 (1974).

14. DiMarco, A. in: Heffter-Heubner:Handbuch der experimentellen Pharmakologie, Vol XXXVIII/2, p. 593. Springer 1975, Berlin-Heidelberg-New York.

15. Druckrey, H. Dtsch. med. Wschr. 77, 1495 + 1534 (1952).

16. Druckrey, H., Preussmann, R., Ivankovic, S., Schmahl, D. Z. Krebsforsch. 69, 103 (1967).

17. Druckrey, H., Steinhoff, D., Nakayama, M., Preussmann, R., Anger, K. Dtsch. med. Wschr. 88, 651 (1963).

18. Goldin, A., Serpick, A.A., Mantel, N. Cancer Chemother. Rep. 50, 173 (1966).

19. Goldin, A., Venditti, J.M., Mantel, N. In:Heffter-Heubner Handbuch der experimentellen Pharmakologie Vol XXXVIII/1, p. 411. Springer 1974, Berlin, Heidelberg, New York.

20. Hartwich, G., Fuchs, H.F. Heidhardt, B. Fortschr, Med. 90, 46, (1972).

21. Hoefer-Janker, H., Scheef, W., Gunther, U., Huls, W. Med. Welt 26, 972 (1975).

22. Hohorst, H.J., Draeger, U. Peter, G., Voelcker, G. Symposium Chester Beatty Research Institute, London July 1975.

23. Ivankovic, S., Zeller, W.J. Blut 28, 288 (1974).

24. Klein, H.O., Lennartz, R.J., Gross, R., Eder, M., Fischer, R. Dtsch. med. Wschr. 97 1273 (1972).

25. Korner, F., Lund, S., Jonas, U. Munch. med. Wschr (in press)

26. Larionov, L.F. Cancer Chemother. Rep. Part 1, 54, 71 (1970).

27. Norpoth, K. 9th Int. Congress of Chemotherapy London July 1975.

28. Potel, J., Brock, N. Z. Rheumaforsch. 31, Supp 2., 339 (1972).

29. Schadel, F.M.Jr., Johnston, T.P., McCales, G.S., Montgomery, J.A., Laster, W.R., Skipper, H.E. Cancer Res. 23, 725 (1963).

30. Schabel, F.M.Jr., Skipper, H.E., Trader, M.W., Laster, W.R.Jr., Cheeks, J.B. Cancer Chemother. Rep. 4, 53 (1974).

31. Voelcker, G., Draeger, U., Peter, G., Hohorst, H.J. Arzneim.-Forsch. (Drug Res.) 24, 1172 (1974).

NEW LEADS TOWARDS ANTITUMOR SELECTIVITY IN THERAPEUTICS[1]

Enrico Mihich

Grace Cancer Drug Center, Roswell Park Memorial Institute

N.Y. State Department of Health, Buffalo, N.Y. 14263, USA

SUMMARY

Four approaches to cancer chemotherapy currently being studied in this Department are discussed: 1) correlations between nucleotide pools in target tumor cells and selective activity of drugs; 2) reversal by a hormone of the host toxicity of an antitumor agent; 3) potential interference with cell division by uses of cyclic nucleotide analogs; and 4) increased antigenicity of leukemic lines resistant to certain drugs.

. . . .

Cancer chemotherapy has achieved some success in the sense that a certain number of patients with different types of cancer can now be brought into complete remission through the use of drugs, and are free of detectable disease five years or later after diagnosis. In most types of tumors, however, chemotherapy alone is relatively ineffective. Failures are essentially related to the fact that the available drugs lack sufficient selectivity of antitumor action. The occurrence of resistance is another factor.

New and better anticancer therapies are sought through development of new compounds and the better utilization of known drugs alone

[1] Results discussed in this contribution were obtained with the partial support of Grants CA-13038, CA-15142, CA-05298, CA-12585 from the National Cancer Institute, USPHS.

or in combination. Information on drug kinetics and disposition and on target determinants of drug action provides the basis for the rational development of treatments with improved selectivity of antitumor action. New approaches are derived from increased knowledge of factors affecting regulation of cell metabolism. The immunological system also offers opportunities for pharmacological intervention. A thorough discussion of current directions in cancer chemotherapy is beyond the scope of this contribution. Instead, four specific areas under study in this Department are briefly described, as examples of the new approaches that are being pursued.

The size of the metabolite pools in tumor cells can be expected to affect the activation of appropriate antimetabolites, their ability to compete successfully for specific enzyme sites, or the sensitivity of biochemical targets susceptible to feed-back control. Therefore, the profile of such pools may be useful in determining whether or not an antimetabolite will ultimately be effective.

The toxicity which an anticancer agent exerts against non-tumor tissues may be reduced through selective manipulation of the metabolism of these tissues. For instance, supplementation of an end-product which is more limiting for a normal than for a tumor cell may protect the normal cell from drug toxicity without affecting its antitumor action. This idea has been applied in the differential reversal of antifolate toxicity by citrovorum factor in animals (Goldin, *et al*., 1954) and in humans (Frei, *et al*., 1975). Thymidine may also reverse methotrexate toxicity (Frei, *et al*., 1975). Modification of host toxicity by metabolites which bear no structural resemblance to the drug can also be achieved. For instance, the dose limiting toxicity of the antileukemic agent 3-deazauridine (3-DU) in mice is reduced by the administration of testosterone (Bloch, *et al*., 1974).

Controls of cell proliferation may provide uniquely sensitive targets in tumor cells. Cytidine 3',5'-monophosphate (cCMP) detected in rapidly proliferating tissues (Bloch, 1974, 1975) was shown to stimulate L1210 cells in culture to progress from G_2 into M (Bloch, 1975). Interference with the formation or function of cCMP may provide novel approaches towards new treatments.

Leukemia L1210 sublines resistant to certain drugs are more antigenic and immunogenic than the parent leukemia (Fuji and Mihich, 1975). Drug-related increases in immunogenicity may offer new possibilities in sequential therapy and in the utilization of highly antigenic cells for immunotherapy (Mihich, 1973).

Adenosine nucleotide pools in tumor cells and selective cytotoxicity of N^6(Δ^2-isopentenyl)adenosine (IPAR). IPAR is an analog of adenosine with antiproliferative action in cell culture and rodent tumor systems, and which can cause complete but short-lasting bone marrow remissions in patients with AML. Background information on IPAR has been described elsewhere (Rustum and Schwartz, 1974, Slocum and Hakala, 1975).

The extent of metabolic activation of IPAR in L1210 and ascitic Taper hepatoma cells in mice was compared to the intracellular profile of nucleotide pools (Rustum, 1975). The ratios of ATP/ADP and ATP/AMP were 10 and 20-fold greater, respectively, in Taper hepatoma than in L1210 cells. In Taper hepatoma cells the drug was phosphorylated to the 5'-mono, di- and triphosphate derivatives and was incorporated into RNA. In contrast, in L1210 cells, IPAR was phosphorylated only to the monophosphate level (Rustum, 1975, Slocum and Hakala, 1975). IPAR treatment markedly increased the survival of mice with Taper hepatoma, whereas the survival of mice with L1210 was only minimally affected, indicating that the differences in the extent of metabolic activation of IPAR in these two tumor lines effects differences in their therapeutic effectiveness (Rustum, 1975). The apparent relationship between IPAR activation and magnitude of ATP/ADP and ATP/AMP ratios found in target cells suggests that these ratios may be useful indicators of the ability of cells to activate analogs of "salvage metabolites." The quantitative differences in the ribonucleotide profiles of L1210, P-288, Taper hepatoma, human AML and ALL cells did not predict the degree to which a tumor relies on "salvage metabolites" for nucleic acid synthesis, but they reflected the relative efficiency of incorporation of such metabolites into nucleic acids (Y. M. Rustum, personal communication).

Reversal by testosterone of the intestinal toxicity caused by 3-DU. The effectiveness of 3-DU against L1210 was significantly greater in male than in female mice, and in castrated than in sham-operated females (Bloch, et al., 1974). The administration of testosterone to either females or males reduced the limiting intestinal toxicity. In tumor cells 3-DU is metabolized to the nucleoside triphosphate derivative without being incorporated into nucleic acid (Wang and Bloch, 1972). Reversal studies suggested that in L1210 cells and in normal mouse tissues the drug interferes with the biosynthesis of cytosine derivatives (Brockman, 1975). Amination of UTP by purified CTP synthetase was inhibited by 3-deazauridine triphosphate competitively with respect to UTP (McPartland, et al., 1974). Glutamine provides the amino group in this reaction. It is of interest, therefore, that α S, 5S- α -amino-3-chloro-4,5-dihydro-5-isoxazole-acetic acid

(U42126) a new antileukemic agent which acts as an antagonist of glutamine (Neil, et al., 1975), is also more effective in male than in female mice bearing L1210, and that the intestinal toxicity of this compound is also reversed by testosterone (G.L. Neil, personal communication). Reversal of the intestinal toxicity of two different inhibitors of the CTP synthetase reaction by testosterone provides an example for the possibility of increasing selectivity of antileukemic action by decreasing the limiting toxicity exerted against normal tissues.

Cyclic CMP and cell proliferation. cCMP was recently isolated from leukemia L1210 cells (Bloch 1974) and was found in about 50-200 fold greater concentration in regenerating than in normal rat liver (Bloch 1975); cCMP was also detected in urines from patients with AML but not in urines from normal individuals (Bloch et al., 1975). This compound accelerated the progression of L1210 cells in culture into mitosis and reversed the decelerating effects of cAMP in this system (Bloch, 1975). Thus inhibitors of cCMP formation and/or function may stop cells from entering mitosis. The therapeutic value of this approach would depend on whether this inhibition would lead to the destruction of arrested tumor cells or merely to a decrease of their growth fraction.

Increased immunogenicity of tumor cells. Immunogenicity of tumor cells may be increased by chemical or enzymatic modification of the plasma membrane (Mihich, 1973). Immunogenicity and antigenicity of leukemic cell populations is also increased subsequent to the development of resistance to certain agents (Fuji and Mihich, 1975). It is not yet clear whether, in either case, this increase is due to the selection of more antigenic cell lines or to drug-induced inheritable changes in antigenic expression. The increased immunogenicity of resistant sublines entails increased sensitivity to drugs unrelated to the one against which resistance was developed and may thus provide a useful basis for sequential chemotherapy. It is also possible that drug-induced increases in the immunogenicity of tumor cells may be exploited to elicit an increased immune response to the cells in the primary host, or that these cells may be used for immunotherapy. The fact that resistance to certain drugs such as guanazole is accompanied by increases in tumor-associated antigens is promising in this regard.

CONCLUDING REMARKS

As outlined in this brief discussion, increases in the selectivity of anti-tumor action may be obtained through modification of the tumor cell metabolism, leading to the increased activity of an antimetabolite or it may be effected through modification of the drug sensitive metabolic target in normal tissues, leading to a reduction in toxicity. Pharmacological modulation of the controls of tumor cell division may represent another approach for intervention. Drug-related increases in tumor immunogenicity may be exploited therapeutically. The ideas discussed require further experimental verification before generalizations applicable to clinical therapeutics can be formulated.

REFERENCES

Bloch, A. (1974). Biochem. Biophys. Research Communications, 58, 652.

Bloch, A. (1975). In Adv. Cyclic Nucleotide Research, G.I. Drummond, P. Greengard and G.A. Robison, eds., Raven Press, New York, 5, 331.

Bloch, A., Dutschman, G., Grindey, G., and Simpson, C.L. (1974). Cancer Research 34, 1299.

Bloch, A., Hromchak, R., and Henderson, E.S. (1975). Proc. Am. Assoc. Cancer Research 16, 191.

Brockman, R.W., Shaddix, S.C., Williams, M., Nelson, J.A., Rose, L.M., and Schabel, F.M.Jr. (1975). Ann. NY Acad Sci 255, 501.

Frei, E., III, Jaffe, N., Tattersall, M.H.N., Pitman, S., and Parker, L. (1975). New England J. Medicine 292, 846.

Fuji, H. and Mihich, E. (1975). Cancer Research 35, 946.

McPartland, R.P., Wang, M.C., Bloch, A., and Weinfeld, H. (1974). Cancer Research 34, 3107.

Mihich, E. (1973). In Drug Resistance and Selectivity: Biochemical and Cellular Basis, E. Mihich, ed., Academic Press, New York, p. 391.

Neil, G.L., Berger, A.E., Blowers, C.L. and Kuentzel, S.L. (1975). Proc. Am. Assoc. Cancer Research 16, 114.

Rustum, Y.M. (1975). Proc. Am. Assoc. Cancer Research 16, 191.

Rustum, Y.M. and Schwartz, H.S. (1974). Biochem. Pharmacology 23, 2469.

Slocum, H.K. and Hakala, M.T. (1975). Cancer Research 35, 423.

Wang, M.C. and Bloch, A. (1974). Biochem. Pharmacol. 21, 1063.

AN EXPERIMENTAL APPROACH TO INCREASE SELECTIVE TUMOUR TOXICITY OF METHOTREXATE

M. H. N. Tattersall

Charing Cross Hospital (Fulham)

Fulham Palace Road, London W6 8RF

Thymidine protects mice bearing leukaemia L1210 and P388 from methotrexate toxicity without impairing antitumour activity. When thymidine containing pellets were implanted subcutaneously in L1210 leukaemia bearing mice, the therapeutic dose range of methotrexate was increased three-fold. The toxic effects of methotrexate in mice may be ascribed to a disturbance of de novo thymidylate synthesis but the antitumour activity must be due to a disturbance of some other folate dependent pathway.

Introduction

The combination of high dose methotrexate and folinic acid rescue has been used clinically for several years (1,2). The enhanced therapeutic index of the combination compared to methotrexate alone has been established in some experimental tumour systems (3) and in patients with head and neck tumours and osteogenic sarcoma (4,5). Delay in administration of folinic acid after methotrexate is necessary for optimal tumour effect in experimental animals but the optimal timing of the rescue in man has not been established. The biological basis for the increased therapeutic effect of methotrexate folinic acid is not known but a number of hypotheses have been advanced (6). Recently an alternative approach to methotrexate rescue has been proposed. When given at appropriate time intervals after methotrexate treatment, asparaginase prevents the bone marrow toxicity of methotrexate and the antitumour effects of the combination are not necessarily similarly reduced. L Asparaginase reduces the cytotoxicity of methotrexate by inhibiting protein synthesis thus preventing the entry of cells into the DNA synthetic phase of the cell cycle during which cells are sensitive to methotrexate (7). The value of this combination in the treatment of acute leukaemia has been reported recently (8). We have studied the effect of thymidine on the toxicity and antitumour activity of methotrexate in leukaemia bearing mice. Our result indicate that thymidine decreases markedly methotrexate toxicity but does not reduce the antitumour effect. Thymidine allows substantially greater doses of methotrexate to be administered to tumour bearing mice and the antitumour activity of methotrexate has been increased.

Materials and Methods

Thymidine was purchased from Nutritional Biochemical Corporation, cholesterol from Aldrich Chemical Co., and methotrexate and folinic acid were obtained from the Division of Cancer Treatment, National Cancer Institute. 250 mg cholesterol pellets and thymidine pellets each containing 60 mg of thymidine and 190 mg cholesterol were pressed using a Wabash hydraulic press. Drugs for injection were dissolved in water and administered intraperitoneally or subcutaneously.

Animal Studies

The toxicity of the drugs in non tumour bearing BDF1 mice was studied by daily weighing and survival of drug treated animals compared to controls. The antitumour activity against rodent ascitic tumours was studied in vivo. The cell lines were carried by weekly serial transplantation. The lines of L1210 and P388 used in the experiments have been maintained for several years in this department. 10^5 cells of L1210 and 10^6 cells of P388 were inoculated routinely intraperitoneally, and drug treatment was started 24 hours later. Thymidine and cholesterol pellets were implanted subcutaneously in the nape of the neck, and left in place for 3 days. In some experiments the pellets were changed every three days for a total of ten days.

Results

Table 1 shows the effect of simultaneous administration of methotrexate (MTX) and thymidine (TdR) or folinic acid (CF) on normal mice. The results indicate that TdR will prevent the toxicity of 250 mg/kg MTX but not 300 mg/kg, whereas CF prevents toxicity of MTX at 300 mg/kg. Chart 1 shows the weight changes in these animals, and indicates that CF is superior to TdR in preventing the weight loss caused by MTX treatment. Tables 2 and 3 show the effect of TdR given intraperitoneally (ip) and subcutaneously (sc) on the toxicity and antitumour activity of MTX in leukaemia L1210. The results indicate that the simultaneous administration of TdR both ip and sc with MTX protects animals to a large degree from the toxicity of MTX and does not inhibit the antitumour activity. The results also show that TdR alone does not have any antitumour or toxic effects. Table 4 indicates that TdR prevents the toxicity of MTX in animals bearing P388 leukaemia, without inhibiting antitumour activity. In this experiment MTX at 200 mg/kg as a single dose was toxic in the majority of mice, but TdR completely prevented toxicity.

Table 1

The Effect of Thymidine and Folinic Acid on the Toxicity of MTX in Normal Mice

Drug	Each Dose mg/kg	Schedule	No. Mice	Number Deaths/ Number Mice	Day of Death
MTX	200	qd x 1	8	1/8	8
	250	qd x 1	8	7/8	7^{8}
	300	qd x 1	8	6/8	$5, 6^{5}$
TdR	500	tid x 4	8	0/8	—
MTX TdR	200 500	qd x 1 tid x 4	8	1/8	6
MTX TdR	250 500	qd x 1 tid x 4	8	1/8	6
MTX TdR	300 500	qd x 1 tid x 4	8	5/8	$6^{4}, 7$
MTX CF	300 500	qd x 1 500 bid x 3	8	0/8	—

Table 2

The Effect of intraperitoneal Thymidine and Folinic Acid on the Toxicity and Antitumour activity of Methotrexate in Leukaemia L1210

	Dose mg/kg	Schedule	No.	Median	Day of Death	% ILS
Control	—		22	9.0	8^{10}, 9^{8}, 10^{2}, 11^{2}	
CF	200	bid x 3	6	8.5	8^{3}, 9^{3}	–6
TdR	500	tid x 4	6	9.0	8, 9^{3}, 10	0
TdR	1000	tid x 4		8.5	8^{3}, 9^{2}, 10	–6
MTX	200	qd x 1	6	11.5	5^{2}, 11, 12, 14, 15	+28
MTX	250	qd x 1	6	5.0	5^{4}, 13^{2}	–45
MTX	275	qd x 1	6	6.0	5^{3}, 7^{2}, 13	–34
MTX	300	qd x 1	6	5.0	5^{4}, 7, 14	–45
MTX TdR	200 500	qd x 1 tid x 4	6	12.5	11, 12^{2}, 13^{3}	+39
MTX TdR	250 500	qd x 1 tid x 4	6	12.0	11, 12^{3}, 13^{2}	+33
MTX TdR	275 500	qd x 1 tid x 4	6	12.0	11, 12^{3}, 13^{2}	+33
MTX TdR	300 500	qd x 1 tid x 4	6	12.0	7, 12^{3}, 13^{2}	+33
MTX TdR	275 1000	qd x 1 tid x 4	6	11.5	10, 11^{2}, 12, 13^{2}	+28
MTX TdR	300 1000	qd x 1 tid x 4	6	12.5	11, 12^{2}, 13^{3}	+39
MTX CF	300 200	qd x 1 bid x 3	6	9.5	9^{3}, 10^{3}	+6

Table 3

The Effect of subcutaneous Thymidine on the Antitumour Activity and Toxicity of Methotrexate in Leukaemia L1210

	Dose mg/kg	Schedule	No.	Median	Day of Death	% ILS
Control			15	12.0	10^2, 11, 12^6, 13^5, 14	
TdR	500	tid qd 1–3	6	11.5	11^3, 11^3	–4
MTX	250	qd x 1	7	15	6, 7, 14, 15, 16, 17, 18	+25
MTX	300	qd x 1	7	7.0	6, 7^3, 8, 16, 20	–42
MTX	400	qd x 1	7	7.0	6^2, 7^4, 20	–42
MTX TdR	250 500	qd x 1 tid qd 1–3	7	16.0	15^3, 16^2, 17, 19	+33
MTX TdR	300 500	qd x 1 tid qd 1–3	7	16.0	8, 14, 15, 16^2, 18, 19	+33
MTX TdR	400 500	qd x 1 tid qd 1–3	7	16.0	13, 14, 15, 16^2, 17, 19	+33

Table 4

The Antitumour Effects of Methotrexate, Thymidine and Folinic Acid in Leukaemia P388

		Dose mg/kg	Schedule	No.	Median	Day of Death	% ILS
	Control	—		13	14	13^2, 14^7, 15^2 16, 18	
	CF	200	qd x 1	6	13.5	13^3, 14^2, 15	-4
	TdR	500	tid qd 1-3	6	14	13^2, 14^3, 16	0
	MTX	200	qd x 1	6	5.5	5^3, 6, 20, 21	-61
	MTX	250	qd x 1	6	5.5	5^3, 6^2, 20	-61
	MTX	275	qd x 1	6	6.5	5, 6^2, 7, 21, 25	-54
	MTX	300	qd x 1	6	5.5	5^3, 6^2, 7	-61
	MTX TdR	200 500	qd x 1 tid qd 1-3	5	20	18, 20^4	+43
	MTX TdR	250 500	qd x 1 tid qd 1-3	6	19.5	19^3, 20^4, 24	+39
	MTX TdR	275 500	qd x 1 tid qd 1-3	6	19.5	6^2, 19, 20^2, 22	+39
	MTX TdR	300 500	qd x 1 tid qd 1-3	6	20.5	6, 19, 20, 21^2, 25	+46
Simult.	MTX CF		qd x 1	6	16.5	16^3, 17, 18, 19	+18
12 hr delay	MTX CF		qd x 1	6	20	17, 20^3, 22, 24	+43
24 hr Delay	MTX CF		qd x 1	6	21	20^2, 21^2, 22 25	+50

Table 5 indicates that the therapeutic effect of MTX is slightly greater if TdR treatment is delayed 12 hours after MTX. In these experiments TdR was superior to CF as a delayed rescue agent. In some experiments the superiority of TdR compared to CF as a rescue agent was less clear. Table 6 shows the effect of TdR pellets implanted subcutaneously on the toxicity and antitumour activity of MTX in L1210 leukaemic bearing mice. The results show that TdR pellets increased threefold the therapeutic dose range of MTX given in the optimal schedule for leukaemia L1210. The antitumour activity of MTX was not compromised by the TdR pellets, but the data do not indicate a clearly increased antitumour activity of MTX at 3 times the usual optimal dose. Experiments with TdR pellets and MTX in the treatment of a MTX-transport resistant subline of L1210 leukaemia will be reported elsewhere.

Discussion

The results reported here indiate that thymidine protects normal tissue in the mouse to a greater extent than malignant tissue against the toxic effects of MTX. This differential effect means that substantially larger doses of MTX can be administered to tumour bearing animals than is possible in the absence of thymidine, and this may permit more effective treatment of "resistant" tumours. The biological bases for these observations are not established, but the results suggest that MTX causes thymidylate starvation in tissues which are usually MTX dose limiting in the mouse, and that these effects are substantially prevented by thymidine which may enter the thymidylate pool via the salvage pathway. The participation of a reduced folate cofactor 5,10-methylene tetrahydrofolate in de novo thymidylate biosynthesis and the block of this reaction in cells treated with methotrexate has been established (9,10). These data indicate that in L1210 and P388 leukaemic cells, methotrexate may have a different site of action which is not bypassed by thymidine.

Reduced folate cofactors are required not only for dTMP synthesis but also for _de novo_ purine biosynthesis, certain amino acid interconversions and possibly the methylation of dopamine (11,12). Clearly any of these reactions could become limiting in tumour cells in the presence of methotrexate and thymidine before similar disturbance occurred in normal tissue.

Whereas any one of these factors may be responsible for the selective reversal by thymidine of MTX toxicity in normal tissue without compromising the antitumour effect, another possibility also must be considered. Bone marrow cells were shown by Lajtha and Vane (13) to utilise purines preformed in the liver for nucleic acid synthesis. Moreover, erythropoietic responses to a 48 hour

Table 5

The Effect of Delayed intraperitoneal Administration of Thymidine and Citrovorum Factor on the Toxicity and Antitumour Activity of Methotrexate in Leukaemia L1210

	Dose mg/kg	Schedule	No.	Median	Day of Death	% ILS
Control	——		15	9.0	8^5, 9^7, 10^3	
TdR	500	tid x 4	6	8.5	8^3, 9^2, 10	-6
CF	200	bid x 3	6	8.0	8^4, 10^2	-11
MTX	200	qd x 1	6	8.5	6^3, 11, 14^2	-6
MTX	250	qd x 1	6	9.5	6^3, 13^3	+5
MTX	275	qd x 1	6	7.0	6^2, 7^2, 13, 14	-22
MTX	300	qd x 1	6	7.0	6^2, 7^3, 8	-22
*MTX TdR	200 500	qd x 1 tid x 4	6	13.0	13^6	+44
MTX *TdR	250 500	qd x 1 tid x 4	6	12.0	11^3, 13^3	+33
MTX *TdR	275 500	qd x 1 tid x 4	6	13.0	11, 13^4, 14	+44
MTX *TdR	300 500	qx x 1 tid x 4	6	13.0	11, 13^4, 15	+44
MTX *CF	300 200	qd x 1 bid x 3	6	10.5	10^3, 11^2, 13	+17

* First dose 12 hrs after MTX

Table 6

The Antitumour Effects of Methotrexate and Thymidine Pellets in L1210 Leukaemia

	Dose mg/kg	Schedule	No.	Median	Day of Death	% ILS
*Control	—		16	10.5	10^8, 11^7, 12	
TdR	60	q3d 1, 4, 7	6	10.5	10^3, 11^3	0
*MTX	7.5	q3d 1, 4, 7	8	17	14, 15, 16^2, 17^2, 19, 21	+61
*MTX	15	q3d 1, 4, 7	8	19	15, 18^2, 19^4, 21	+81
*MTX	30	q3d 1, 4, 7	6	20	7, 11, 19, 21, 22, 37	+90
*MTX	60	q3d 1, 4, 7	6	11.5	9^2, 11, 12, 13, 18	+10
*MTX	90	q3d 1, 4, 7	6	8.5	7^2, 8, 9, 10, 11	−19
*MTX	120	q3d 1, 4, 7	6	8.0	7^2, 8^3, 9	−24
MTX TdR	7.5 60	q3d 1, 4, 7	8	17	14, 16, 17^4, 19	+61
MTX TdR	15 60	q3d 1, 4, 7	8	17.5	15, 16, 17^2, 18^2, 19, 20	+67
MTX TdR	30 60	q3d 1, 4, 7	6	19.0	18^2, 19^3, 25	+81
MTX TdR	60 60	q3d 1, 4, 7	6	21	19^2, 21^3, 22	+100
MTX TdR	90 60	q3d 1, 4, 7	6	22.5	18^2, 21, 24, 25, 27	+114
MTX TdR	120 60	q3d 1, 4, 7	5	9.0	9^4, 10	−14

* Animals given cholesterol pellets (250 mg)
Thymidine pellets contained 60 mg TdR & 190 mg cholesterol

thymidine infusion have been reported in human megaloblastic anaemia (14). These data suggest that a disturbance of purine biosynthesis may not occur in bone marrow cells due to folate depletion or antifolate treatment because the bone marrow cells do not synthesise purines de novo. Since the dose limiting toxicity of MTX in rodents is the bowel, the results reported here that thymidine reduces substantially MTX toxicity in mice suggest that gut cells may also not depend on de novo purine biosynthesis but utilise purines either in the diet or preformed in the liver for nucleic acid synthesis.

Following intravenous administration, thymidine removal from the blood in mice occurs in two phases. One with a half-time of less than a minute, the other with a half-time of about 8 minutes (15). It is therefore surprising that the subcutaneous and intraperitoneal administration of thymidine reported here was so

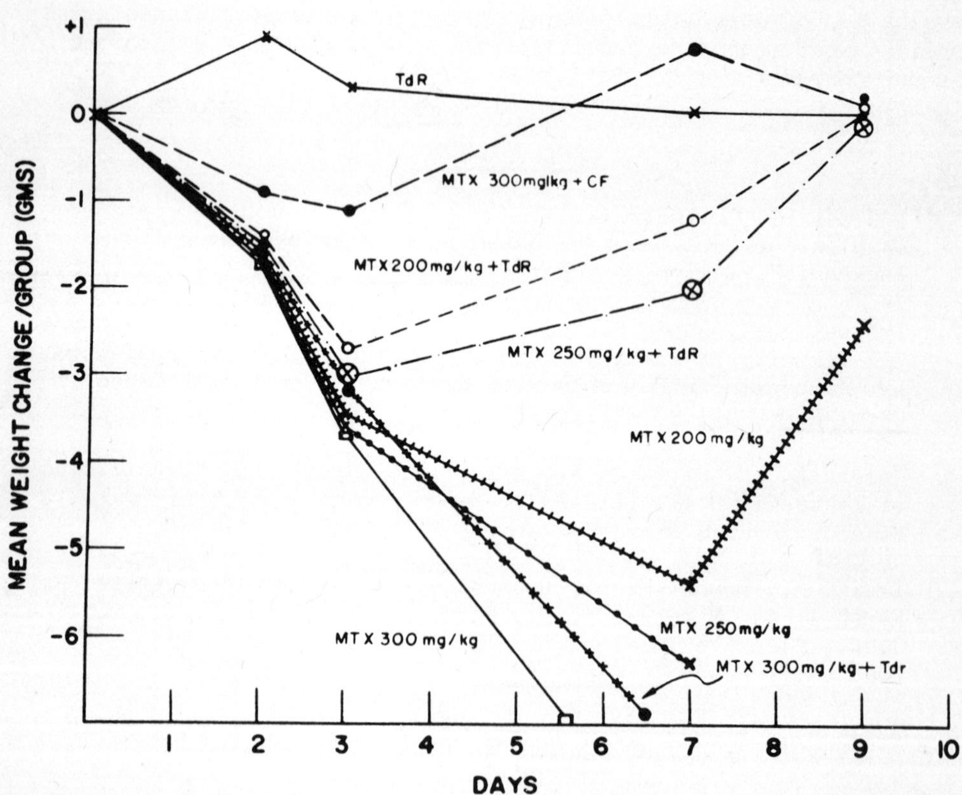

Fig. 1. The effect of thymidine and citrovorum factor on methotrexate treated mice.

effective at preventing MTX toxicity. The thymidine pellets used in these experiments were modelled on those reported by Lee and Prensky (16) who found that serum concentrations of thymidine in the mouse were maintained between 3 and 20 times normal for up to 48 hours after subcutaneous implantation in CDF mice. We have not measured the serum thymidine concentration following the implantation of our pellets but the results indicate that the toxicity of MTX has been substantially reduced by the pellet, presumably due to thymidine release.

Some tumour cells have been noted to be extremely sensitive to thymidine, and it is reported that this sensitivity correlates with the cellular level of thymidine phosphorylase (17). L1210 cells do not belong to the group of thymidine sensitive tumours, and no antitumour effects of thymidine alone were observed in these experiments. It is possible however that manipulation of the serum thymidine level may lead to selective antitumour effects in special circumstances, and since thymidine infusions have been administered in man without side effects, it is possible that this approach should be explored. We have recently started a phase I evaluation of methotrexate-thymidine in patients with disseminated solid tumours, and the results of these studies will be reported in due course.

References

1. Djerassi I.,"Methotrexate Infusions and Intensive Supportive Care on the Management of Children with Acute Lymphcytic Leukaemia", follow up report Cancer Res., 27, 2561-2564 (1967).

2. Lefkowitz E., Papac R. C., Bertino J. R., "Head and Neck Cancer III Toxicity of 24 hr Infusions of Methotrexate and Protection by Leucovorin in Patients with Epidermoid Concinoma, Cancer," Chem. Rep., 51, 305-311 (1967).

3. Goldin A., Venditti J. M., Kline I., Mantel N., "Eradication of Leukaemia Cells (L1210) by Methotrexate and Methotrexate Plus Citrovorum Factor", Nature, 212, 1548-1550 (1966).

4. Levitt M., Mosher M. B., DeConti R. C., Farber L. R., Skeel R.T., Marsh J. C., Mitchell M. S., Papac R. J., Thomas E. D., Bertino J. R., "Improved Therapeutic Index of Methotrexate with Leucovorin Rescue", Cancer Res., 33, 1729-1734 (1973).

5 Jaffe N., "Recent Advances in the Chemotherapy of Metastatic Osteogenic Sarcoma", Cancer, 30, 1627-1631 (1972).

6. Tattersall M. H. N., Jaffe N., Frei Emil III, "The Pharmacology of Methotrexate Rescue Studies". The University of Texas,

M. D. Anderson Hospital and Tumor Clinic Synposium. The Pharmacologic Basis of Cancer Chemotherapy, Monograph (in press, 1974.

7. Capizzi R. L., Summers W. P., Bertino J. R., "L-Asparaginase Induced Alteration of Amethopterin (Methotrexate) Activity in Mouse Leukaemia L51784", Annals of the N. Y. Acad. Sci., 186, 302-311 (1971).

8. Capizzi R. L., Castro O., Aspnes G., "Treatment of Acute Lymphocytic Leukaemia with Intermittent High Dose Methotrexate and Asparaginase", Proc. Amer. Asso. Cancer Res, 15, 182 (1974).

9. Wahba A. J., Friedkin M., "The enzymatic Synthesis of Thymidylate", J. Biol. Chem., 237, 3794-3801 (1962).

10. Osborn M. J., Freeman M., Huennekens F. M., "Inhibition of Dihydrofolic Reductase by Aminopterin and Amethopterin", Proc. Soc. Exp. Biol., 97, 429- , (1958).

11. Laduron P. "N-Methylation of Dopamine to Epinine in Brain Tissue Using N methyl Tetrahydrofolic Acid as the Methyl Donor", Nature New Biol., 238, 212-213 (1972).

12. Laduron P. M., Gommeren W. R., Leysen J. E., "N-Methylation of Biogenic Amines I", Biochem. Pharmacol, 23, 1599-1608 (1974). (1974).

13. Lajtha L. G. Vane R. J., "Dependence of Bone Marrow Cells on the Liver for Purine Supply", Nature, 182, 191-192 (1958).

14. Killman S-A., "Erythropoietic Response to Thymidine in Pernicious Anaemia", Acta Medica Scandinavica, 175, 489-496 (1964).

15. Hughes W. L., Christine M., Stollar B.D., "A Radioimmunoassay for Measurement of Serum Thymidine", Analyt. Biochem., 55, 468-478 (1973).

16. Lee D. J., Prensky W., "Measurements of DNA Turnover: Suppression of IUdR Reutilization in vivo by Long-acting Thymidine Pellets", Fed. Proc., 31, 6737, (1972).

17. Lazarus H., Oppenheim S. O., Barett E. F., submitted for publication.

Acknowledgments: Supported in part by NIH Grants No. 2 PO2-CAO 651612. M.H.N. Tattersall is a Medical Research Travelling Fellow.

ALTERATIONS IN INTRACELLULAR CYCLIC AMP AS A POTENTIAL FORM OF ANTI-TUMOUR CHEMOTHERAPY

M.J. TISDALE and B.J. PHILLIPS

Department of Biochemistry, St. Thomas's Hospital Medical School, London SE1 7EH, UK., Chester Beatty Research Institute, London, SW3 6JB, UK

SUMMARY

The possibility of using cyclic AMP either as an inhibitor of cell proliferation, or to facilitate the reversal of the abnormally differentiated state of neoplastic tumours has been considered. The parameters involved in regulation of intracellular levels of cyclic AMP have been defined. The anti-tumour akylating agents have been given as an example of tumour growth-inhibitors the mechanism of action of which may involve cyclic AMP.

The discovery of adenosine 3',5'-monophosphate (cyclic AMP) by Sutherland and Rall, and the elucidation of its role in cellular function provide an opportunity to use this system for the development of new drugs. Cyclic AMP is an important intracellular mediator which is involved in the control of cell growth (Eker 1974; Kurtz et al. 1974), morphology (Prasad and Sheppard 1972) and in the regulation of mitosis (Millis et al. 1974). Malignant transformation is often accompanied by defects in the metabolism of cyclic AMP in cells either chemically (Murray and Verma 1973) or virally transformed (Carchman et al. 1974). This is reflected in a lowered basal intracellular level of the cyclic nucleotide in malignant cells compared with the tissue of origin (Oler et al. 1973). Furthermore, addition to transformed cells of cyclic AMP, or agents which elevate the intracellular level of cyclic AMP, cause morphological reversion and differentiation in many cases (Edstrom et al. 1974). Thus one approach to cancer chemotherapy would be the design of agents which selectively alter the concentration of cyclic AMP in neoplastic tissues.

The intracellular level of cyclic AMP is a balance between

its rate of synthesis from ATP by membrane bound adenylate cyclase, its rate of degradation by cyclic nucleotide phosphodiesterase, and its loss to extracellular fluid. In many cases alteration in the activity of the adenylate cyclase is responsible for the lowered intracellular level of cyclic AMP (Pastan and Johnson 1974). In view of this and also in view of the highly specific discriminative nature of the cyclase which appears to be primarily designed to distinguish only the natural information transferring molecules (hormones), drug-induced alteration of cyclase activity in neoplastic tissue would appear unlikely. Loss of cyclic AMP to the extracellular fluid is also an important factor in determining the intracellular levels of the cyclic nucleotide. Little is known of this process however, e.g. whether it is active or passive, or whether it is affected by hormones or drugs.

The hydrolysis of cyclic AMP by phosphodiesterase appears to provide the best possibility for altering the intracellular levels of the cyclic nucleotide via the use of drugs. In a number of tissues this enzyme has been shown to exist in multiple forms differing in their Michaelis-Menten constants (Km values), stability, drug sensitivity, substrate specificity, electrophoretic and chromatographic behaviour, and subcellular localization (Appleman *et al*. 1973). This tissue specificity of the cyclic nucleotide phosphodiesterase may facilitate the design of agents which specifically affect the enzyme in neoplastic tissue.

The anti-tumour alkylating agents and *cis*-dichloro diammine Pt II (cis $Cl_2(NH_3)_2$Pt II) have been shown to cause a rise in intracellular cyclic AMP in Walker carcinoma *in vitro* at doses which produce an inhibition of cell growth (Tables 1 and 2) (Tisdale and Phillips 1975). This effect is restricted to those agents acting by an alkylating type mechanism as other commonly used anti-tumour drugs have no effect on basal levels of the cyclic nucleotide at doses which produce a comparable degree of growth inhibition (Table 2). Also the corresponding N-ethyl analogue of an active difunctional agent (chlorambucil) which is therapeutically inactive has no effect on cyclic AMP levels even at a dose which produces 98% inhibition of cell growth. This dose is 36 times that of the corresponding difunctional agent (Table 1). With chlorambucil the increase in intracellular cyclic AMP reaches a peak within 1 hour. This precedes the inhibition of thymidine incorporation into DNA which reaches 50% by 7 hours.

In contrast chlorambucil causes no increase in cyclic AMP levels in Walker cells with a ten fold resistance to this agent (Table 3).

The cyclic nucleotide phosphodiesterase from Walker carcinoma shows evidence either of two isoenzymic forms or a single enzyme showing negative cooperativity. To investigate the mechanism by which chlorambucil causes a rise in cyclic AMP only

Table 1. Effect of Alkylating Agents on the Intracellular Level of Cyclic AMP and Viability of Walker Carcinoma Cells

Compound	Dose (μg / ml)	Increase in cyclic AMP level %	Growth inhibition %
Merophan*	0.5	118	99
	0.1	76	83
	0.05	18	63
HN2⁄	0.1	108	100
	0.05	68	97
Chlorambucil*	5.0	114	99
	1.0	72	80
	0.5	21	50
CB 1954*	1.0	96	100
	0.4	67	100
	0.05	22	97
N-ethyl analogue* of chlorambucil	250.0	0	98

* Cyclic AMP values 8 hr after treatment
⁄ Cyclic AMP values 24 hr after treatment

in sensitive Walker cells the effect of this agent on the phosphodiesterase has been investigated. Table 4 shows the specific activity of the enzyme in total cell sonicated suspensions of sensitive and resistant cells 8 hours after treatment with various doses of chlorambucil. The specific activity has been measured either at 1 mM cyclic AMP (which measures mainly the high Km form of the enzyme) and at 3.3μM cyclic AMP (for the low Km form). The results shown in Table 4 indicate that the specific activity of the high Km form of the phosphodiesterase is similar in sensitive and resistant tumour, and that the activity of this form of the enzyme is unaffected by any of the doses of chlorambucil employed. For the low Km form of the phosphodiesterase the activity in the resistant tumour is only 50% of that in the sensitive. Moreover, whereas this form of the enzyme in the resistant tumour shows no inhibition by any of the doses of chlorambucil employed, that in the sensitive line is inhibited by 74, 35 and 12% at doses of chlorambucil of 5, 1 and 0.5 μg / ml respectively. Since the Km value (1.1 μM) of this

Table 2. Effect of other Anti-tumour Agents on the Intracellular Level of Cyclic AMP and Cell Viability of Walker Carcinoma

Compound	Dose (μg / ml)	Cyclic AMP (μM)	Growth inhibition (%)
cis $Cl_2(NH_3)_2PtII$*	0.5	2.9	96
	0.25	2.65	88
	0.1	2.1	56
	0.05	1.95	40
	0.00	1.95	-
ICRF 159⨍	100	1.98	94
	50	1.95	92
	25	1.90	79
	10	1.76	46
	0	1.96	-
BCNU⨍	100	1.24	100
	20	1.26	99
	10	1.25	96
	0	1.22	-

* Cyclic AMP values 8 hr after treatment
⨍ Cyclic AMP values 24 hr after treatment

Table 3. Cyclic AMP Content of Resistant Walker Carcinoma Cells 8 hours after Treatment with Chlorambucil

Culture conditions	Cyclic AMP p mole / mg protein
No additions	41.0
5.0μg / ml chlorambucil	42.0
1.0μg / ml chlorambucil	40.0
0.5μg / ml chlorambucil	40.0

Table 4. Cyclic AMP Phosphodiesterase Activities of Sensitive and Resistant Walker Carcinoma 8 hours after Treatment with Chlorambucil

	Cyclic AMP Phosphodiesterase Activity			
	Resistant		Sensitive	
Treatment	"High Km" activity	"Low Km" activity	"High Km" activity	"Low Km" activity
Control	1.55±0.05	0.25±0.01	1.60±0.05	0.6±0.02
5μg/ml chlorambucil	1.54±0.05	0.23±0.01	1.45± 0.06	0.16± 0.03
1μg/ml chlorambucil	1.53±0.05	0.22±0.01	1.50±0.05	0.39±0.03
0.5μg/ml chlorambucil	1.45±0.05	0.25±0.01	1.55±0.05	0.53±0.03

Table 5. Specific Activity of Cyclic AMP Binding Protein (p mole/mg protein) in Walker Carcinoma Sensitive (WS) and Resistant to CB 1954 (WR)

Cell Type*	Binding Activity at pH 4.0⁄
WS	13.3
WR_1	7.5
WR_2	4.7
WR_3	4.4
WR_4	4.2

* WR_1 shows a 16 fold, WR_2 a 64 fold, WR_3 a 500 fold and WR_4 a 2000 fold resistance to CB 1954.

⁄ Binding activity was measured at a ligand concentration of 100nM.

form of the phosphodiesterase approximates to the intracellular level of cyclic AMP (1.96 μM) it is considered that it plays an important role in regulating cyclic AMP levels under physiological conditions.

Resistance of the Walker tumour to alkylating agents is accompanied by changes in the low Km form of the phosphodiesterase manifested by a lower enzyme activity, a shift in pH optima (pH 8.0 in the sensitive to pH 8.4 in the resistant) and a different inhibition constant for the competitive inhibitor theophylline (Ki 2.35 mM for the sensitive and 0.32 mM for the resistant). These results suggest a change in the tertiary structure of the enzyme with the acquisition of resistance. Resistance to CB1954 is also accompanied by a decrease in the cyclic AMP binding protein in Walker tumour (Table 5).

Thus the difunctional alkylating agents which are effective anti-tumour agents cause a rise in the intracellular level of cyclic AMP in Walker cells sensitive to the cytotoxic effects of these agents. This rise in cyclic AMP may play a role in tumour growth inhibition by these agents.

Acknowledgement

M.J. Tisdale wishes to thank the Cancer Research Campaign for the receipt of a research grant.

References

Appleman, M.M., Thompson, W.J. and Russel, T.R. (1973), Advan. Cyclic Nucleotide Res., 3, 65.
Carchman, R.A., Johnson, G.S. and Pastan, I. (1974), Cell, 1, 59.
Edström, A., Kanje, M. and Walum, E. (1974), Expl. Cell Res.,85,217.
Eker, P. (1974), J. Cell Sci., 16, 301.
Johnson, G.S., Morgan, W.D. and Pastan, I. (1972), Nature New Biol., 235, 54.
Johnson, G.S. and Pastan, I. (1972), Nature New Biol., 236, 247.
Kurtz, M.J., Polgar, P., Taylor, L. and Rutenburg, A.M. (1974), Biochem. J., 142, 339.
Millis, A.J.T., Forrest, G.A. and Pious, D.A. (1974), Expl. Cell Res., 83, 335.
Murray, A.W. and Verma, A.K. (1973), Biochem. Biophys, Res. Commun. 54, 69.
Oler, A., Iannaccone, P.M. and Gordon, G.B. (1973), In vitro, 9,35.
Pastan, I. and Johnson, G.S. (1974), Adv. Cancer Res., 19, 303.
Prasad, K.N. and Sheppard, J.R. (1972), Expl. Cell Res., 73, 436.
Tisdale, M.J. and Phillips, B.J. (1975), Biochem. Pharmac. 24, 211.

THE DRUG-CARRIER POTENTIAL OF LIPOSOMES IN CANCER CHEMOTHERAPY

Gregory Gregoriadis

Clinical Research Centre

Watford Road, Harrow, Middx. HA1 3UJ, U.K.

INTRODUCTION

The treatment of cancer is associated with a variety of problems which, to various extents, contribute to the failure of most therapeutic attempts. The outstanding cause of our present difficulties in treating cancer derives from the absence of specificity in the action of available antitumour drugs which in most cases will kill malignant and normal cells alike. Because of this lack of discrimination, a variety of side effects can harass or even threaten the life of treated patients.

Equally important, perhaps, to the pursuit of the ideal antitumour drug is that efforts should be made to employ existing drugs in a manner which will greatly augment their efficacy. To this end I wish to describe our progress towards the development of a universal drug-carrier which upon injection could transport relevant therapeutic agents in isolation from the environment precisely to the site of action.

THE LIPOSOMAL CARRIER

Liposomes have been described as assemblages of phospholipids and other lipids.[1] They form when water insoluble polar lipids are confronted with water and undergo a sequence of conglomerations. The highly ordered structures which finally emerge (liposomes) persist in the presence of excess water which being associated with unfavourable entropy leads to a system of concentric closed membranes each one of which represents an unbroken bimolecular sheet of molecules (Fig. 1). Multilamellar liposomes

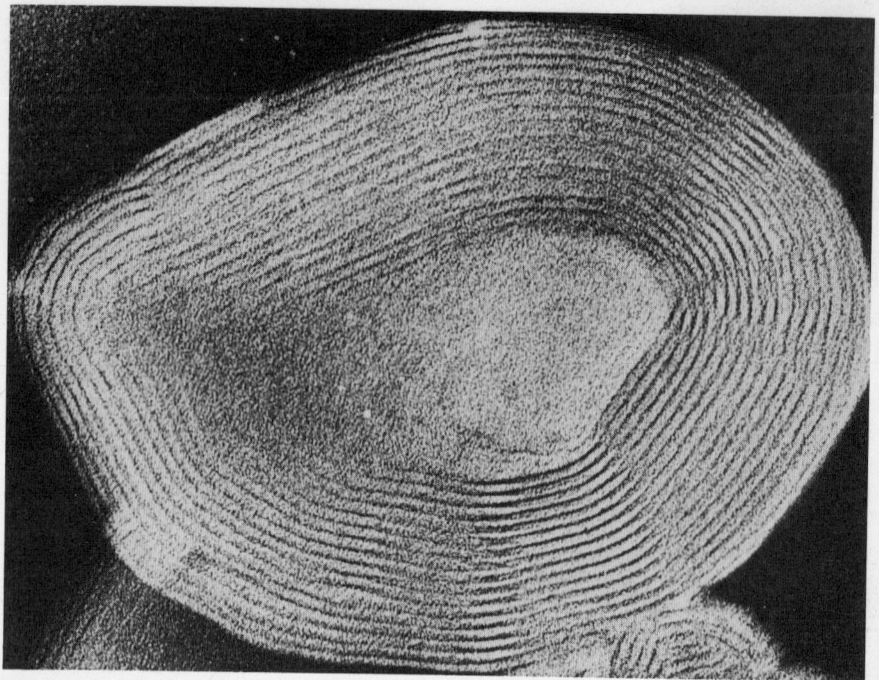

Fig. 1. Multilamellar liposome. Sodium silico-tungstate X 136,000⁹.

consisting of several phospholipid bilayers can upon sonication break up to form smaller monolamellar structures of approximately 250 Å in diameter. These can penetrate basement and endothelial membranes.

The usefulness of liposomes as vehicles for the administration of therapeutic agents is related to the fact that as lipids undergo rearrangements prior to the formation of closed structures, there is unrestricted entry of solutes (e.g. drugs) in between the planes of polar head groups. It is therefore possible to accommodate in the aqueous phase of liposomes a variety of water-soluble substances. Alternatively some lipid soluble substances can be entrapped in between the lipids thus becoming part of the structure of the liposomal membrane. Although lecithin alone is sufficient for the formation of liposomes, some of the properties of the latter can improve by the presence of other lipids. For instance, the addition of cholesterol can augment the stability of the bilayers and the inclusion of charged amphiphiles can not only increase the volume of entrapped drug solution, hence the absolute amount of entrapped drug, but also confer a negative or positive charge on the liposomal surface.

Recent work[3] has shown that liposomes can satisfy many of the criteria of an ideal carrier. Thus liposomes, being composed of simple lipids, are non-toxic and non-antigenic. For instance, repeated intravenous injections of rats with large amounts of liposomes have not resulted in loss of health or in any measurable change in the microscopic appearance of a large number of tissues (C.D.V. Black and G. Gregoriadis, unpublished observations). Liposomes are biodegradable and therefore do not accumulate in the body. At the same time, biodegradation guarantees the eventual liberation of entrapped drugs in the site of action. The easiness and the principles governing the preparation of liposome-entrapped materials warrants the use of liposomes as carriers of an almost unlimited variety of agents. Since it is possible to control the lipid components of liposomes, reactive lipid groups can be accommodated in or on the outermost lipid bilayer. These can interact through ionic or hydrophobic bonding with specific homing devices which could then direct liposomes (and their contents) to target sites.[3]

Experiments with liposome-entrapped agents presented to cells *in vitro* or *in vivo* has led to a number of observations: following their injection into the bloodstream of rats or other experimental animals liposomes, while in circulation, remain intact thus preventing contact of blood with the entrapped agents.[4,5] Liposomes are subsequently endocytosed[2,3,6] by both parenchymal and Kupffer cells of the liver and by the spleen macrophages. A very small proportion is taken up by kidney and lungs.[3] The rate of uptake by tissues is controlled by both the size[7,8] and charge[9] of liposomes. *In vitro*, a variety of cells have been shown to take up liposomes.[10-12]

LIPOSOME-ENTRAPPED ANTITUMOUR DRUGS

A number of cytotoxic drugs have been entrapped in liposomes and their fate studied in vivo.[13-16] The first observation to be made on entrapment itself is that the proportion of the drug which can be associated with liposomes depends on the nature of the drug. For instance 5-fluorouracil[17] or actinomycin D[15] can be passively entrapped in the water phase of liposomes and the extent of entrapment (usually up to 10%) depends on the volume of the entrapped drug solution. On the other hand bleomycin[18] or asparaginase (G. Gregoriadis and E.D. Neerunjun, unpublished observations) can be entrapped to the extent of up to 80 and 50% respectively and, unlike 5-fluorouracil and actinomycin D, bleomycin which is also a small molecule does not diffuse out of liposomes upon exhaustive dialysis. Indeed, even disruption of bleomycin-containing liposomes with an organic solvent (acetone) does not lead to the liberation of bleomycin and it is therefore possible that substances such as bleomycin or asparaginase can interact with lipids to form stable complexes. It is a prerequisite however that such interaction is not detrimental to the formation of the liposome structure and that it does not alter the carrier qualities of liposomes.

Fate of Injected Liposome-Entrapped Drugs

Ideally, the rate of elimination from the circulation of a liposome-entrapped drug should be identical to that of its carrier. However, this can be true only in cases where the drug remains associated with liposomes in the presence of blood. For instance, it has been found that tritiated 5-fluorouracil or actinomycin D entrapped in the aqueous phase of liposomes attain, a few minutes after injection a rate of clearance which is much more rapid than that of the carrier.[17] This could be attributed to an accelerated diffusion of the drug in the presence of plasma proteins such as albumin which possesses an affinity for these drugs. Indeed, diffusion of 5-fluorouracil and actinomycin D from liposomes in water in the absence of serum is much slower. Entrapment of actinomycin D, which is lipid soluble as well, in the lipid phase of liposomes prevents such diffusion from occurring *in vivo* and the rate of the drug elimination from the plasma is identical to that of the liposomal carrier.[15] Similar results are obtained with ^{111}In-labelled bleomycin entrapped in the aqueous phase of liposomes, probably because of the firm association of the drug with the liposomal lipids. Further, the liposomal carrier succeeds in imposing a drug tissue distribution which reflects that of the carrier i.e. pronounced hepatic and splenic uptake and diminished localisation in cells (e.g. intestinal mucosa) to which free drugs can be toxic.[15,17] Studies[11] at the intracellular level have shown that radioactivity from injected liposome-entrapped actinomycin D localises in the lysosome-rich fraction (54% of the total in the liver). However, by 24h following administration radioactivity in the nuclei-rich fraction has doubled to 24%. This is in contrast with the free drug which localises in the nuclear fraction (60%) and to a very small extent (2%) in the lysosome-rich fraction. In experiments[11] with partially hepatectomised rats, it was shown that the passage of actinomycin D through the lysosomes as a necessary step for its liberation from liposomes did not affect its inhibitory properties: both entrapped and free actinomycin D inhibited DNA directed RNA synthesis. Similar results have been recently obtained with bleomycin and asparaginase (C.D.V. Black and G. Gregoriadis, unpublished observations). In the case of asparaginase which because of its molecular weight cannot escape from the lysosomes, it is assumed that hepatic cell asparagine enters the lysosomes where it is attacked by asparaginase. This could deplete the liver of asparagine and prevent cell regeneration.

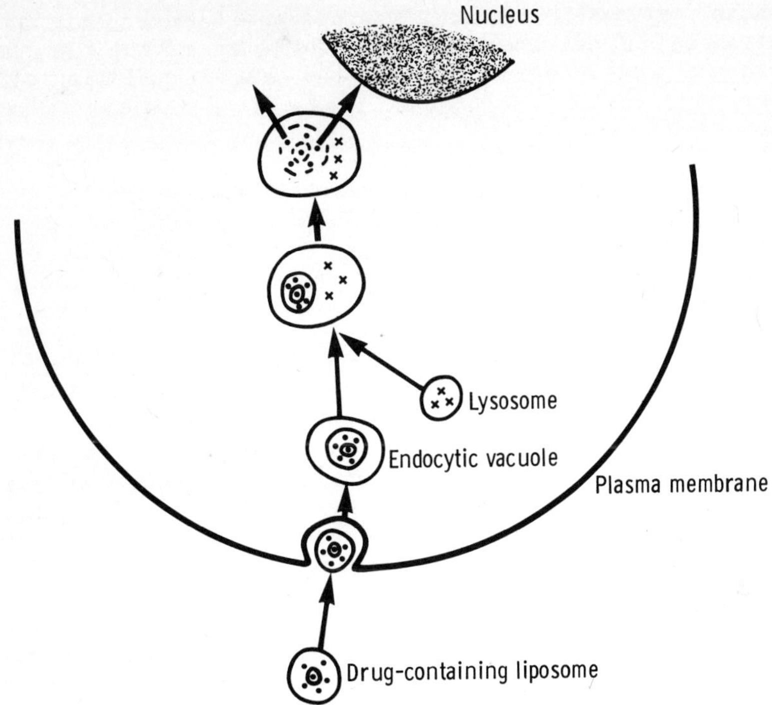

Fig. 2. Cellular uptake and lysosomotropic action of liposome-entrapped drugs. A liposome containing drug molecules ( ) is taken up into a cell by endocytosis. The endocytic vacuole fuses with a lysosome, the hydrolases (X) of which disrupt the lipid bilayers of the liposome, releasing the entrapped drug, which can then diffuse out and act in other cellular compartments (e.g., nucleus).[19]

Mode of Action of Liposome-Entrapped Drugs

Findings with liposome-entrapped cytotoxic drugs injected into normal,[15] partially hepatectomised[11] and tumour-bearing animals,[12] suggests a mode of drug action which in its main lines could be universal for all agents introduced into cells via the liposomal carrier (Fig. 2). Following endocytosis of the carrier by the cell, the endocytic vacuole containing the liposome fuses with a primary or secondary lysosome. This brings liposomes in contact with the lysosomal hydrolases and it is assumed here that the observed disruption of liposomes and subsequent liberation of the entrapped drug is carried out by the lysosomal phospholipases. The freed drug, provided it remains intact in the lysosomal milieu can then act either from within the lysosomes (asparaginase?) or, after its diffusion from lysosomes, in other cell compartments, e.g. nucleus[11]. At present it is not known whether the mode of introduction of a liposomal drug into the site of action is exclusively lysosomotropic. Others[13] have suggested that liposomes can under certain conditions, fuse with cell membranes and expel their contents into the cell's cytoplasm.

INTERACTION OF LIPOSOME-ENTRAPPED DRUGS WITH MALIGNANT CELLS

In vitro[13,14,18] and in vivo[12,19] experiments have shown that liposomes can enter malignant cells. Intravenous or intra-arterial administration into cancer patients of liposome-entrapped radiolabelled albumin was followed by the localisation of radioactivity in tumour cells and in most instances uptake by tumours was higher than by the surrounding normal tissue.[19] Similar observations have been recently made using a number of transplanted carcinomas in mice and rats which received liposomes containing ^{111}In-labelled bleomycin. It also appeared that tumour localisation of liposomes could be improved upon by diminishing the size of the carrier (G. Gregoriadis and E.D. Neerunjun, unpublished observations).

Intraperitoneal administration of therapeutic doses of free and liposome-entrapped actinomycin D to AKR-A mice inoculated with AKR-A cells showed that survival of treated mice was longer when the entrapped drug was used.[12] This was attributed to a more efficient uptake of the drug via the liposomal carrier and also to the decreased toxicity of the entrapped drug.

HOMING OF LIPOSOMES TO TARGET CELLS

The almost exclusive uptake of liposomes by cells of the liver and spleen would hardly allow any significant portion of a therapeutic dose to reach the diseased target area. It therefore follows that any strategy for homing could only be successful if at the same time one could prevent or even delay premature clearance of the injected dose by these tissues. We have found that such delay can be achieved by the simultaneous administration of a large quantity of "empty" liposomes[9] or by the use of positively charged liposomes which exhibit a slower rate of elimination from plasma.[9]

It has now been established[18] that homing of liposomes by the use of molecular probes which possess a specific affinity for the surface of target cells is possible. When IgG immunoglobulins raised against a variety of normal and malignant cells are co-entrapped (in their radiolabelled form) with ^{111}In-labelled bleomycin in liposomes, the latter appear to possess on their surface immunologically active portions of the entrapped IgG

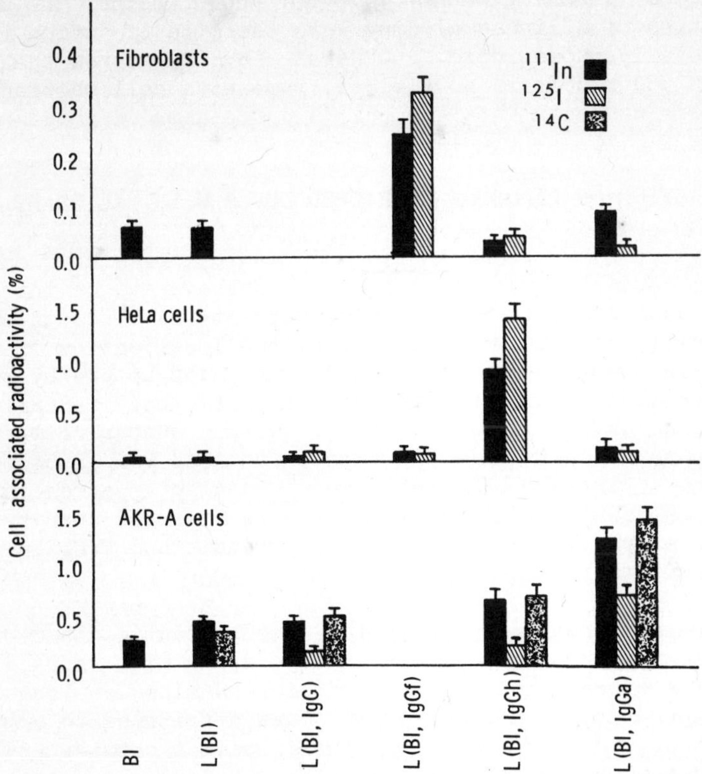

Fig. 3. Homing of liposomes by IgG immunoglobulins. Cells were exposed to media containing ^{111}In-labelled bleomycin, free (Bl) or entrapped in liposomes containing: PBS,(L,Bl); non-specific IgG, L(Bl,IgG); anti-human fibroblasts IgG, L(Bl,IgGf); anti-HeLa cells IgG, L(Bl,IgGh); anti-AKR-A cells IgG, L(Bl,IgGa). Values are expressed as percent (mean ± standard error) of added radioactivity associated with cells.[18]

molecules. Indeed, when cells are exposed to such liposomes, judging from radioactivity measurements, uptake of bleomycin and IgG and of the liposomal carrier (^{14}C-labelled cholesterol) is most pronounced when liposomes are associated with the IgG corresponding to the cell type studied (Fig. 3). These results suggest that following their attachment to the respective antigenic sites, IgG molecules mediate uptake of the associated liposomal carrier and its drug contents.

Present experiments in my laboratory are now carried out in tumour bearing animals and it is hoped that the appropriate combination of both blocking of hepatic uptake of liposomes and of homing techniques will lead to a pharmacologically effective drug action.

ACKNOWLEDGMENTS

I thank Mrs. E.Diane Neerunjun for technical assistance and Mrs. Dorothy Seale for secretarial work.

REFERENCES

1. Bangham, A.D., Hill, M.W. and Miller, N.G.A. (1974) in "Methods in Membrane Biology" (E.D. Korn, ed.) p.1, vol. 1, Plenum Press
2. Segal, A.W., Wills, E.J., Richmond, J.E., Slavin, G., Black, C.D.V. and Gregoriadis, G. (1974) Br. J. Exp. Pathol. 55, 320
3. Gregoriadis, G. (1974) in "Enzyme Therapy in Lysosomal Storage Diseases" (J.M. Tager, G.J.M. Hooghwinkel and W.Th. Daems, eds.) p.131, North-Holland Publishing Company, Amsterdam.
4. Gregoriadis, G. and Ryman, B.E. (1972) Biochem. J. 129, 123
5. Gregoriadis, G., Putman, D., Louis, L. and Neerunjun, E.D. (1974) Biochem. J. 140, 323
6. Rahman, V.-E. and Wright, B.J. (1975) J. Cell Biol. 65, 112
7. Juliano, R.L. and Stamp, D. (1975) Biochem. Biophys. Res. Comm. 63, 651
8. McDougall, I.R., Dunnick, J.K., McNamee, M.G. and Kriss, J.P. (1974) Proc. Nat. Acad. Sci. U.S.A. 71, 3487
9. Gregoriadis, G. and Neerunjun, E.D. (1974) Eur. J. Biochem. 47, 179
10. Gregoriadis, G. and Buckland, R.A. (1973) Nature 244, 170
11. Papahadjopoulos, D., Mayhew, E., Poste, G. and Smith, S. (1974) Nature 252, 163
12. Magee, W.E., Goff, C.W., Schoknecht, J., Smith, M.D. and Cherian, K. (1974) J. Cell Biol. 63, 492
13. Black, C.D.V. and Gregoriadis, G. (1974) Biochem. Soc. Trans. 2, 869
14. Gregoriadis, G. and Neerunjun, E.D. (1975) Res. Comm. Chem. Pathol. Pharm. 10, 351
15. Gregoriadis, G. (1973) FEBS Lett. 36, 292
16. Colley, C.M. and Ryman, B.E. (1975) Biochem. Soc. Trans. 3,157
17. Gregoriadis, G. (1973) Biochem. Soc. Trans. 2, 117
18. Gregoriadis, G. and Neerunjun, E.D. (1975) Biochem. Biophys. Res. Comm. In press
19. Gregoriadis, G., Swain, C.P., Wills, E.J. and Tavill, A.S. (1974) Lancet i, 1313

SIGNIFICANCE OF PROSTAGLANDINS IN TUMOUR GROWTH

Jennifer A.C. Sykes

Department of Physiology, The Medical School
University of Bristol, Bristol BS8 1TD

In recent years, attention has been focused on the possible role of prostaglandins (PGs) in tumour physiology. They have been implicated in such aspects as cell replication, bone resorption and hypercalcaemia as well as being potentially responsible for many of the symptoms associated with malignancy.

1. OCCURRENCE OF PROSTAGLANDINS IN TUMOURS

In 1968, Williams, Karim and Sandler reported elevated levels of both PGE_2 and $PGF_2\alpha$ in tumour tissue & plasma of patients with medullary carcinoma of the thyroid. Later in the same year they showed that tumours that secreted peptides and amines were also able to secrete PGs (Sandler, Karim and Williams, 1968). It is now recognised that a variety of human tumours can secrete PGs, including

- *Medullary carcinoma of the thyroid
- Carcinoma of the bronchus
- Lung metastases
- Breast tumours
- *Neuroblastoma
- *Phaeochromocytoma
- Liver metastases
- *Ileal carcinoid
- Rectal carcinoid
- *Kaposi's sarcoma
- *Renal cell carcinoma
- Islet cell tumours

(For a fuller report of such tumours, see Karim & Rao, 1975.) When PGs are detected in the peripheral plasma of patients with tumours (marked with *) it suggests that these tumours secrete very large amounts of PGs since 97% of PGs are removed in one circulation through the lungs (Ferreira & Vane, 1967).

A variety of animal tumours have also been shown to contain PGs, but in contrast to human tumours, these usually only contain PGE_2, which has been positively identified by gaschromatography - mass spectrometry in some instances (Sykes & Maddox, 1972). PGs can also be detected in the peripheral plasma of mice bearing the $HSDM_1$ fibrosarcoma (Tashjian, Voelkel, Goldhaber & Levine, 1973) and in the blood directly draining the Walker carcinosarcoma where the PG release from this tumour was 0.26ngPGE_2/min/ml blood (Sykes, unpublished). PGs are not only released from tumours in vivo, they can be released into the media when cells are grown in culture; included amongst these are BP8/P_1 and Lewis lung cells (Sykes & Maddox, 1974), $HSDM_1$ fibrosarcoma cells (Levine, Hinkle, Voelkel & Tashjian, 1972), neuroblastoma, glioma, HeLa, HEp-2 and L cell lines (Cohen & Jaffe, 1973; Jaffe, Philpott, Hamprecht & Parker, 1973; Hamprecht, Jaffe & Philpott, 1973). Human colon carcinoma cells in culture have also been shown to release PG, eight times as much as did normal colonic mucosa cells obtained from the same surgical specimen (Jaffe, Parker & Philpott, 1972). The finding that PG synthesis can be shown in vivo and in vitro shows that such synthesis is not dependent on any host-tumour interaction but is a property of the cells themselves.

PGs are formed from essential fatty acid precursors such as arachidonic acid which is incorporated in membrane phospholipids. This synthesis can be inhibited by non-steroidal anti-inflammatory compounds such as aspirin and indomethacin (Vane, 1971). Several tumour lines show an increased PG synthesis on addition of arachidonic acid including Sarcoma 180, BP8/P_1 (Sykes & Maddox, 1972), Kaposi's sarcoma (Bhana, Hillier & Karim, 1971), HeLa, L and HEp-2 (Cohen & Jaffe, 1973) DMBA mammary tumour (Tan, Privett & Goldyne, 1974).

Many different tumours and cell lines are capable of synthesising large amounts of PG and the question arises as to the significance of this synthesis : is it another form of inappropriate hormone secretion or do the PGs play some important role in cell growth?

2. PROSTAGLANDINS AND CELL REPLICATION

The involvement of PGs in cell replication appears to be closely related with the effects of cyclic adenosine 3^1 - 5^1 monophosphate (cAMP).

a: cAMP decreases cell proliferation and there are low levels of cAMP in rapidly dividing and transformed cells (Sheppard, 1972). If the exogenous level of cAMP is raised, transformed cells revert to their pretransformed state and stop dividing. As these cellular alterations can be mimicked by PGE_1 and PGE_2, it seems possible that PGs may act through altered cAMP levels.

b: cAMP increases PG synthesis in many cells and PGs themselves increase adenylate cyclase activity in many cell lines (Peery, Johnson & Pastan, 1971; Makman, 1971; Hamprecht & Schultz, 1973).

c: Some animal tumours have been shown to contain high levels of PGs as well as cAMP which also suggests a link between these two compounds. However treatment of mice bearing Moloney sarcomas with a prostaglandin synthesis inhibitor such as indomethacin reduced the tumour PG levels without any concomitant effect on the tumour cAMP levels. (Humes, Cupo & Strausser, 1974).

d: In some cells both PG and cAMP activity appears to be linked with the process of transformation. Otten, Johnson & Pastan (1971) have investigated the cAMP levels in a temperature sensitive mutant fibroblast which is transformed at 36°C but not at 40.5°C. They found that the cellular cAMP levels fell dramatically with a fall in temperature and so a decrease in cAMP levels preceded the establishment of the transformed state. SV 40 viral transformation of medullary carcinoma of the thyroid cells leads to a production of PGs by the cells in monolayer culture (Grimley, Deftos, Weeks & Rabson, 1969). More recently, Hammarström, Samuelsson & Bjursell (1973) showed that polyoma virus transformation of baby hamster kidney fibroblasts led to a considerable increase in PGE_2 production by these cells.

As both cAMP and PGs decrease cell proliferation, it might be expected that inhibition of PG synthesis would result in an increase in cell growth. This has certainly been demonstrated _in vitro_ by Thomas, Philpott & Jaffe (1974); indomethacin inhibited HEp-2, L and HeLa cell PG synthesis by as much as 85% and stimulated cell growth by up to 37%. _In vivo_ however, indomethacin produces variable results. Sykes & Maddox (1972) have shown that inhibition of tumour PG synthesis in the sarcoma 180, $BP8/P_1$ and Lewis lung tumours was not accompanied by any significant alteration in tumour growth: these results were supported by Powles, Clarke, Easty, Easty & Neville (1973) using the Walker carcinosarcoma but in direct contrast Humes et al (1974) and Tashjian, Voelkel, Goldhaber & Levine (1973) showed that _in vivo_ indomethacin inhibited both PG synthesis and tumour growth in the Moloney sarcoma and HSDM tumours. The interrelationship between PGs and cAMP in the control of cell growth is still uncertain and more work is needed to clarify the relationship.

3. PROSTAGLANDINS AND HYPERCALCAEMIA

In 1960, Goldhaber first described a transplantable mouse fibrosarcoma ($HSDM_1$) which synthesised a bone resorpting factor *in vitro* Klein & Raisz (1970) showed that both parathyroid hormone (PTH) and PGE were capable of stimulating bone resorption *in vitro* but *in vivo* only PTH was capable of raising serum calcium levels. Levine, Hinkle, Voelkel & Tashjian (1972) found that the $HSDM_1$ cells were capable of synthesising PGs. Later the same year, Tashjian, Voelkel, Goldhaber & Levine (1972) proved conclusively that the bone resorpting substance secreted by the $HSDM_1$ cells was PGE_2. In addition they were able to demonstrate that mice bearing these tumours had elevated serum calcium levels which could be reduced by treatment of the animals with indomethacin. More recently, Powles et al.(1973) have shown that rats bearing the Walker carcinosarcoma have hypercalcaemia as well as bony and soft tissue metastases. Treatment of such animals with indomethacin and/or aspirin lowered the serum calcium levels, reduced the bony metastases but had no effect on the development of soft tissue metastases. Indomethacin has no antimetastatic effect in the Lewis lung tumour where implantation of the primary in the flank leads to the development of pulmonary metastases (Ketcham, Wexler & Minton, 1966).

Human breast cancer is often associated with osteolytic bone metastases and bone resorption as well as a hypercalcaemia which is not due to PTH. Bennett, McDonald, Simpson & Stamford (1975) recently found that tissue from human malignant breast cancer contained and synthesised more PG-like material than normal breast tissue. They speculated that bone metastases were usually associated with tumours containing high levels of PGF-like material although no definitive analysis of the PGs involved was carried out. Treatment with indomethacin lowered serum calcium levels in a patient with renal cell adenocarcinoma (Brereton, Halushka, Alexander, Mason, Keiser & DeVita, 1974). Furthermore Blum (1975) found that hypercalcaemia of unknown origin could be lowered by treatment with indomethacin. Unfortunately neither group measured the blood PG levels before and after treatment which might have provided direct evidence that hypercalcaemia is related to excess PG production by some human tumours. Hypercalcaemia caused by tumour metastases in bone which is not due to excess PTH secretion may be due to a local release of PG from the tumour cells. This PG could then cause bone resorption.

4. CONCLUSIONS

A wide range of animal and human tumours can synthesise and release PGs both *in vivo* and *in vitro*. The PGs are usually of the E-series. The high levels of PGs may be simply due to biochemical aberrations in the tumour cells as a result of transformation to a malignant type of cell. The exact inter-relationship with cAMP in the control of cell proliferation is still uncertain. The PG production by tumours may be classed as another form of inappropriate hormone secretion also seen with hormones such as PTH, antidiuretic hormone, adrenocorticotrophic hormone, etc. Although the synthesis may be inappropriate, many of the symptoms associated with malignancy may be due to excessive PG production. It is likely that drugs which will inhibit the synthesis of PGs or their actions will prove useful additions to standard cancer therapy.

REFERENCES

Bennett, A., McDonald, A.M., Simpson, J.S. & Stamford, I.F. (1975) Lancet i 1218-1220.

Bhana, D., Hillier, K. & Karim, S.M.M. (1971) Cancer 27, 233-237.

Blum, I. (1975) Lancet i 866.

Brereton, H.D., Halushka, P.V., Alexander, R.W., Mason, D.M., Keiser, H.R. & DeVita, V.T. (1974) New Engl. J. Med. 291 83-85.

Cohen, F. & Jaffe, B.M. (1973) Biochem. Biophys. Res. Comm. 55 724-729.

Ferreira, S.H. & Vane, J.R. (1967) Nature, 216 868-873.

Goldhaber, P. (1960) Proc. Am. Ass. Canc. Res. 3 113.

Grimley, P.M., Deftos, L.J., Weeks, J.R. & Rabson, A.S. (1969) J. Nat. Canc. Inst. 42 663-680.

Hammarström, S., Samuelsson, B. & Bjursell, G. (1973) Nature New Biology 243 50-51.

Hamprecht, B. & Schultz, J. (1973) FEBS Letters 34 85-89.

Hamprecht, B., Jaffe, B.M. & Philpott, G.W. (1973) FEBS Letters, 36 193-198.

Humes, J.L., Cupo, J.J. & Strausser, H.R. (1974) Prostaglandins 6 463-473.

Jaffe, B.M., Parker, C.W. & Philpott, G.W. (1972). In: Prostaglandins in Cellular Biology. Ed. P.W. Ramwell & B.B. Phariss. Plenum Press. N.Y. p. 207.

Jaffe, B.M. Philpott, G.W., Hamprecht, B. & Parker, C.W. (1973) Adv. Biosci. 9 179-182.

Karim, S.M.M. & Rao, B. (1975) Prostaglandins - Progress in Research, MTP Oxford & Lancaster. Ed. S.M.M. Karim. To be published.

Ketcham, A.S., Wexler, H. & Minton, J.P. (1966) J. Am. med. Ass., 198 157-164.

Klein, D.C. & Raisz, L.G. (1970) Endocrinology 86 1436-1440.

Levine, L., Hinkle, P.M., Voelkel, E.F. & Tashjian, A.H. (1972) Biochem. Biophys. Res. Comm. 47 888-897.

Makman, M.H. (1971) Proc. Natl. Acad. Sci. U.S.A. 68 2127-2130.

Otten, J., Johnson, G.S. & Pastan, I. (1971) Biochem. Biophys. Res. Comm. 44 1192-1198.

Peery, C., Johnson, G.S. & Pastan, I. (1971) J. Biol.Chem. 246 5785-5790.

Powles, T.J., Clarke, S.A., Easty, D.M., Easty, G.C. & Munro-Neville, A. (1973) Br. J. Cancer 28 316-321.

Sandler, M., Karim, S.M.M., & Williams, E.D. (1968) Lancet ii 1053-1055.

Sheppard, J.R. (1971) Nature New Biology 236 14-16.

Sykes, J.A.C. & Maddox, I.S. (1972) Nature New Biology 237 59-61.

Sykes, J.A.C. & Maddox, I.S. (1974) Pol.J.Pharmacol.Pharm. 26 83-91.

Tan, W.C., Privett, O.S. & Goldyne, M.E. (1974) Cancer Res. 34 3229-3231.

Tashjian, A.H., Voelkel, E.F., Levine, L. & Goldhaber, P. (1972) J. Exp. Med. 136 1329-1343.

Tashjian, A.H., Voelkel, E.F., Goldhaber, P. & Levine, L. (1973) Prostaglandins 3 515-524.

Thomas, D.R., Philpott, G.W. & Jaffe, B.M. (1974) Exp.Cell.Res., 84 40-46.

Vane, J.R. (1971) Nature New Biol., 231 232-235.

Williams, E.D., Karim, S.M.M. & Sandler, M. (1968) Lancet i 22-23.

OESTROGEN BINDING AS A PREDICTIVE TEST FOR DMBA-INDUCED TUMOUR RESPONSE TO TAMOXIFEN THERAPY

V.C. Jordan & T. Jaspan

Department of Pharmacology

School of Medicine, Leeds LS2 9NL

INTRODUCTION

Jensen *et al.* (1971) have suggested that oestrogen receptor assays may be a useful predictive test to determine the oestrogen dependency of breast tumours. In the laboratory, the 7,12-dimethylbenz(a)anthracene (DMBA)-induced rat mammary carcinoma (Huggins *et al.* 1961) provides a model for the study of this theory, since oestrogen binding in the tumour has been reported to be related to oestrogen dependency (Mobbs 1966, McGuire & Julian 1971, Mobbs & Johnson 1974).

Tamoxifen (ICI 46,474), an anti-oestrogen used clinically in the treatment of breast cancer (Cole *et al.* 1971; Ward 1973), inhibits the growth of DMBA-induced rat mammary tumours (Jordan, 1974; Jordan & Koerner, 1976) with a simultaneous inhibition of oestrogen binding (Jordan & Dowse 1976). In the present study we report our investigation of oestrogen binding as a predictive test for DMBA-induced tumour response to tamoxifen therapy.

METHODS

Tumours were induced in 50 day old female Sprague Dawley rats by the intragastric administration of 20 mg DMBA (Sigma). One hundred days after DMBA administration, suitable tumours (2-5 cm^2) were biopsied, the tumour tissue frozen in liquid N_2, powdered and homogenized in phosphate buffer (pH 7.3) 1:5 w/v. Cytosols (100,000 x *g* supernatants) were used for determinations of oestrogen binding by an adaptation of the methods described by Ginsberg *et al.* (1974). Cytosol (150 μl) was incubated (30°C for 30 min) with 50 μl buffer and 50 µl buffer containing a saturating dose (0.2 pmole) of [2,4,6,7-^{3}H] oestradiol-17β (110 Ci/mmole NEN Corp.). Diethylstilboestrol (BDH), 25 pmole in 50 µl buffer, was used to determine non-specific binding in parallel incubates (in place of 50 µl buffer). Bound and free oestradiol were separated on Sephadex LH20 columns (Pharmacia) at 4°C and after counting in a Packard Tricarb Liquid Scintillation Spectrometer (3320) results were expressed as fmole/mg cytosol protein. Protein was determined according to Lowry et al. (1951).

Each biopsied rat was immediately treated with 50 µg Tamoxifen (ICI Ltd. see below) daily for 3 weeks. Tumour areas were determined with calipers before and after 3 weeks of therapy.

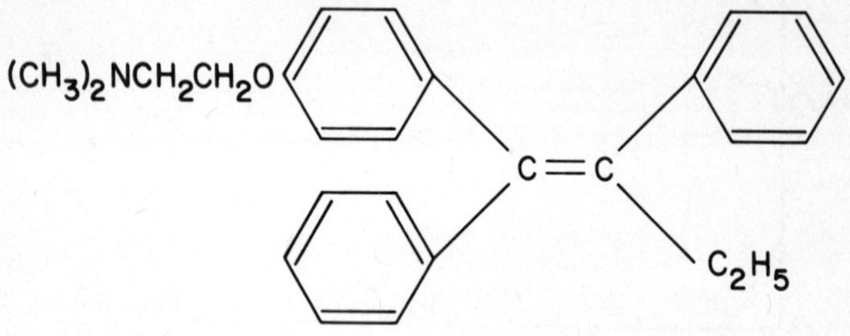

$(CH_3)_2NCH_2CH_2O$ — $C=C$ — C_2H_5

ICI 46,474 (trans)

(Tamoxifen, Nolvadex®)

RESULTS & DISCUSSION

We have found three types of tumour response to tamoxifen therapy based on the oestrogen binding of biopsy samples (Fig 1 & 2). In tumours with low oestrogen binding ($<$11 fmole/mg cytosol protein) there was either stasis or tumour growth (Group A). At intermediate levels of oestrogen binding (11-36 fmole/mg cytosol protein) an increased oestrogen binding concentration was found to be related to an increased tumour regression (Group B) but at high levels of oestrogen binding ($>$36 fmole/mg cytosol protein) the expected 100% regression was not attained and often $<$ 50% regression was observed (Group C). Amalgamation of data from Groups A, B & C : $r = 0.515$ $P < 0.01$, whereas data from Groups A & B : $r = 0.82$ $P < 0.001$. The reason for the partial response of Group C remains obscure although a larger daily dose of tamoxifen may have been more effective.

The present investigation is the first to our knowledge, of the successful use of an oestrogen receptor assay as a predictive test for anti-oestrogen therapy in this animal model. Tamoxifen

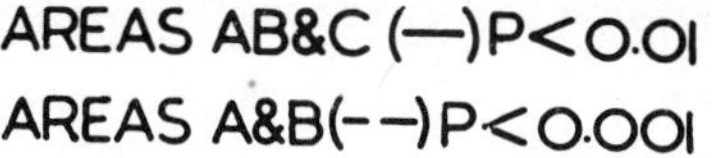

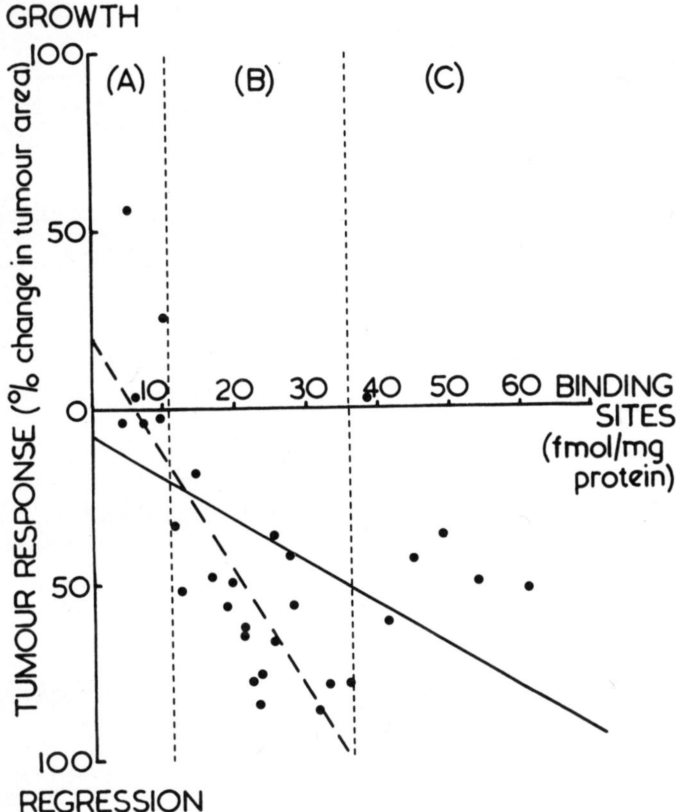

Fig. 1. Correlation of oestrogen binding in DMBA-induced tumour biopsies with response to 3 weeks of tamoxifen therapy (50 µg/day) (Jordan & Jáspan, 1976. Journal of Endocrinology).

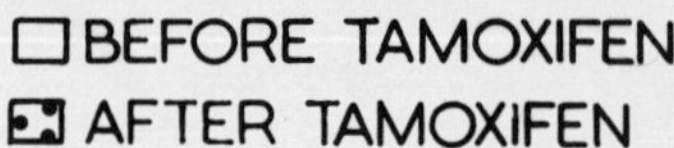

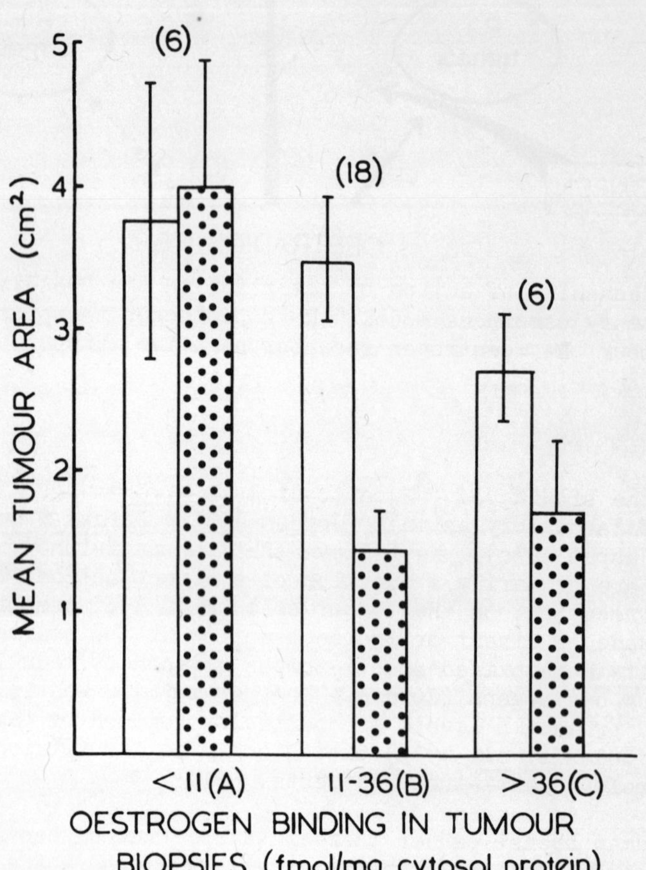

Fig. 2. DMBA-induced tumour areas before and after 3 weeks of tamoxifen therapy (50 μg/day). Tumours are classified by oestrogen binding assay prior to therapy. Group B: area before vs area after therapy $P < 0.001$. Other groups $P > 0.05$ (by Student's *t* test) (Jordan & Jaspan, 1976. Journal of Endocrinology).

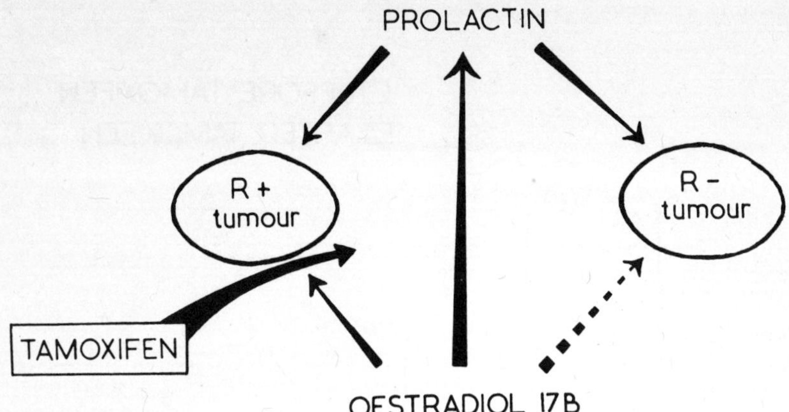

Fig. 3. Mechanism of action of tamoxifen in the DMBA-induced rat mammary carcinoma model. R + = oestrogen receptor positive tumour R- = oestrogen receptor negative tumour.

inhibits the binding of [^{3}H]oestradiol *in vivo* to the target tissues of laboratory animals (Jordan 1975; Jordan & Dowse 1976; Jordan & Jaspan 1976). We believe that the anti-tumour effects of tamoxifen are primarily a function of a direct action, via the oestrogen receptor, on the tumour cell (Fig. 3). Associated with this blockade, a direct or indirect action at the ovarian level may facilitate tamoxifen's anti-tumour actions by reducing circulating oestrogens (Jordan & Koerner 1976). Oestrogen-stimulated prolactin levels are partially reduced by tamoxifen therapy (Jordan *et al.* 1975) but this may be insufficient to produce profound anti-tumour effects.

In human breast cancer there is a spectrum of oestrogen receptor concentrations (Feherty *et al.* 1971) and where present, tamoxifen inhibits the binding of [^{3}H]oestradiol *in vitro* to 8S oestrogen binding components (Jordan & Koerner 1975). It may therefore be useful to preselect breast cancer patients for anti-oestrogen therapy based on oestrogen receptor determinations.

SUMMARY

We have demonstrated the practicality of using an oestrogen receptor assay as a predictive test for DMBA-induced tumour response to tamoxifen therapy. Although a high oestrogen receptor concentration group failed to respond as fully as expected, the results were such as to suggest that a similar approach in the treatment of human breast cancer may be useful.

Acknowledgements We wish to thank Mr K. Heald for equipment used in the oestrogen receptor assay and Mr P. Rylett for drawing the figures. We also thank ICI for a grant for the study.

REFERENCES

Cole, M.P., Jones, C.T.A. & Todd, D.H. (1971). British Journal of Cancer 25 270.

Feherty,P., Farrer-Brown, G. & Kellie, A.E. (1971). British Journal of Cancer 25 697.

Ginsberg, M. Greenstein, B.D., Maclusky, N.H., Morrison, I.D. & Thomas, P.J. (1974). Steroids 23 773.

Huggins, C., Grand, L.C. & Brillantes (1961). Nature (London) 189 204.

Jensen, E.V., Block, G.E., Smith, S., Kyser, K. & De Sombre, E.R. (1971). NCI Monograph 34 55.

Jordan, V.C. (1974). Journal of steroid Biochemistry 5 354. (Abstr.)

Jordan, V.C. (1975). Journal of Reproduction & Fertility 42 251

Jordan, V.C. & Dowse, L.J. (1976). Journal of Endocrinology. (in press).

Jordan, V.C. & Jaspan, T. (1976). Journal of Endocrinology (submitted for publication)

Jordan, V.C. & Koerner, S. (1975). European Journal of Cancer 11 205.

Jordan, V.C. & Koerner, S. (1976). Journal of Endocrinology (in press)

Jordan, V.C., Koerner, S. & Robison, C. (1975). Journal of Endocrinology 65 151.

Lowry, O.H., Rosebrough,N.J., Farr, A.L. & Randall, R.J. (1951) Journal of biological chemistry 193 265.

McGuire, W.L. & Julian, J.A. (1971). Cancer Research 31 1440.

Mobbs, B.G. (1966). Journal of Endocrinology 34 409.

Mobbs, B.G. & Johnson, I.E. (1974). European Journal of Cancer 10 757.

Ward, H.W.C. (1973). British Medical Journal 1 13.

ACTION OF ANTICANCER DRUGS ON THE CELL CYCLE. CHROMOSOME DAMAGE AND DIFFERENTIAL STAGE SENSITIVITY

David Scott

Paterson Laboratories
Christie Hospital & Holt Radium Institute, Manchester
M20 9BX, United Kingdom

In spite of the fact that the relative sensitivities of different phases of the cell cycle to the cytotoxic effects a large number of anticancer drugs is known[1] the *mechanisms* of differential stage sensitivity are, in general, poorly understood. A better understanding of these mechanisms should allow a more rational approach to the practical application of these drugs. As a cytogeneticist I am struck by the high proportion of anticancer drugs which produce chromosome structural damage; Table 1 gives a list of such drugs taken from a survey by Shaw[2] in 1970 so it is by now certainly incomplete but is nevertheless an impressive list and includes many anticancer drugs in common use. I hope to show that at least for one class of drugs, the alkylating agents, chromosome aberration frequencies play an important part in determining differential stage sensitivity.

It is now well established that the major cause of radiation-induced lethality in mammalian cells is the induction of chromosome damage[3,4,5]. Recently it has become apparent that this may also be the case for a number of anticancer drugs and related compounds[5,6]. A rather striking example of this relationship has come from studies in our laboratory of the Yoshida lymphosarcoma of rats. This transplantable tumour is particularly sensitive to treatment with difunctional alkylating agents and Fox[7] has shown that a single dose of 10mg/kg methylene dimethane sulphonate (MDMS) will cure over 90% of animals carrying this tumour. Those tumours which recur prove to be resistant to MDMS and when cells from MDMS-sensitive (YS) and MDMS-resistant (YR) tumours are put into *in vitro* culture they retain their differential sensitivity to this drug and also exhibit a differential sensitivity to nitrogen mustard[8].

Table 1

Some Anticancer Drugs Which Produce Chromosome Structural Aberrations in Human Cells

Alkylating Agents	Antimetabolites
Busulphan	Amethopterin
Cyclophosphamide	Aminopterin
Nitromin	Cytosine arabinoside
Nitrogen mustard	6-Azauridine
Trenimon	5-Fluorodeoxyuridine
TEPA	Thioguanine
ThioTEPA	6-Mercaptopurine
Hexamethylmelamine	
Hexamethylphosphoramide	**Alkaloids**
Imuran	
	Demecolcine
Antibiotics	Podophyllotoxin
	Heliotrine
Actinomycin D	
Daunomycin	**Misc**
Mitomycin C	
Phleomycin	Hydroxyurea
Streptonigrin	Urethane
Bleomycin	

We have now shown that this pair of cell lines show a very striking differential sensitivity to the lethal effect of sulphur mustard (Fig 1) even though both cell lines incorporate similar amounts of the drug into their DNA, RNA and protein[5]. The reason for choosing to use this alkylating agent, in spite of the fact that it is not used in tumour therapy, is that it has a half-life of only a few minutes in aqueous solution[9]. This is a great advantage in studies on differential stage sensitivity since, after treatment, the drug is not retained in the cells as they pass from one stage to another; differential stage sensitivity is therefore not blurred as it often is with many other more stable drugs.

When exponentially growing populations of YS and YR cells are treated with 20 ng/ml of sulphur mustard (SM) very much more chromosome damage is induced in YS cells (Figs 2,3,4). Thus there is a positive correlation between chromosome structural aberrations and lethality in this pair of cell lines, suggesting a causal relationship.

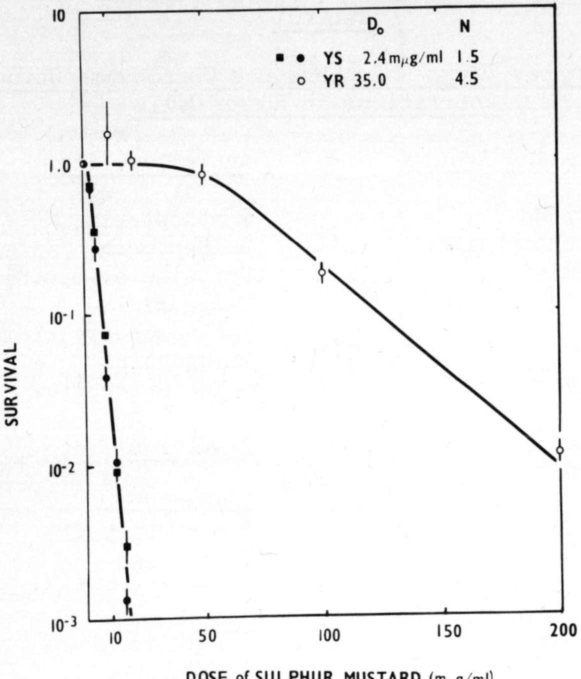

Fig. 1. Survival of YS and YR cells treated with sulphur mustard.

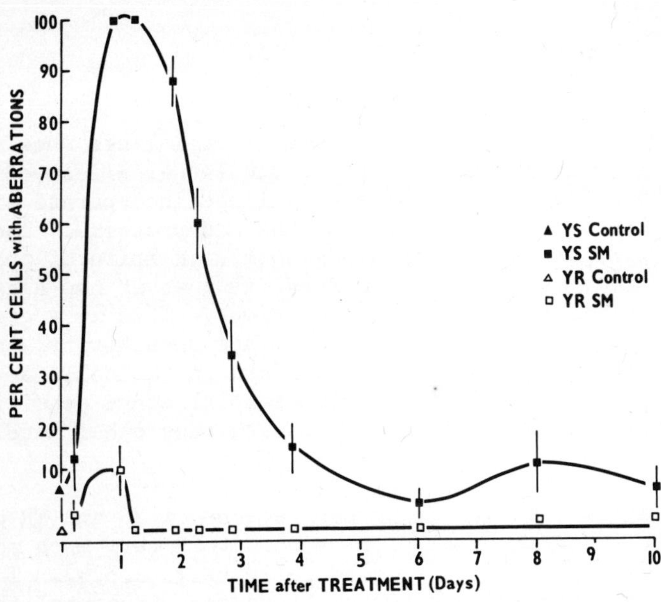

Fig. 2. Frequency of cells with chromosome aberrations after treatment of YS and YR cells with 20 ng/ml SM.

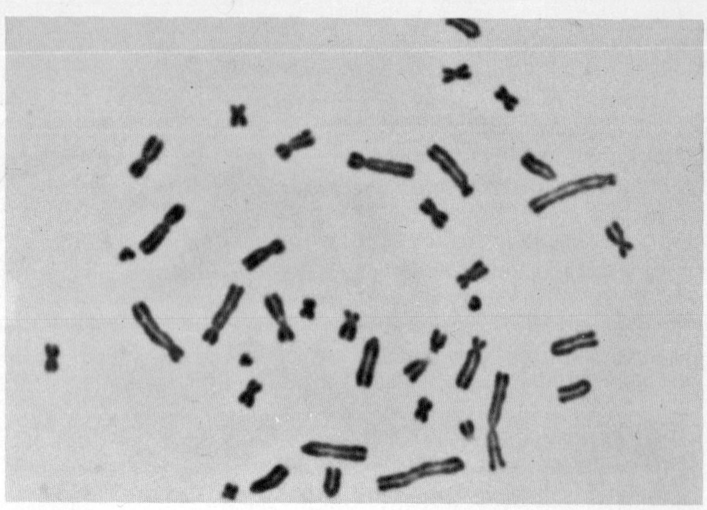

Fig. 3. Metaphase preparation of a YR cell fixed 24h after treatment with 20 ng/ml SM; no visible chromosome damage.

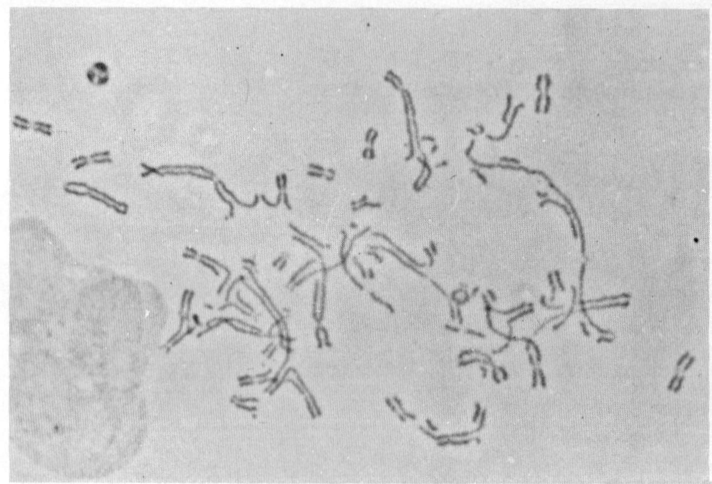

Fig. 4. Metaphase preparation of a YS cell fixed 24h after treatment with the same dose of SM (20 ng/ml) as the YR cell in Fig. 3; note extensive chromosome damage.

These Yoshida lymphosarcoma cells grow in suspension culture <u>in vitro</u> and are therefore not amenable to the most satisfactory form of artificial synchronisation, that of mitotic shake-off[10]. Therefore in order to determine the relative sensitivities of the different stages of the cell cycle to the chromosome-damaging action of SM we have subjected asynchronous populations of Yoshida cells to a one hour treatment of SM + tritiated thymidine and fixed cells at various intervals up to 63 hours after treatment. Autoradiographs were prepared in order to obtain labelled mitosis curves, and metaphase cells were analysed for chromosome aberrations. A maximum frequency of aberrations was found in cells which were at the G_1/S boundary at the time of SM treatment, with a declining frequency in cells nearer to the end of S (Figs 5,6). This confirms earlier observations on PHA-stimulated lymphocytes[11].

If chromosome damage does play an important role in cell lethality after SM then there should be a correlation between stage sensitivity to lethality and to chromosome aberrations. Unfortunately, since we have not yet satisfactorily synchronised the Yoshida cells we have no data on survival as a function of cell cycle stage. However, a comparison of our cell cycle data for chromosome damage (Figs 5,6) with published survival data on synchronised HeLa and Chinese hamster cells after SM shows a remarkably good correlation. Roberts, Brent and Crathorn[12] observed maximum killing by SM at the G_1/S boundary in HeLa cells and a decreasing sensitivity as cells progressed through S (Fig 7). Cells in early G_1 and G_2 were increasingly more resistant. Chinese hamster cells, with a short G_1 phase, were most sensitive whilst in G_1, less so as cells progressed through S, and least sensitive in G_2[13]. Thus there is good evidence that chromosome aberrations are of importance in determining differential cell stage lethality after SM.

The reason for the different frequencies of chromosome aberrations at different stages of the cycle is a reflection of the mechanism of formation of aberrations after treatment of cells with alkylating agents. Evans and Scott[14] first demonstrated the need for cells treated with alkylating agents to pass into S before aberrations could be formed, presumably by some error in DNA synthesis. This has since been confirmed for a number of other alkylating agents[15,16]. Scott and Bigger[11] showed, in cultured lymphocytes treated with SM, that pre-aberration lesions could be repaired before cells reached the S phase. Cells just about to pass into S will have least time for repair and will therefore carry the highest frequencies of aberrations. This repair process is likely to be a combination of excision repair[17] and the "unhooking" of one arm of an alkylation cross-link in the DNA[18]. We have found that YS and YR cells have the same capacity for excision repair after SM treatment[5] so their differential sensitivity cannot be explained in terms of this repair process. YS and YR

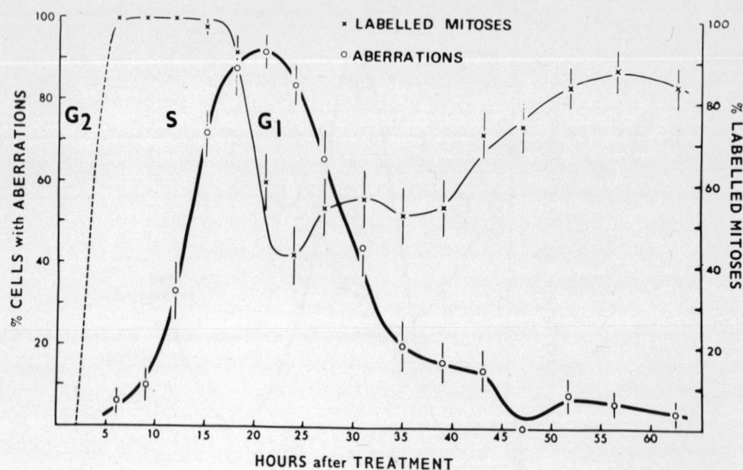

Fig. 5. Labelled mitosis curve and frequency of cells with chromosome aberrations after treatment of YR cells for 1 hour with a mixture of 80 ng/ml SM and tritiated thymidine.

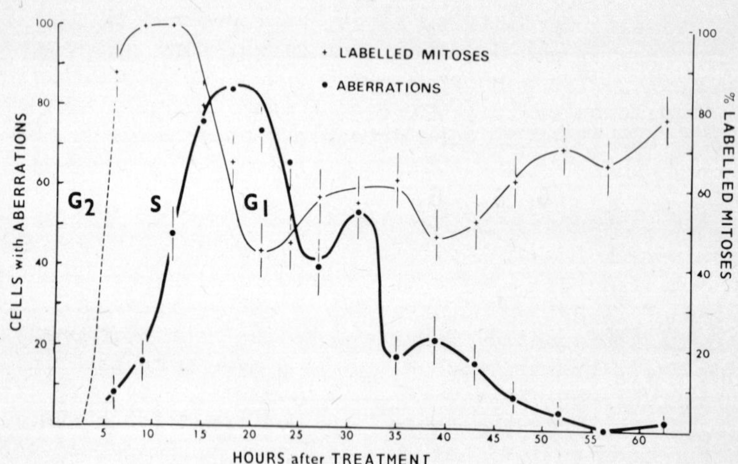

Fig. 6. Labelled mitosis curve and frequency of cells with chromosome aberrations after treatment of YS cells for 1 hour with a mixture of 7 ng/ml SM and tritiated thymidine.

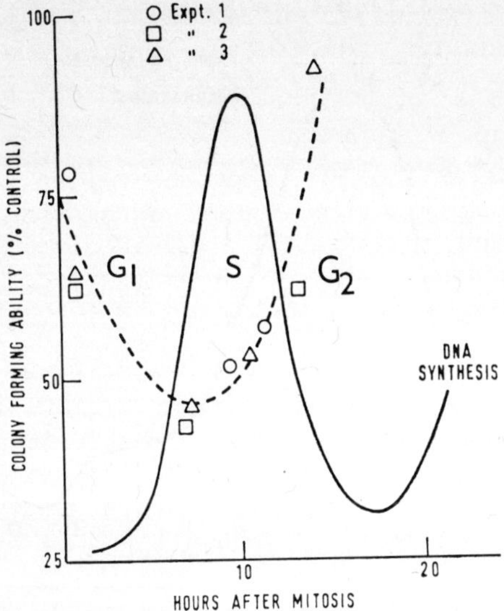

Fig. 7. Survival of HeLa cells treated with 75 ng/ml SM at various times after mitotic synchronisation. Modified from Roberts, Brent and Crathorn.[12]

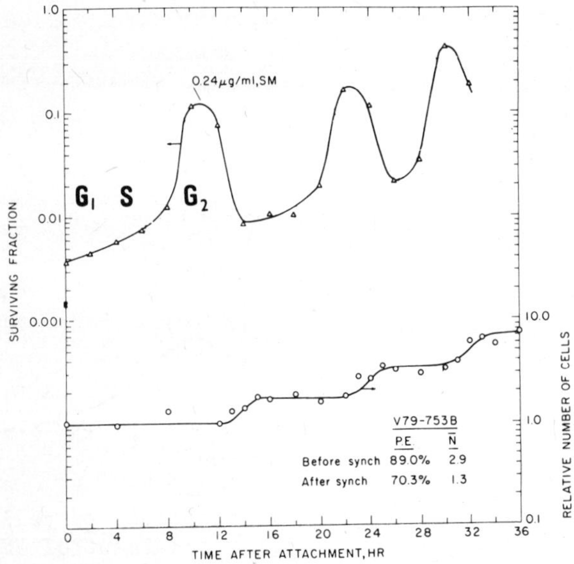

Fig. 8. Survival of Chinese hamster cells treated with 240 ng/ml SM at various times after mitotic synchronisation. Lower curve shows growth of the synchronised cell population. Modified from Mauro and Elkind.[13]

cells do, however, appear to differ in their capacity for post-replication DNA repair[19] which occurs during the S phase[20]. A reduced capacity for this type of repair leads to an increase in chromosome aberrations and cell killing[21].

These results on Yoshida lymphosarcoma cells treated with SM provide a good example of the role of chromosome damage in differential stage sensitivity and of the involvement of cellular repair processes in determining the aberration frequencies. Since many more alkylating agents, including those used in cancer therapy (Table 1), have been shown to induce chromosome structural aberrations the conclusions derived from these studies with SM may well apply to alkylating agents in general. Furthermore, the ubiquity of chromosome aberrations after treatment of cells with a wide range of anticancer drugs (Table 1), not just the alkylating agents, perhaps indicates a greater role of chromosome damage in differential stage lethality than has hitherto been suspected.

REFERENCES

1) MADOC-JONES, H. and F. MAURO. In "Handbook of Experimental Pharmacology Vol 38(1)" p.205. Eds. A.C. Sartorelli and D.G. Johns. Springer-Verlag, Berlin, 1974.

2) SHAW, M.W. Ann.Rev.Med. 21, 409 (1970).

3) GROTE, S.J. and S.H. REVELL. Current Topics in Radiation Research 7, 303 (1972).

4) CARRANO, A.V. Mutation Res. 17, 355 (1973).

5) SCOTT, D., M. FOX and B.W. FOX. Mutation Res. 22, 207 (1974).

6) KOLLER, P.C. Mutation Res. 8, 199 (1969).

7) FOX, B.W. Intern.J.Cancer 4, 54 (1969).

8) FOX, M. and B.W. FOX. Chem.-Biol. Interactions 4, 363 (1971/2).

9) ROSS, W.C.J. Biological Alkylating Agents. Butterworth and Co. London, 1962.

10) TERASIMA, T. and L.J. TOLMACH. Biophys.J. 3, 11 (1963).

11) SCOTT, D. and T.R.L. BIGGER. In "Chromosomes Today Vol 3"p162. Eds. C.D. Darlington and K.R. Lewis. Longmans, London, 1972.

12) ROBERTS, J.J., T.P. BRENT and A.R. CRATHORN. In "The interaction of drugs and subcellular components in animal cells" p5.

Ed. P.N. Campbell. Churchill Limited, London,(1968).

13) MAURO, F. and M.M. ELKIND. Cancer Res. 28, 1150 (1968).

14) EVANS, H.J. and D. SCOTT. Proc.Roy.Soc. B 173, 491 (1969).

15) STURELID, S. Hereditas 68, 255 (1971).

16) KELLY, F. and M. LEGATOR. Mutation Res. 10, 237 (1970).

17) PAINTER, R.B. Current Topics in Radiation Res. Vol 7, p45. Eds. M. Ebert and A. Howard. North-Holland, Amsterdam, (1970).

18) REID, B.D. and I.G. WALKER, Biochem.Biophys.Acta. 179, 179 (1969).

19) SCOTT, D. Unpublished observations.

20) LEHMAN, A.R. Life Sciences 15, 2005 (1975).

21) KIHLMAN, B.A., S. STURELID, B. HARTLEY-ASP and K. NILSSON. Mutation Res. 26, 105 (1974).

ADRIAMYCIN METABOLISM IN MAN

Nicholas R. Bachur

Baltimore Cancer Research Center, NCI

3100 Wyman Park Drive, Baltimore, Maryland 21211, U.S.A.

Over the past eight years, adriamycin, the outstanding representative of the anthracycline antibiotics, has demonstrated a remarkable activity against human and animal malignancies (1,2). Whereas adriamycin's sibling, daunorubicin, has been impressive for remission induction in acute myelogenous and acute lymphocytic leukemias, adriamycin has a wider spectrum of activity and is useful against solid tumors. Clinical investigators in Europe, the Americas, Asia, and Africa find adriamycin has anticancer activity against soft tissue sarcomas, breast cancer, lung cancer, hepatomas, lymphomas, acute leukemias, etc. Against some malignancies, adriamycin has no useful pharmacologic activity. Complicating the usage of both adriamycin and daunorubicin are the toxic effects: myelosuppression, stomatitis, nausea, vomiting, alopecia, electrocardiographic changes, and a serious cumulative dosage related myocardiopathy.

For an agent that has such potential utility to alleviate human suffering and disease, we felt it very important to pursue the causes of the inadequacies and shortcomings of this drug Therefore we studied various aspects of adriamycin's pharmacokinetics and pharmacodynamics with emphasis on mechanism of action and drug disposition and metabolism. Early studies on adriamycin depicted the drug as a relatively simple agent that was taken into tissues, retained for a period of time, and then slowly excreted unchanged. However this is a very dynamic substance with untold potential for interaction in biologic systems.

Adriamycin is a complex molecule having surface-active properties because of its bifunctional physical chemical nature (Fig. 1). One end of the adriamycin molecule is hydrophobic and the other end is hydrophilic. The hydrophobic A, B, and C resonating ring system

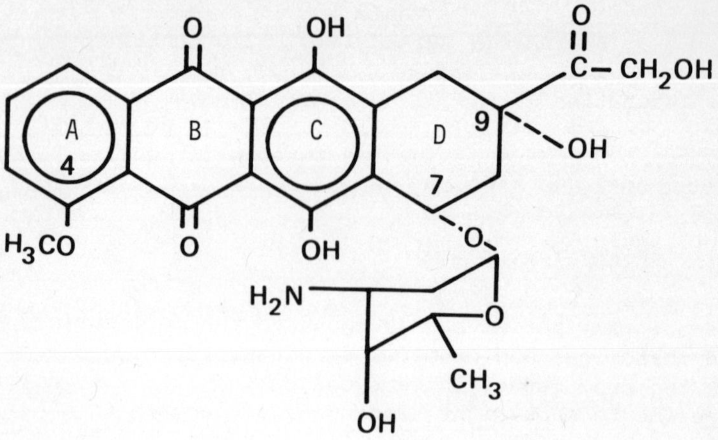

Fig. 1. Adriamycin

interacts quite readily with lipids and other hydrophobic biologic materials. This resonating planar system according to Pigram et al, Waring, and other investigators intercalates readily into the helical structure of DNA and displaces the base stacking so that unwinding of the double helical chains occurs (3,4). The other end of the molecule, the hydroxylated D ring with attached amino sugar, is hydrophilic. The amino sugar is theorized by Pigram et al as necessary for stabilization for drug intercalation into DNA. We have found binding of the drug to plasma proteins and cell membranes (5) and I am certain we will find many more interactions of this elaborate system with other biologic components. In addition to the hydrophobic-hydrophilic physical characteristics, adriamycin is amphoteric, containing both positive and negative charges. The basic amino group is positively charged, and the acidic phenolic hydroxyls on the anthracycline ring have the potential for negative charges. These further increase the interaction potential of adriamycin. Besides these physical properties, adriamycin has an availability of biotransformable groups throughout the molecule.

When adriamycin is administered intravenously to humans or to animals, the molecule is rapidly absorbed into cells and is localized mainly in the cell nucleus. Transport of the drug across the cell membrane is temperature sensitive, but binding of drug to the cell membrane is a rapid, nontemperature-sensitive, phenomenon (Table 1) (6). This membrane binding is identified in the 0 time samples. Subsequent to binding, uptake ensues which is ultimately against a gradient to give a high tissue to plasma ratio. In some tissues such as spleen, in vivo, this ratio approaches a level of 300 to 1 (7).

Table 1
ADRIAMYCIN UPTAKE INTO L1210 CELLS

Incubation	Minutes				
	0	15	30	60	120
	(nmoles per 1 x 10^6 cells)				
0°	0.30	0.25	0.32	0.30	0.35
37°	0.30	0.45	0.56	0.58	0.90

Evidence that adriamycin is bound to the cell nucleus comes from good anatomical and chemical findings. Cytological evidence indicates the drug causes chromosomal damage (8). In addition, *in vitro* experiments show tight binding of adriamycin to DNA. Since adriamycin is highly fluorescent, the drug can be detected readily in tissues by fluorescence microscopy (9). This fluorescence is not common to other biological structures. When adriamycin containing cells are excited with the appropriate light wavelength, the drug fluorescence appears as a unique orange-yellow that is localized in the nuclear structures. Shortly after dosing, adriamycin appears in nuclei of most tissues; and only transient cytoplasmic fluorescence is seen in the kidney. No mitochondrial fluorescence is seen.

On entering the cell, adriamycin (I) (Fig. 2) is subject to extensive metabolism by both constitutive and inducible enzyme systems. The major metabolic transformation occurs in the cytoplasm via the keto reduction reaction of aldo-keto reductase (7,10)(Fig. 2) (I ➤ II, IV ➤ V). Aldo-keto reductase reduces the carbonyl group at the 13 carbon position of the side chain attached to the anthracycline ring system. The enzymatic product of this reaction, adriamycinol (II), has inhibitory activity against L1210 tumor cells and inhibits DNA synthesis and RNA synthesis of these cells as does the parent compound. The metabolite has different physical-chemical characteristics from the parent compound caused by the addition of the polar group. Aldo-keto reductase is a constitutive enzyme that requires NADPH as a cofactor and has a molecular weight of about 39,000. This enzyme is ubiquitous in mammals and is found in all tissues that we have analyzed. In fact, aldo-keto reductase even occurs in human erythrocytes and platelets.

The impact of *in vivo* adriamycin metabolism is easily seen in rabbits that are administered 5 mg/kg adriamycin and sacrificed and analyzed 8 hours later. Their tissues contain predominantly the parent drug but adriamycinol stands out as a metabolite (Table 2) (7). This supports the finding of widespread distribution and activity of the aldo-keto reductase. Several human tissues were analyzed for aldo-keto reductase activity (Table 3) (11). All the tissues analyzed contained the enzyme. Since the aldo-keto reductase produces a pharmacologically active metabolite which differs from

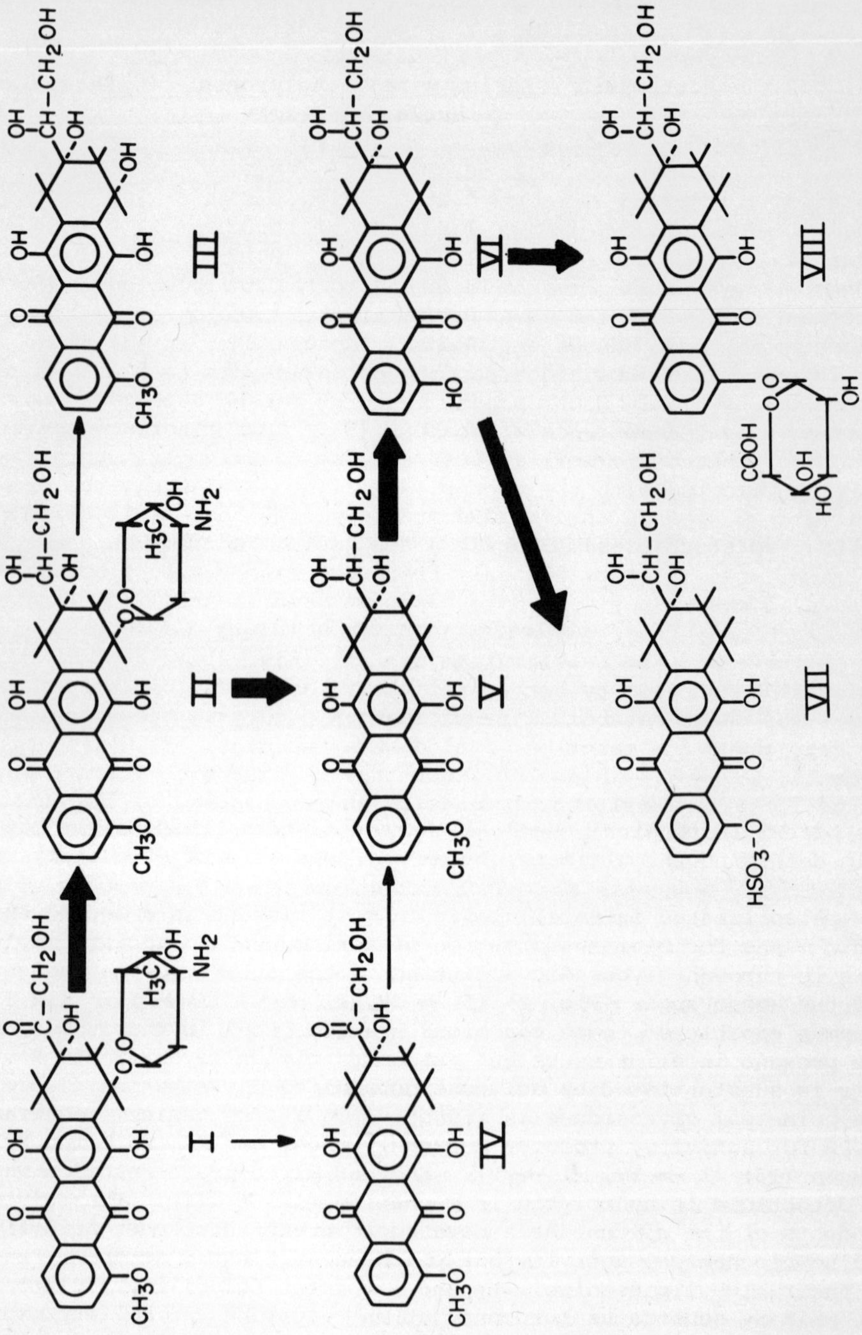

Figure 2

Table 2
ADRIAMYCIN AND METABOLITES IN RABBIT TISSUES
(8 hours after I.V. 5 mg/kg adriamycin)

	Adriamycin	Adriamycinol	Aglycones	P. Metabolites
		μg/g wet weight		
Brain	N.D.	0.08	N.D.	0.07
Heart	2.63	0.25	0.01	0.01
Lung	6.13	1.03	0.03	0.04
Liver	1.95	1.97	0.85	0.07
Kidney	16.80	13.80	0.94	0.45
Pancreas	2.40	0.92	0.05	0.02
Spleen	14.70	4.30	0.12	0.26
Sm. Intes.	4.63	1.79	0.13	0.44
Sk. Muscle	1.12	0.18	0.04	0.01
Adipose	0.37	0.04	0.03	N.D.

Table 3
ALDO-KETO REDUCTASE ACTIVITIES OF HUMAN TISSUES

Tissue	Adriamycinol nmoles/mg protein/30 min. ± S.E.M.
Liver	0.1 ± 0.08
Kidney	0.4 ± 0.2
Heart	0.2 ± 0.1

the parent in physical chemical characteristics, this enzyme may help determine the ultimate pharmacodynamic effects of adriamycin.

Also located intracellularly in most tissues is a second enzymatic means for biotransformation of adriamycin and adriamycinol. This is through glycosidic splitting of the anthracycline nucleus and the amino sugar (Fig. 2) (I → IV, II → V, II → III) (12,13). Enzymes capable of these reactions are localized in microsomes and are present in all tissues but predominantly in liver (Table 4). This is substantiated by aglycone metabolite distribution (Table 2). The principal glycosidase is reductive in its mechanism, requires NADPH for activity, produces deoxyaglycones, and is inhibited by oxygen (13) (I → IV, II → V). Another glycosidase reaction which is detectable is hydrolytic in mechanism (II → III). The aglycone products of the glycosidases have no apparent anticancer activity, and no biochemical activity has yet been attributed to them. Because of their high lipid solubility and low water solubility, aglycones are primary substrates for conjugation reactions and biliary excretion.

Table 4
MICROSOMAL GLYCOSIDASE OF HUMAN TISSUES

Tissue	Adriamycin Aglycones nMoles/mg protein/30 min. ± S.E.M.
Liver	165.7 ± 68.2
Kidney	8.0 ± 0.9
Heart	12.5 ± 4.1

To prepare suitable conjugation sites the aglycones are 4-O demethylated (Fig. 2) (V → VI) exposing an aryl hydroxyl group (14). The 4-O-hydroxy aglycones are then sulfated (VI → VII) or β-glucuronidated (VI → VIII). Demethylation, O-sulfation, and β-glucuronidation are catalyzed presumably by the classical microsomal enzyme systems. The 4-O-sulfate conjugate (VII) and the 4-O-beta glucuronide (VIII) conjugate are excreted in human bile and human urine. Other identified metabolites are detectable in human urine, bile, and plasma indicating further expansion of this scheme is necessary.

These metabolic biotransformations are reflected in adriamycin disposition in humans. Studies in the human pharmacokinetics of adriamycin show the rapid appearance in plasma of numerous adriamycin metabolites and degradation products. Some of these are identifiable as adriamycinol and several aglycones but the resultant pharmacokinetics are extremely complex. In one well studied case, about 40% of administered adriamycin is excreted in human bile over a seven day period as parent drug and fluorescent metabolites (15). Parent drug excretion amounted to 17% and adriamycinol 9% of the administered dose. The remainder consisted of polar metabolites and aglycones. However, counting the urinary excretion, only 53% of the administered adriamycin was recovered in bile and urine. This suggests more extensive interactions of the drug than presented here with prolonged tissue retention and biotransformation to nonfluorescent metabolites.

Because of the large number of adriamycin metabolites present *in vivo*, it is possible that some metabolites may be biologically active and produce pharmacologic effects and/or toxicity. We are continuing our study of the complex interactions of this exciting drug with biologic systems.

1. International Symposium on Adriamycin. Ed. S.K. Carter, A. DiMarco, M. Ghione, I.H. Krakoff, and G. Mathe, Milan 1971, Springer-Verlag, Berlin, 1972.

2. Adriamycin New Drug Symposium. Ed. N.R. Bachur, R.S. Benjamin, and T.C. Hall, San Francisco 1975, Cancer Chemother. Rep., in press.

3. Pigram, W.J., Fuller, W., and Hamilton, L.D.: Nature, New Biol. 235, 17 (1972).

4. Waring, M: Progress in Molecular and Subcellular Biology. Ed. F.E. Hahn, Springer-Verlag, Berlin 2, 216 (1971).

5. Axelrod, M., Kaber, M., Bachur, N.R.: Unpublished observations

6. Meriwether, W.D. and Bachur, N.R.: Cancer Res. 32, 1137 (1972).

7. Bachur, N.R., Hildebrand, R.C., and Jaenke, R.S.: J. Pharmacol. Exp. Ther. 191, 331 (1974).

8. Whang Peng, J., Leventhan, B.G., Adamson, J.W., and Perry, S.: Cancer 23, 113 (1969).

9. Egorin, M.J., Hildebrand, R.C., Cimino, E.F., and Bachur, N.R.: Cancer Res. 34, 2243 (1974).

10. Felsted, R.L., Gee, M., and Bachur, N.R.: J. Biol. Chem. 249, 3672 (1974).

11. Bachur, N.R., Takanashi, S., Arena, E.: Proc. XI Inter. Cancer Congress, Florence (1974).

12. Bachur, N.R. and Gee, M.: J. Pharmacol. Exp. Ther. 177, 567 (1971).

13. Bachur, N.R. and Gee, M.: Fed. Proc. 31, 835 (1971).

14. Takanashi, S. and Bachur, N.R.: Proc. Amer. Assoc. Cancer Res. 15, 76 (1974).

15. Benjamin, R.S., Riggs, C.E., Jr., Serpick, A.A., and Bachur, N.R.: Clin. Res. 22, 483 (1974).

[illegible] APPLICATIONS [illegible]

[illegible]

School of Pharmacy, [illegible]

Kinetic processes during [illegible] [illegible]

[illegible]

PHARMACOKINETICS OF ANTICANCER DRUGS

Wolfgang Sadée

School of Pharmacy, University of California, and
Western Cancer Study Group, San Francisco, California
94143

Kinetic processes during absorption, distribution, metabolism and excretion determine the extent of drug activity. The success of cancer chemotherapy is particularly dependent upon a series of dynamic events, such as pharmacokinetics, cell cycle kinetics, target enzyme activities, dosage schedule and sequence in combination therapy, and kinetics of endogenous metabolites. Pharmacokinetics therefore, should represent an integral part of pharmacological and clinical studies. Anticancer drugs present special problems in pharmacokinetic investigations. The very nature of their mechanism of action often requires interaction of the drug with specific anabolic and catabolic enzymes in addition to interaction with the hepatic microsomal drug metabolizing enzyme system. Exploitation of enzyme differences between normal and neoplastic tissue may be important in drug efficacy. This demonstrates the complexity frequently encountered in pharmacokinetics of antineoplastic agents. Every single agent may require an entirely different approach to yield useful data. The following information can result from pharmacokinetic studies.

1. Description and prediction of drug and metabolite concentations. Plasma and target tissue levels can be simulated using pharmacokinetic models. Many linear and non-linear systems are now available and can readily be applied using digital computation methods. In cancer chemotherapy, knowledge of the active drug level in target tissues may be necessary for predicting pharmacological response. Therefore, kinetic models are suitable, which include variables such as blood flow to the target tissues and their enzyme activities, diffusion parameters, active transport and drug binding constants. Experimental confirmation of kinetic simulations is difficult in patient studies. Upscaling of animal data to humans often remains the only method to obtain tissue level estimates in cancer

patients.

2. Correlation to Pharmacodynamics. The time course of drug action or toxicity (Pharmacodynamics) can be correlated with pharmacokinetic parameters in order to evaluate the active principle of chemotherapy. Pharmacokinetic determinants of drug activity can then be defined as total amount of drug administered, area under the plasma concentration-time curve, peak drug levels, duration of exposure above a threshold drug level, amount of metabolite formed in the body or target tissue or other parameters. Identification of efficacy determinants is important in Pharmacokinetics of anticancer agents.

3. Bioavailability, route of administration and dosage schedule Pharmacokinetic analysis is necessary to define the proper dose and route of administration.

4. Drug-drug interactions. It appears that drug-drug interactions at the pharmacokinetic level are relatively infrequent in cancer chemotherapy when compared to other mechanisms of interaction. Depletion or enhancement of endogenous substrate pools, *e.g.* purines and pyrimidines, may play a more prominent role. Thus, enhanced efficacy of combination therapy or its lack can be investigated only to a limited extent by Pharmacokinetics.

5. Clinical Pharmacokinetics. Clinical application of Pharmacokinetics results in monitoring drug kinetics in individual patients undergoing cancer chemotherapy. Variables between patients, *i.e.*, differences in absorption, distribution, excretion and metabolism caused by genetic, environmental and patho-physiological factors, might be determinants of drug efficacy in the individual. Measured drug levels, concentrations predicted by pharmacokinetic models or both in combination can be applied to optimize individual therapy. Cancer chemotherapy is a prime candidate for Clinical Pharmacokinetics, since interindividual variability in drug response and toxicity are high. However, application is still limited by our lack of knowledge of efficacy and toxicity determinants.

Some antineoplastic agents are discussed below to illustrate application of pharmacokinetic methods. Also, analytical methods for the measurement of drug and metabolites in biological samples should be mentioned, since methodological requirements in cancer chemotherapy are high. We have extensively utilized isotope dilution-mass fragmentography due to its specificity, sensitivity and potential to apply stable isotope labeling techniques (W. Sadée, C. Finn and J. Staroszik, Gas Chromatography-Mass Fragmentography in Pharmacokinetics of Antineoplastic Agents, Abstracts, 2nd Int. Symp. on Mass Spectrometry in Biochemistry and Medicine, Milano, June 1974).

PLASMA LEVELS OF ICRF-159

The dioxopiperazine, (±)-1,2-bis-(3,5-dioxopiperazinyl)propane (ICRF-159) is under clinical evaluation as a chemotherapeutic agent against various neoplasms (K. Hellmann and K. Burrage, Nature 224,

273 (1969); K. Hellmann et al., Brit. Med. J. 1, 822 (1969)). The mechanism of pharmacological activity remains unknown. The drug is given orally in tablet form, while an intravenous preparation is not yet available due to the limited solubility of the racemic mixture. Pharmacokinetic analysis has, thus, to be primarily focused on bioavailability and exposure time measured by plasma concentration-time curves and metabolism. Specific assay methods were developed to measure ICRF-159 plasma levels by gas chromatography and mass fragmentography (W. Sadée, J. Staroszik, C. Finn, and J. Cohen, J. Pharm. Sci. 64, 998 (1975)). Significantly higher total ^{14}C levels compared to intact ICRF-159 in plasma following doses of ^{14}C-ICRF-159 to rats and rabbits indicated rapid biotransformation to unknown metabolites. Lack of significant differences between ICRF-159 plasma disappearance half-life measured by bioassay techniques ($t_{1/2}$ ∿ 30 min., E.O. Field, F. Mauro and K. Hellmann, Cancer Chemother. Rep. (I) 55, 527 (1971)) and by our specific assay ($t_{1/2}$ ∿ 40 min.) suggested, that the parent drug and not its metabolites represents the active principle in plasma. The oral bioavailability of ICRF-159 appeared to be limited in both rat and rabbit relative to intravenous administration. Two patients receiving 3 g ICRF-159/m^2 orally showed ICRF-159 plasma levels similar to those obtained after equivalent oral doses in rats and rabbits with peak concentrations of 3.8 μg/ml at two hours after the dose and still measurable levels of 0.4 μg/ml 12 hours after the dose. In another study using ^{14}C-ICRF-159 in patients it was shown that oral bioavailability is inversely related to the amount administered as judged by ^{14}C urinary excretion (P. J. Creaven, L. M. Allen, and D. A. Alford, Abstract, APhA Meeting, San Diego, Cal., Nov. 1973). Further studies will serve to evaluate treatment with ICRF-159 in the individual patient.

5-FLUOROURACIL (5-FU) PHARMACOKINETICS

The metabolism of 5-FU can be divided into hepatic degradative pathways initiated by reduction to dihydro-5-FU and anabolic metabolism to nucleosides and nucleotides, the latter representing the active principle of the drug. A simplified overall model for 5-FU disposition in the body can be depicted as follows.

Schematic 1

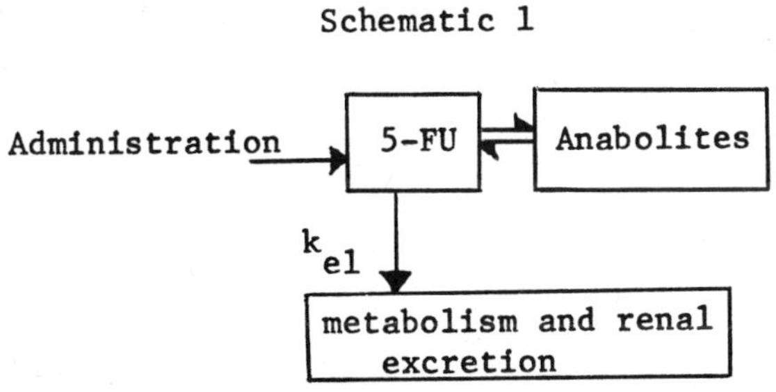

A major difficulty in the pharmacokinetic analysis of pyrimidine and purine antimetabolites is the mostly intracellular distribution of the corresponding active nucleotides, while the biochemically usually inactive bases and nucleosides are distributed throughout the body. Measured half-lives of base and nucleoside plasma disappearance are in the order of 10-20 min., although pharmacological activity may persist for several hours or days. Thus, determinants of pyrimidine and purine antimetabolites are not readily available in patients.

Assuming that the model in Schematics 1 describes 5-FU disposition in plasma, one has to expect a biexponential decay curve of 5-FU plasma levels. The terminal log-linear phase of 5-FU elimination (β-phase) should then provide an indirect relative measure of the anabolic pool size and thus, the amount of active metabolite formed. Prerequisite for this approach is a highly sensitive and specific 5-FU assay, which we have developed using mass fragmentography (C. Finn and W. Sadée, Cancer Chemother. Rep. (I) 59, 279 (1975). Indeed, a β-phase of 5-FU plasma elimination with a half-life of about 20 hrs. was found following high intravenous doses of 5-FU in rats. Further studies with this assay technique in patients receiving intravenous, oral and intrahepatic artery doses of 5-FU showed that hepatic 5-FU metabolism is saturable at therapeutic doses depending on route of administration. Oral 5-FU doses are non-equivalent to intravenous doses, even assuming complete gastrointestinal absorption.

Measurements of endogenous pyrimidine kinetics may provide another approach to define determinants of 5-FU efficacy. We have developed mass fragmentographic methods to measure endogenous uracil and thymine plasma levels and are working on the assay of their corresponding ribosides and deoxyribosides. These methods will be applied in animal studies and clinical trials of the Western Cancer Study Group.

5-AZACYTIDINE (5-AZA-C) KINETICS

The chemical instability of 5-Aza-C presents additional difficulties in its pharmacokinetic analysis. The 5-azacytosine ring moiety readily hydrolyzes at N_1-C_6 to form an open chain formyl intermediate, which undergoes further degradation by loss of formic acid derived from the original C_6 position. We have synthesized ^{14}C-6-5-aza-C in order to study the significance of this decomposition *in vivo* and *in vitro* (K. K. Chan, J. Staroszik, and W. Sadée, to be published). The half-life of *in vitro* 5-Aza-C decomposition in pH 7.4 phosphate buffer and human plasma at 37°C was in the order of 4 hrs., while the *in vivo* plasma half-life in rabbits following intravenous administration of 5-Aza-C was 25 min. which was measured by HPLC analysis. Total ^{14}C-activity curves in rabbit plasma suggested rapid *in vivo* metabolite formation, one of which being possibly identical to the formyl intermediate degradation product. Further studies are in progress.

CLINICAL PHARMACOKINETICS OF METHOTREXATE

Few examples are yet available in cancer chemotherapy, where monitoring drug levels in individual patients can directly contribute to optimize individual patient care. Large doses of methotrexate in combination with citrovorum factor rescue are now being used in the treatment of osteogenic sarcoma and other neoplasms. It has been shown that patients with sustained methotrexate plasma levels above 10^{-6}M over 60 hrs following single large doses of methotrexate were destined to have high marrow toxicity and that this toxicity could in part be reversed by a prolonged administration of citrovorum factor (E. Frei *et al*., New England J. Med. 292, 846 (1975)). Therefore, measurements of methotrexate plasma levels are necessary to at least partially prevent drug toxicity. We are now in process of establishing this assay with a turn-over time of less than 8 hrs. in the Clinical Pharmacokinetics Laboratory at UC San Francisco.

These studies were supported by Grants No. CA. 05186-13 from the NCI and No. 16496-06 from the NIH.

PHARMACOKINETICS AND METABOLISM OF ANTICANCER DRUGS

Ti Li Loo

The University of Texas System Cancer Center
M.D. Anderson Hospital and Tumor Institute
Houston, Texas U.S.A.

The design of cancer chemotherapeutic agents would already have evolved from empiricism to rationalism if a unique structural feature exists that specifically confers anticancer activity on a chemical substance. In reality, the structures of anticancer drugs vary widely; this structural diversity dictates a similar diversity in the pharmacokinetics and metabolism of these drugs. Generally however, the pharmacological disposition and metabolism of a particular class of anticancer agents, the antimetabolites, closely mimic those of their natural counterparts, and a reasonable extrapolation can frequently be made.

Except for the nitrosoureas, the majority of anticancer drugs are poorly and varyingly absorbed. As an example, the important antimetabolite 5-fluorouracil (5-FU) is incompletely absorbed in man (1), although it is apparently actively transported *in vivo* across the intestinal epithelium (2). In view of the steep dose-response of anticancer drugs, their erratic and inconsistent gastrointestinal absorption makes it difficult to predict clinical response and toxicity. In addition, "first-pass" hepatic degradation of the orally administered drug materially reduces the effective drug level. These disadvantages seriously offset the convenience of oral administration of an antitumor agent.

In common with any other drug, an anticancer agent that is highly lipid-soluble, not appreciably ionized at body pH, and not extensively bound to proteins, tends to penetrate plasma membranes with ease. But too high a lipid solubility may prove to be a disadvantage since the drug will remain localized in the membrane lipoprotein and fail to diffuse intracellularly. Besides passive diffusion, many anticancer agents are transported by a variety of carrier-mediated mechanisms such as active transport and facilitated diffusion. One must be aware, however, that concentrative uptake is not always an active process. Frequently an antitumor drug is biotransformed inside the cell to a metabolite that effluxes only with difficulty resulting in intracellular trapping; the concentrative uptake of ribosyl-6-methylthiopurine by human leucocytes exemplifies this (3).

An anticancer drug with a close structural relationship to a natural metabolite often shares with it a common transport mechanism; for instance, methotrexate (MTX) and folate (4), mechlorethamine (HNZ, nitrogen mustard) and choline (5), 5-fluorouracil and uracil (1).

One of the distressing clinical problems confronting the chemotherapist in the treatment of cancer is the failure of most anticancer agents to reach malignant cells sequestered in the so-called anatomical sanctuaries such as the central nervous system (CNS); 6-mercaptopurine (6-MP) (3), MTX (6), dacarbazine (DIC) (7), and thiopurine nucleosides (8) are typical examples of antitumor agents that do not noticeably penetrate the blood-brain barrier. In contrast, 5-FU (9) and ftorafur, the 1-(2-tetrahydrofuranyl)-derivative of 5-FU (10), can achieve a significant level in the CSF after intravenous administration. As expected, large protein molecules, like L-asparaginase with a molecular weight of about 140,000 daltons are denied entry to the CNS (11). By virtue of their lipid-solubility, the nitrosoureas cross the blood-brain barrier with ease (12, 13). But besides lipid-solubility, other factors also influence the entry of an antitumor drug to the CNS. Though extremely soluble in lipids, the di-n-amyl ester of MTX is not detectable in the CNS of dogs injected with this drug, most likely because of its quick metabolism to an ionizable product that fails to cross the blood-brain barrier (14).

When an agent is directly introduced into the systemic circulation, the plasma is the only body compartment immediately permeable to the drug, and it is also the only tissue in which <u>in vivo</u> drug concentration and distribution can be readily assessed with some certainty. Nevertheless, plasma drug levels are rarely representative of those in other body compartments. Yet the sampling of tissues other than the plasma normally involves considerable risk except post mortem; consequently, information on drug distribution therein must be inferred indirectly. To this end elegant mathematical models have been constructed, which have shown promise to predict tissue drug levels at different intervals (15, 16).

Once in the systemic circulation, the drug will be removed by a number of processes, including excretion, biotransformation, and storage in body depots. Traditionally the efflux rate of the drug from the plasma is expressed in terms of its "half-time". Such an expression presupposes that there is a single body compartment, in which the drug is immediately permeable, and from which it exists by simple first-order kinetics. Actually these conditions seldom hold, and the drug efflux follows complex kinetics. In most cases after intravenous administration, the plasma concentration, Cp, of a drug is best described as the sum of several exponential terms, thus

$$Cp = Ae^{-\alpha t} + Be^{-\beta t} + Ge^{-\gamma t} + \ldots, \text{ in which the constants}$$

$$A > B > G > \ldots > 0, \text{ and } \alpha > \beta > \gamma > \ldots > 0.$$

A plot of Cp versus time, t, on a semilogarithm scale often reveals a curve, the slope of which is not constant but a function of time. Clearly, the "half-time" of the drug in the plasma connotes very little unless qualified by the time interval during which the segment of the Cp-t curve is nearly "log-linear" or exponential. At the early part of the experiment, for small values of t, Cp is principally governed by the first term of the above equation. Toward the later part of the experiment, however, Cp is almost entirely determined by the term with the least exponential. In place of the conventional "half-times" of a drug, a more appropriate way to describe the rate of drug disappearance from the plasma is perhaps by the time required for the drug concentration to fall below an arbitrary level, for example, the minimal effective level, if known.

Many anticancer drugs bind nonspecifically to proteins, the so-called "silent receptors", plasma albumin in particular. It is likely that drugs bound to protein cannot cross cell membranes under normal circumstances. At therapeutic plasma concentrations most nucleoside analogues such as arabinosylcytosine (ara-C) and ribosyl-6-mercaptopurine are bound to human plasma albumin only to a limited extent (17). MTX is about 50% bound but its 3',5'-dichloro derivative, dichloromethotrexate (DCM), is 90% bound (18). Extensive protein binding of anticancer drugs appears to be associated with high lipid-solubility; for instance, 1,3-bis(2-chloroethyl)-1-nitrosourea (BCNU) (12) and dichloroallyl lawsone (DCL) (19), both soluble in lipids, are almost completely bound to human plasma albumin. Plasma albumin is not the only protein that binds to anticancer drugs: Both vincristine (VCR) and vinblastine (VLB) exhibit a higher affinity for α- and β-globulins than for γ-globulin or albumin (20).

Like other drugs, anticancer drugs are excreted primarily in the urine. However, hepatobiliary excretion plays a significant part in the elimination of many important anticancer drugs, especially those soluble in lipids. In man, adriamycin (ADR), daunorubicin (DRC), and their metabolites are largely excreted in the bile (21). The folate antagonist DCM is excreted in the bile (22), although its parent drug MTX is not. The hepatobiliary excretion of DIC in the rat is concentrative; at steady state the DIC concentration in the bile is twice as high as that in the plasma; however, less than 3% of the administered dose is so excreted in 2 hr. (23). Also in the rat, 25%-35% of an intravenously administered dose of tritiated VCR is found in the bile in 4 hr. in concentrations 10-50 times those in the blood (24). In the dog, DCL is concentratively excreted in the bile to attain an average concentration 50-fold of the plasma level (19). The new folate antagonist BAF (Baker's antifolate, (1-[3-chloro-4-(m-dimethylcarbamoylbenzyloxy)]phenyl-4,6-diamino-1,2-dihydro-2,2-dimethyl-*s*-triazine ethanesulfonate) is concentratively excreted in the bile of rats and dogs to attain a high steady-state bile to plasma concentration ratio of 300-1,000 (25). An anticancer drug may persist in the body if its hepatobiliary excretion is accompanied by entero-hepatic cycling. Principally depending upon the mode of action of the drug and its selective toxicity, this persistence may or may not be desirable. In cancer patients with severe liver dysfunction, the plasma levels of ADR and metabolites are much higher than expected, with a corresponding delay in drug elimination. In these patients, to avoid serious toxicity dosage reduction of ADR is mandatory (21).

We have already alluded to the observation that the pharmacologic disposition and metabolism of antimetabolites are nearly indistinguishable from those of their natural counterparts. It is well established for instance, that analogous to folate, MTX is hardly metabolized *in vivo*. Further, the biotransformation of purine and pyrimidine antimetabolites such as 6-MP, 5-FU, and ara-C differs little from that of the natural metabolites hypoxanthine, uracil, and deoxycytidine. The enzyme systems involved in these biotransformations are those essential for normal body function and metabolism.

Although hepatic microsomal enzymes perform a critical function in drug metabolism, hitherto their participation in the biotransformation of anticancer drugs has been less than conspicuous; corticosteroids, thiopurines, cyclophosphamide (CTX), procarbazine appear to be the few metabolized by these enzymes. But as more anticancer drugs with novel chemical structures are discovered, hepatic microsomal enzymes have gained increasing prominence in the biotransformation of these new drugs. Recently it has been demonstrated that DIC (26), iphosphamide (27), the nitrosoureas (28,29), and the anthracycline antibiotics (30,31), are substrates of these enzymes. Moreover, BAF (32) and DCL (19) are most likely metabolized by them also. Unquestionably this list will expand rapidly.

It is well recognized that *in vivo* drug metabolism is not necessarily a detoxification process. This holds true particularly for anticancer drugs. The purine and pyrimidine antimetabolites 6-MP, 6-thioguanine, 5-FU, and ara-C must be converted to the nucleotides to exert their cytotoxic action. Other anticancer drugs that are metabolically "activated" in vivo include, CTX, DIC, and the nitrosoureas. Nonetheless, in the majority of cases, the metabolites are less active than the parent anticancer agents. Modification of drug metabolism with a view to increasing the activation or decreasing the inactivation of an anticancer drug cannot be expected to influence its therapeutic index simply because the sensitive normal cells and the susceptible malignant cells would be affected alike.

In experimental animals neoplasia impairs drug metabolism (33, 34), including the metabolism of anticancer drugs, for example, that of DIC (35). Such an impairment is difficult to demonstrate clinically. However, using plasma antipyrine half-time as an index for hepatic microsomal enzyme activity, we have shown that this $t\frac{1}{2}$ is 13.5 ± 1.3 hr. (mean ± standard error) in 13 patients with various neoplastic diseases, and 13.5 ± 1.6 hr. in 9 patients with advanced cancer; in contrast, it is 10.8 ± 0.5 hr. in 7 normal subjects. In 5 acute leukemic patients with a positive diagnosis of hepatitis, the plasma antipyrine $t\frac{1}{2}$ is 28.6 ± 6.7 hr., significantly longer than in normal subjects. This serves to alert the clinician that the disposition and metabolism of anticancer and other drugs in patients with cancer may be markedly abnormal.

Finally, patients with cancer are inevitably treated with numerous supportive therapeutic agents and adjuvants; further, anticancer drugs are seldom used alone but frequently in combination. These practices introduce the possibility of drug interactions as manifested in alterations in pharmacokinetics and drug metabolism. The transport of hydrolyzed HN2 in L5178Y murine lymphoblasts is significantly stimulated by atropine, morphine, and cocaine but not by phenobarbital (PB) (36). On the other hand, the in vitro uptake and retention of MTX, 6-MP, ara-C, and 5-FU by the same cells in mice implanted with this tumor are inhibited by the intraperitoneal (i.p.) administration of L-asparaginase (37). In L1210 murine leukemia, the cellular transport and antitumor activity of MTX are markedly influenced by anticancer agents; hydrocortisone and L-asparaginase inhibit the transport and antagonize the antitumor activity of MTX, while VCR and VLB exhibit the opposite effects (38). The renal clearance of MTX in man is generally suppressed by the simultaneous administration of weak organic acids (39). In the rabbit pretreatment with MTX lowers plasma levels of 6-MP, presumably as a result of pharmacokinetic interference (40). Like X-irradiation, CTX and HN2 administered i.p. inhibit the development of hepatic microsomal enzymes in young rats; further, they reduce the activities of these enzymes in adult animals (41). Similar inhibition has been reported in the same species by MTX, 5-FU, DRC, and thalicarpine (42-45). Also in the rat, the immunostimulants Bacillus Calmette-Guérin and Corynebacterium parvum significantly decrease the hepatic microsomal enzyme activities, including the DIC N-demethylation activity (46). Undoubtedly, anticancer drugs, supportive therapeutic agents and adjuvants will interact among themselves and with each other to cause marked modifications in their pharmacokinetics and metabolism.

References

1. B. Clarkson, A. O'Connor, L. Winston, and D. Hutchinson: The physiologic disposition of 5-fluorouracil and 5-fluoro-2'-deoxyuridine in man. Clin. Pharmac. Therap., 5, 581 (1964).

2. L. S. Schanker and J. J. Jeffrey: Active transport of foreign pyrimidines across the intestinal epithelium. Nature, 190, 727 (1961).

3. T. L. Loo, J. K. Luce, M. P. Sullivan, and E. Frei, III: Clinical pharmacologic observations on 6-mercaptopurine and 6-methylthiopurine ribonucleoside. Clin. Pharmac. Therap., 9, 180 (1968).

4. I. D. Goldman, N. S. Lichtenstein, and V. T. Oliverio: Carrier-mediated transport of the folic acid analogue, methotrexate, in the L1210 leukemic cells. J. Biol. Chem., 243, 5007 (1968).

5. R. M. Lyons and G. J. Goldenberg: Active transport of nitrogen mustard and choline by normal and leukemic human lymphoid cells. Cancer Res., 32, 1679 (1972).

6. D. P. Rall, R. E. Rieselbach, V. T. Oliverio, and E. Morse: Pharmacology of folic acid antagonists as related to brain and cerebrospinal fluid. Cancer Chemoth. Rep., 16, 187 (1962).

7. T. L. Loo, J. K. Luce, J. H. Jardine, and E. Frei, III: Pharmacologic studies of the antitumor agent 5-(dimethyltriazeno)-imidazole-4-carboxamide. Cancer Res., 28, 2448 (1968).

8. T. L. Loo, K. Lu, and J. A. Gottlieb: Disposition and metabolism of thiopurines. II. Arabinosyl-6-mercaptopurine and ribosyl-6-mercaptopurine. Drug Met. Disp., 1, 645 (1973).

9. R. S. Bourke, C. R. West, G. Chheda, and D. B. Tower: Kinetics of entry and distribution of 5-fluorouracil in cerebrospinal fluid and brain following intravenous injection in a primate. Cancer Res., 33, 1735 (1973).

10. K. Lu, T. L. Loo, J. A. Benvenuto, R. S. Benjamin, M. Valdivieso, and E. J Freireich: Pharmacologic disposition and metabolism of ftorafur. Pharmacologist, 17, (1975).

11. D. H. W. Ho, B. Thetford, C. J. K. Carter, and E. Frei, III: Clinical pharmacologic studies of L-asparaginase. Clin. Pharmacol. Therap., 11, 408 (1970).

12. T. L. Loo, R. L. Dion, R. L. Dixon, and D. P. Rall: The antitumor agent, 1,3-bis(2-chloroethyl)-1-nitrosourea. J. Pharm. Sci., 55, 492 (1966).

13. M. D. Walker: Physiologic barriers to pharmacologic efficacy. Proc. 5th Int. Congr. Pharmac., 3, 354 (1973).

14. D. G. Johns, D. Farquhar, and T. L. Loo: Physiologic disposition of the di-amyl ester of 3',5'-^{3}H-methotrexate in the dog. Pharmacologist, 16, 231 (1974).

15. K. B. Bischoff, R. L. Dedrick, D. S. Zaharko, and J. A. Longstreth: Methotrexate Pharmacokinetics. J. Pharm. Sci., 60, 1128 (1971).

16. R. L. Dedrick, D. D. Forrester, and D. H. W. Ho: In vitro in vivo correlation of drug metabolism - Deamination of 1-β-D-arabinofuranosylcytosine. Biochem. Pharmacol., 21, 1 (1972).

17. T. L. Loo, D. H. W. Ho, G. P. Bodey, and E. J Freireich: Pharmacological and clinical studies of some nucleoside analogues. Ann. N. Y. Acad. Sci. (1975).

18. E. S. Henderson, R. H. Adamson, and V. T. Oliverio: The metabolic fate of tritiated methotrexate. II. Absorption and excretion in man. Cancer Res., 25, 1018 (1965).

19. T. L. Loo and S. E. Sugarek: Unpublished work.

20. D. W. Donigian and R. J. Owellen: Interaction of vinblastine, vincristine, and colchicine with serum proteins. Biochem. Pharmac., 22, 2113 (1973).

21. R. S. Benjamin, P. H. Wiernik, and N. R. Bachur: Adriamycin chemotherapy - efficacy, safety, and pharmacologic basis of an intermittent single high-dose schedule. Cancer, 33, 19 (1974).

22. V. T. Oliverio and J. D. Davidson: The physiological disposition of dichloromethotrexate - ^{36}Cl in animals. J. Pharmac. Exp. Ther., 137, 76 (1962).

23. N. B. Kuemmerle: Hepatobiliary excretion of 5-(3,3-dimethyl-1-triazeno)-imidazole-4-carboxamide (DIC) in the rat. M.S. Thesis, The Univ. of TX System Health Sci. Ctr. at Houston Grad. Sch. of Biomed. Sci., 1975.

24. R. J. Owellen and D. W. Donigian: [^{3}H] Vincristine. Preparation and preliminary pharmacology. J. Med. Chem., 15, 894 (1972).

25. D. R. Brand: Hepatobiliary excretion of Baker's folate antagonist in the rat. M.S. Thesis, The Univ. of TX System Health Sci. Ctr. at Houston Grad. Sch. of Biomed. Sci., 1975.

26. J. L. Skibba, D. D. Beal, G. Ramirez, and G. T. Bryan: N-demethylation of the antineoplastic agent 4(5)-(3,3-dimethyl-1-triazeno)imidazole-5(4)-carboxamide by rats and man. Cancer Res., 30, 147 (1970).

27. D. L. Hill, W. R. Laster, Jr., M. C. Kirk, S. El Dareer, and R. F. Struck: Metabolism of iphosphamide [2-(2-chloroethylamino)-3-(2-chloroethyl)tetrahydro-2H-1,3,2-oxazaphosphorine-2-oxide] and production of a toxic iphosphamide metabolite. Cancer Res., 33, 1016 (1973).

28. H. E. May, R. Boose, and D. J. Reed: Hydroxylation of the carcinostatic 1-(2-chloroethyl)-3-cyclohexyl-1-nitrosourea (CCNU) by rat liver microsomes. Biochem. Biophys. Res. Comm., 57, 426 (1974).

29. D. L. Hill, M. C. Kirk, and R. F. Struck: Microsomal metabolism of nitrosoureas. Cancer Res., 35, 296 (1975).

30. N. R. Bachur and M. Gee: Daunorubicin metabolism by rat tissue preparations. J. Pharmac. Exp. Ther., 177, 567 (1971).

31. M. A. Asbell, E. Schwartzbach, F. J. Bullock, and D. W. Yesair: Daunomycin and adriamycin metabolism via reductive glucosidic cleavage. J. Pharmac. Exp. Ther., 182, 63 (1972).

32. T. L. Loo and J. Friedman: Unpublished work.

33. R. Kato, A. Takanaka, A. Takahashi, and K. Onoda: Drug metabolism in tumor-bearing rats. Jap. J. Pharmac., 18, 245 (1968), and subsequent papers.

34. R. Rosso, M. G. Donelli, G. Franchi, and S. Garattini: Impairment of drug metabolism in tumor-bearing animals. Europ. J. Cancer, 7, 565 (1971).

35. G. E. Housholder and T. L. Loo: Disposition of 5-(3,3-dimethyl-1-triazeno)imidazole-4-carboxamide, a new antitumor agent. J. Pharmac. Exp. Ther., 179, 386 (1971).

36. G. J. Goldenberg: Drug-induced stimulation of nitrogen mustard and choline transport and other systems in L5178Y lymphoblasts *in vitro*. Cancer Res., 34, 2511 (1974).

37. A. Nahas and R. L. Capizzi: Effect of *in vivo* treatment with L-asparaginase on the *in vivo* uptake and retention of some anti-

leukemic agents. Cancer Res., 34, 2689 (1974).

38. R. F. Zager, S. A. Frisby, and V. T. Oliverio: The effects of antibiotics and cancer chemotherapeutic agents on the cellular transport and antitumor activity of methotrexate in L1210 murine leukemia. Cancer Res., 33, 1670 (1973).

39. D. G. Liegler, E. S. Henderson, M. A. Hahn, and V. T. Oliverio: The effect of organic acids on renal clearance of methotrexate in man. Clin. Pharmac. Ther., 10, 849 (1969).

40. F. Pannuti, A. Ligabue, and F. Trasarti: Interferenza farmacologica in oncologia: Variazioni della cinetica della 6-mercaptopurina (6-MP) in animali pretrattati con methotrexate (MTX). Boll. Soc. Ital. Biol. Sper., 48, 574 (1972).

41. R. G. Tardiff and K. P. DuBois: Inhibition of hepatic microsomal enzymes by alkylating agents. Arch. Int. Pharmacodyn., 127, 445 (1969).

42. M. G. Donelli, G. Franchi, and R. Rosso: The effect of cytotoxic agents on drug metabolism. Europ. J. Cancer, 6, 125 (1970).

43. P. Klubes and I. Cerna: Effect of 5-fluorouracil on drug-metabolizing enzymes in the rat. Cancer Res., 34, 927 (1974).

44. P. J. Creaven, L. M. Allen, and C. P. Williams: The interaction of the antineoplastic drug thalicarpine with aniline hydroxylase and microsomal cytochrome of rat liver. Xenobiotica, 4, 255 (1974).

45. T. K. Basu and D. C. Williams: Effects of methotrexate and phenobarbital on the hepatic microsomal drug-metabolizing enzymes in normal rats. Chemoth., 21, 33 (1975).

46. D. Farquhar and T. L. Loo: BCG-induced impairment of drug-metabolizing enzyme activities of the rat liver. Pharmacologist, 16, 239 (1974).

THE ACTIVITY OF NEW DRUGS AGAINST MOUSE TUMOURS*

John M. Venditti and Mary K. Wolpert-DeFilippes
Drug Evaluation Branch
Drug Research and Development
Division of Cancer Treatment
National Cancer Institute
Bethesda, U.S.A.

In 1974, more than 39,000 synthetic compounds and 8,000 crude natural product extracts were submitted to the National Cancer Institute for evaluation of their antitumour activity in laboratory models. For more than 75% of the synthetic materials, the amount received was 2.0 g. or less. Testing of a large number of new materials available in limited quantity requires the use of an initial biological screen which is rapid, reproducible, inexpensive and above all, predictive for clinical utility.

Retrospective studies of correlations of activity among various animal tumor models and clinical efficacy led to the selection of mouse leukemia L1210 as our current initial screen for synthetic agents (1,2). Mouse leukemia P388 is used for initial *in vivo* screening of

*With the exceptions noted below the data shown in the tables and figures resulted from studies conducted under contract to the Division of Cancer Treatment, NCI, at Arthur D. Little Inc., Battelle Memorial Institute, Hazelton Laboratories, Microbiological Associates, Inc., and the Wisconsin Alumni Research Foundation. In addition, the authors wish to thank Drs. J.A.R. Mead and L.C. Mishra, National Cancer Institute, forthe use of their data on 5-methyl-tetrahydrohomofolic acid and Mrs. L.M. Hummer for her aid in preparing this manuscript.

crude natural products because it responds to many L1210-active drugs, but is quantitatively more sensitive than L1210 (2,3). It was reasoned that a crude natural product extract might contain an active material in a concentratio too low to be effective against the less sensitive L1210, but that minimal activity might be observed using the more sensitive P388 and lead to the isolation of an L1210-activ drug (2,3). The value of P388 for identifying active natural products has been demonstrated (3,4). Drugs emerging as active from initial screens are evaluated against a number of additional animal tumors selected on the basis of their growth characteristics; e.g., slower-growing tumors, or because they may represent laboratory models of specific human malignancies (2). Active materials are studied also with respect to factors that may influence their usefulness; e.g., route and treatment schedule (5), in combination chemotherapy (6,7), and in combined treatment modalities (8-12); and with respect to their cellular and biochemical sites of action (13-16). New active structural congeners of known antitumour drugs are investigated in models designed to determine whether the new agent is qualitatively similar to the parent in its biological, biochemical andpharmacological effects and if so, whether it may be superior in some way (17,18). The potential advantage of a new active structural congener may be suggested, for example, because it is considerably more effective than the parent drug against animal tumors, because it retains activity against a tumor variant developed for resistance to the parent suggesting a difference in pharmacological or biochemical actions, because it is easier to synthesize or to formulate for clinical use, or because it produces less of some specific toxicity that limits the use of the parent drug. The last instance is represented by Chlorozotocin (NSC 178248), a structural congener of Streptozotocin (NSC 85998) and the nitrosoureas. Against L1210, Chlorozotocin is much more effective than Streptozotocin and as effective as clinically active nitrosoureas. Interest in Chlorozotocin stems from the observation that it produces considerably less bone marrow toxicity than the nitrosoureas (19) and is considerably more water soluble.

This report summarizes pertinent experimental antitumour results for five drugs that are either in early clinical trial or in development toward clinical trial in the NCI program. The general experimental methods used have been published. (20).

<u>Maytansine (NSC 153858, Fig. 1)</u> was isolated from the bark root of the East African plant, Maytenus ovatus (later

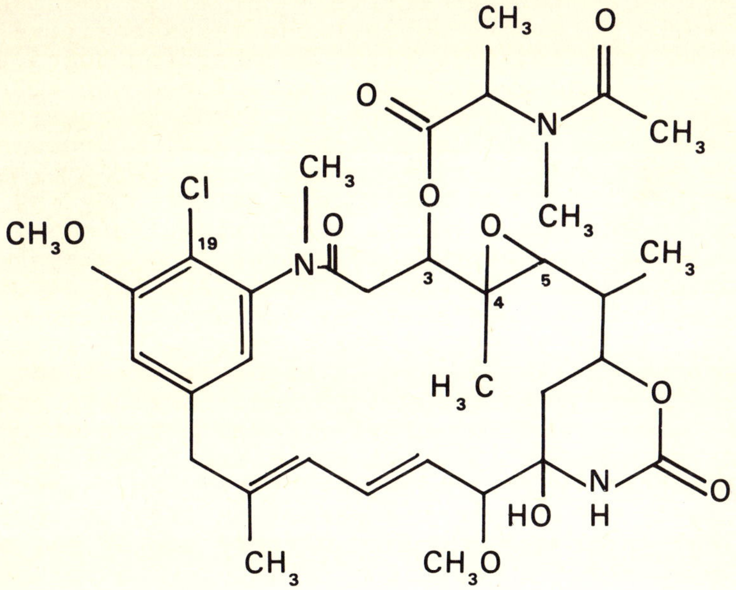

FIGURE 1 : Structure of Maytansine, NSC 153858.

TABLE 1

MAYTANSINE. NSC 153858. CYTOTOXICITY AGAINST KB CELLS IN CULTURE*

	ED50 (μg/ml.)
Experiment 1	$<1.0 \times 10^{-5}$
Experiment 2	$<3.9 \times 10^{-5}$

*Data of Thayer et al, Arthur D. Little, Inc.

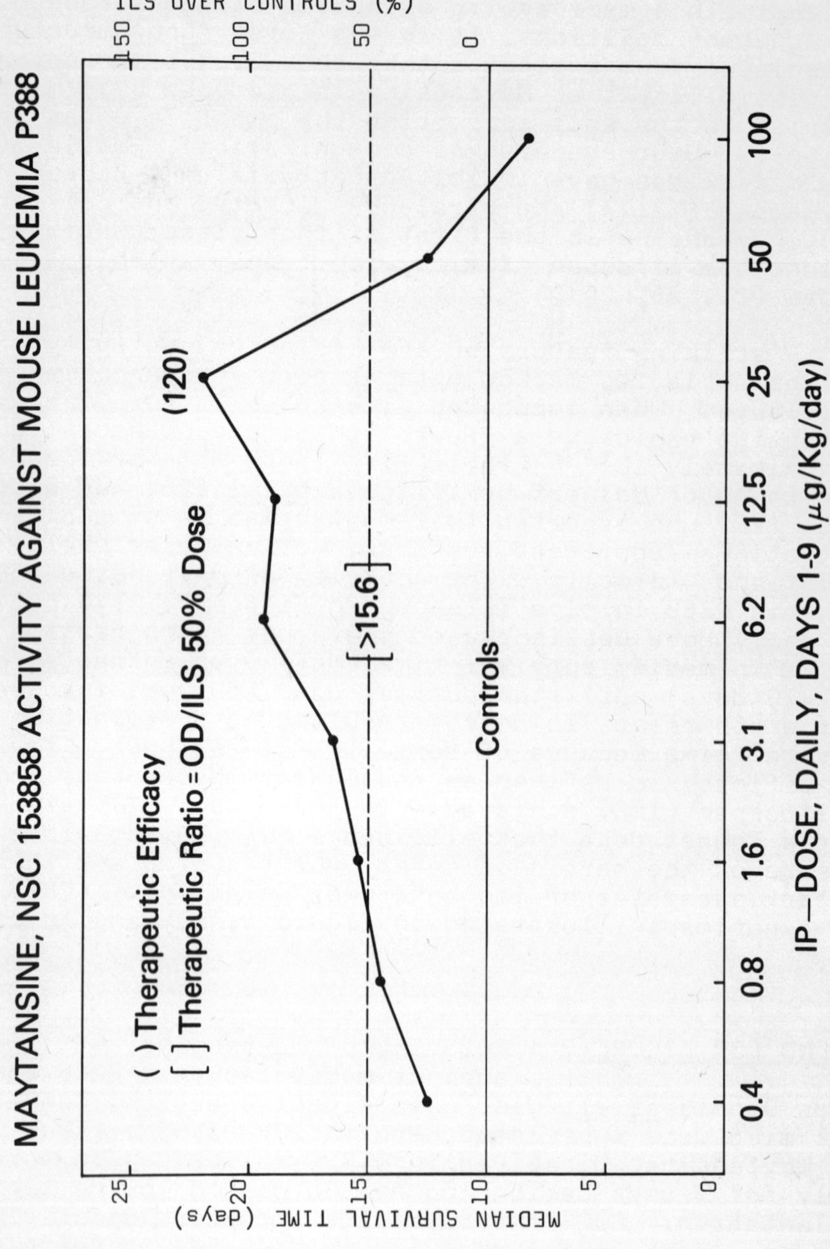
MAYTANSINE, NSC 153858 ACTIVITY AGAINST MOUSE LEUKEMIA P388
( ) Therapeutic Efficacy
[ ] Therapeutic Ratio = OD/ILS 50% Dose
(120)
[>15.6]
Controls
ILS OVER CONTROLS (%)
150
100
50
0
MEDIAN SURVIVAL TIME (days)
25
20
15
10
5
0
0.4
0.8
1.6
3.1
6.2
12.5
25
50
100
IP—DOSE, DAILY, DAYS 1-9 (μg/Kg/day)

re-identified as M. serrata) and identified by Kupchan _et al_ (21). Maytansine appears to be related structurally to the ansamycin antibiotics in that it contains an aromatic nucleus with a macrocyclic aliphatic bridge attached at two non-adjacent positions. It is the first such structure to be isolated from a plant rather than from a microorganism. The possibility that Maytansine is produced by a microorganism in the soil supporting the plant is under investigation (J. Douros, personal communication). While other ansa macrolides have inhibited bacterial DNA-dependent RNA polymerase (22,23) and viral-RNA directed DNA polymerase (24), Maytansine is the first of this class observed to prolong the lifespan of mice with transplantable lethal tumors (21, 25, 26).

A striking feature of the biological activity of Maytansine is its marked cytotoxicity for mammalian cells in culture. When incubated with KB cells for 72 hours, Maytansine exhibited a growth inhibitory ED50 of $<10^{-5}$ µg/ml, approximately 10^{-10}M (Table 1). These data are consistent with those of Wolpert-DeFillippes _et al_ (26) and O'Connor _et al_ (27) who reported that Maytansine in nanomolar concentrations suppressed the growth of cultured L1210, P388, L5178Y and 3T3 cells. The activity of Maytansine against Leukemia P388 in mice is shown in figure 2. Typically, as the daily dose was increased there was a progressive increase in median survival time (MST) over untreated controls (MST=10 days) until the optimal dose (OD) was reached. Further increases in dosage resulted in a diminution of survival time because of toxicity for the host. Therapeutic efficacy is defined as the maximum percentage increase in lifespan (ILS) achieved - in this case, 120% at the OD to the lowest dose that elicited a 50% ILS, provides a measure of the margin of safety for the drug and is an ancillary parameter of its antitumor selectivity (28). In the experiment illustrated in figure 2, Maytansine provid-

---

LEGEND FOR FIGURE 2 : Activity of Maytansine, NSC 153858 against mouse leukemia P388 (data of de Dennis _et al_, Wisconsin Alumni Research Foundation). BDF1 mice were inoculated ip with 10^6 P388 cells on day 0. Maytansine, dissolved in 0.85% saline was injected ip daily for 9 days beginnning on the day following tumor implantation. OD = the optimally effective dose. ILS 50% dose = the lowest dose providing a 50% increase in lifespan over controls.

TABLE 2

MAYTANSINE. NSC 153858. INFLUENCE OF ROUTE AND SCHEDULE ON ACTIVITY AGAINST MOUSE LEUKEMIA P388*

Treatment Route-Schedule	Experiment 1 Dose Range (μg/Kg/Injection)	OD	ILS (%)	Experiment 2 Dose Range (μg/Kg/Injection)	OD	ILS (%)
IP-Once; Day 1	1.0-256	128	54	128-1024	512	54
IP-qd; D1-9	0.3-64	16	86	2.0-32	8.0	59
IP-q4d; D1,5,9	0.5-128	128	90	128-1024	128	63
IP-q8d; D1+9	1.0-256	256	81	128-1024	256	81
IP-q3h; D1 only	0.1-32	32	100	16-128	32	81
IP-q3h; D1+9	0.1-32	16	90	8.0-128	16	81
IP-q3h; D1,5,9	--	--	--	16-128	16	95
SC-qd. D1-9	--	--	--	64-512	256	72

*Data of Wodinsky *et al*, Arthur D. Little, Inc.
Tumor inoculum - 10^6 cells (IP).

ed a therapeutic ratio of 15.6. Table 2 summarizes two experiments designed to determine the influence of variations in drug route and treatment schedule on the therapeutic efficacy of Maytansine. Although the differences were not profound, it appeared that intensive-intermittent intraperitoneal (ip) treatment (q3hrs x 8 on day 1, every 4th day, or on days 1 and 9) or two widely spaced treatments (once on days 1 and 9) may be more effective than daily treatment. Subcutaneous (sc) daily treatment appeared to be as effective as ip daily treatment. In experiments carried out to this time, Maytansine has been ineffective when given orally against P388; nor has ip Maytansine shown important activity against L1210. However, it has produced moderate increases in the survival of mice with ip implanted melanoma B16 (Table 3).

In preliminary studies of the biochemical sites of Maytansine action, Wolpert-DeFillippes et al (26) observed inhibition of DNA and RNA synthesis. Although the degree of DNA inhibition exceeded that of RNA inhibition, these investigators examined effects on RNA polymerase in view of the sensitivity of that enzyme to other ansa macrolides and found that *E. coli* RNA polymerase was not inhibited at Maytansine concentrations up to 10^{-4} M. However, they did observe, in L1210 cell cultures, that Maytansine, at the irreversibly cytotoxic conentration of 10^{-8} M, produced a ten fold increase over controls in the number of cells with mitotic figures (26). Remillard, working in the laboratory of L.I. Rebhun and S.M. Kupchan, observed that Maytansine irreversibly inhibited cell division in eggs of two species of sea urchins and one species of clam (29). Such observations prompted the investigation of the activity of Maytansine against a Vincristine resistant variant of P388 (P388/VCR)(26) and cross-resistance was found (Table 4). O'Connor et al (27) observed that Maytansine produced a 50% inhibition of focus formation in murine sarcoma virus (MSV) infected 3T3 cells at about one-fourth the concentration required to inhibit the growth of non-infected cells by 50%. The foci inhibitory ED50 concentration permitted 100% growth of non-infected cells. In the same studies, the ansa macrolide, Geldanamycin (NSC 122750), produced a 50% inhibition of MSV focus formation at about one-fifth the cytotoxic ED50 concentration for non-infected 3T3 cells. Neither Maytansine nor Geldanamycin depressed the enzymatic activity of simian sarcoma virus DNA polymerase or RNA polymerases from BALB/C mouse embryo cells (27). These findings suggest that Maytansine may exert antiviral activity by some specific, but as yet unknown action. The

TABLE 3: Maytansine. NSC 153858. Activity against mouse melanoma B16 (IP)

IP-Dose qd, Days 1-9 (μg/Kg/Day)	Increase in Median Survival Time Over Controls (%) Expt. 1	Expt. 2
32	0	0
16	45	57
8.0	40	55
4.0	5	32

*Data of Gargus *et al*., Hazelton Laboratories.

specific action of Maytansine against mammalian tumor cells leading to its selective toxicity against P388 and B16 *in vivo* is also unknown, but the observed ability to arrest progression through the mitotic phase of the cell cycle suggests a potentially fruitful area for further study.

The crystalline antibiotic, NSC 135758, a piperazinedione (Fig. 3) was isolated from *Streptomyces griseoluteus* and shown to inhibit the growth of human tumour cells on embryonated eggs by Gitterman *et al* (30). Subsequent *in vivo* screening against a number of animal tumors showed a high level of activity against L1210, P388 and rat carcinoma W256. The activity against L1210 is summarized

TABLE 4: Activity of Maytansine or Vincristine against Vincristine sensitive or resistant P388 Leukemia*

Drug	Dose Range (Mg/Kg/Day-IP-D1-9)	OD	ILS (%)
	(Leukemia P388)		
Maytansine	0.025-0.10	0.025	95
Vincristine	0.25 -0.50	0.25	125
	(Leukemia P388/VCR)		
Maytansine	0.025-0.10	-	0
Vincristine	0.25 -0.50	-	0

*Wolpert-Defilippes *et al*. (26).

TABLE 5: NSC 135758*. Activity against ip planted L1210 Leukaemia (10^5 cells/mouse)+

IP-Treatment Schedule	Dose Range (Mg/Kg/Injection)	OD	ILS (%)	60 Day Survivors
Once, Day 1	2.0 -32	8.0	>501	6/10
Q3 hr. X 8, D1 only	0.5 -8.0	2.0	>354	4/10
Q4d.; D1,5,9	1.0 -16	4.0	221	0/10
Q 3 hr. X 8, q4d; D1,5,9	0.25-4.0	1.0	>299	2/10
Q8d.; D1 and 9	1.0 -16	8.0	>415	3/10
Q3 hr. X 8; D1 and 9	0.25-4.0	1.0	252	0/10
Qd.; D1-9	0.5 -8.0	2.0	223	0/10

*3,6-Bis-(5-chloro-2-piperidinyl)-2,5-piperazinedione,dihydrochloride
+Data of Wodinsky et al., Arthur D. Little, Inc.

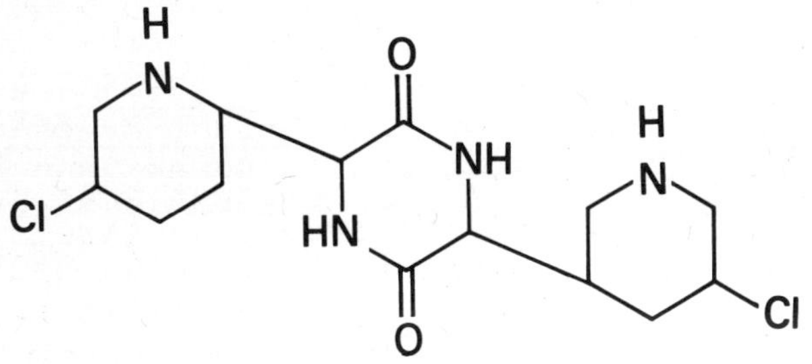

FIGURE 3: Structure of the crystalline antibiotic, NSC 135758 (Merck Antibiotic - 593A) Crystalline isolate from Streptomyces griseoluteus
3,6-bis-(5-Chloro-2-piperidinyl)2,5-piperazinedione

in Table 5. When given ip to mice with ip implanted L1210, NSC 135758 produced an ILS of 200% on a variety of treatment schedules. It was most effective as a single treatment on day 1 only or days 1 and 9; and when given q3 hrs on day 1 or on days 1,5, and 9. On these schedules long term survivors were observed. The antibiotic retained its anti-L1210 activity when it was given orally, sc, or intravenously (iv) to mice with ip implanted L1210. Its activity against ip implanted P388 was comparable to its anti-L1210 activity; i.e., optimal single ip treatment resulted in 40% long term survivors while optimal daily ip treatment produced a marked extension in survival, but no "cures". Non-lethal daily ip doses inhibited the growth of intramuscularly implanted W256 by 100%. R.L. Dion and V.H. Bono (personal communication), using flow microfluorometric techniques, reported that NSC 135758 selectively blocked cell cycle progression of L1210 cells in culture at the G_2 phase. Cells were prevented from entering mitosis and giant cells were formed.

5-Methyl-tetrahydrohomofolic acid (MeH^{4}HF, NSC 139490; Fig. 4.) is an example of a drug designed and developed on the basis of a biochemical pharmacological rationale. Steps leading to its development have been recently reviewed by J.A.R. Mead (31). M.E. Friedkin had proposed that the high dihydrofolate reductase levels in an antifolate resistant variant of L1210 might be used to produce a reduced substrate with minimal dihydrofolate reductase inhibitory activity, but which might be a potent inhibitor of thymidylate synthetase (31,32). Dihydrohomofolate seemed to be a suitable substrate for dihydrofolate reductase, and the product, tetrahydrohomofolate, was tested *in vivo* (33). It was quite effective against a Methotrexate (MTX)-resistant subline of L1210 which had high dihydrofolate reductase levels, but it was minimally effective against the parent tumor. Tetrahydrohomofolate did inhibit *E. coli* thymidylate synthetase, but *in vivo* inhibition of this target enzyme was not marked (34). This was attributed to the spontaneous oxidation of tetrahydrohomofolate back to dihydrohomofolate *in vivo* and establishment of a redox cycle between the two forms. The ensuing search for an analog of tetrahydrohomofolate which would be stable *in vivo* resulted in the synthesis of the 5-methyl derivative, MeH^{4}HF (35). MeH^{4}HF was nearly as active as MTX against the parent line, L1210/0 (Table 6). More important however, was the observation that MeH^{4}HF retained its activity over a wide dose range against L1210/FR-8, a MTX resistant variant characterized by high dihydrofolate reductase levels (34). MeH^{4}HF has little effect on dihydrofolate reductase, but also little effect on *E. coli* thymidylate synthetase (31). Elucidation of its site of action will be interesting. It exemplifies how the application of a biochemical rationale can lead to the development of a new drug worthy of clinical trial even though its activity may not be related directly to that rationale.

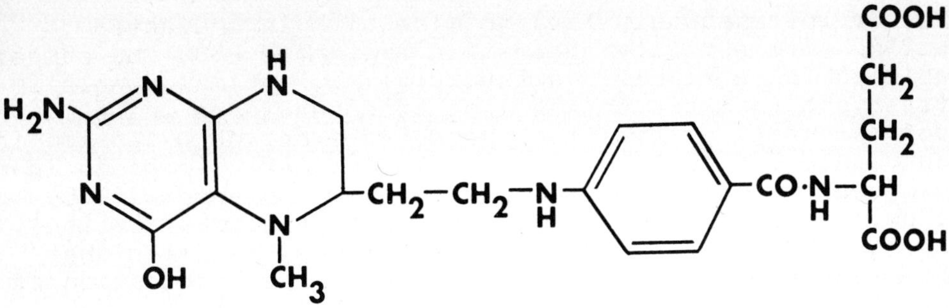

FIGURE 4: Structure of 5-Methyl-D,L-tetrahydrohomofolic acid, MeH[4] HF, NSC 139490.

TABLE 6: Activity of 5-methyl-D,L-Tetrahydrohomofolate and methotrexate (MTX) against L1210 and L1210/FR-8*[†].

Durg	Dosage (Mg/Kg/Day)	L1210/0 (ILS %)	L1210/FR-8 (ILS %)
Me-H4F	400	55	100
	200	50	83
	100	33	78
	50	33	72
MTX	3.0	72	0
	1.5	50	0
	0.75	33	0

*IP treatment, qd., days 1-9, to mice with SC inoculated tumor.
†Data of Mishra et al (34).

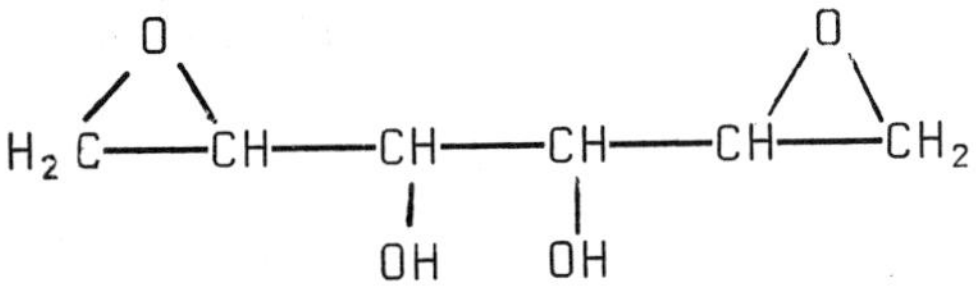

$$H_2C(O)CH-CH(OH)-CH(OH)-CH(O)CH_2$$

FIGURE 5 : Structure of Dianhydrogalactitol 1,2:5,6 NSC 132313

Maytansine; the antibiotic, NSC 135758; and MeH[4] HR are representative of drugs whose initial activities were discovered in the NCI Drug developmental program. The two drugs discussed below were reported from other programs and were studied further by us because of the interesting biological and pharmacological activities reported.

Dianhydrogalactitol (NSC 132313, Fig. 5) also known as dianhydrodulcitol, was synthesized by Institoris in Hungary (36) and its biological activity was described by Elson _et al_ (37), Nemeth _et al_ (38) and Kellner _et al_ (39) who reported the _in vivo_ activity of this diepoxyhexitol against a variety of animal tumors including L1210. The point was made (38) that dianhydrogalactitol was superior to Dibromodulcitol (NSC 104800; DBD) for the treatment of mouse tumours L1210, NK/Ly, Ehrlich ascites, and S180 ascites. DBD was more effective than dianhydrogalacitol against Harding-Passey melanoma and a number of rat solid tumors (38). Our own experiments (Table 7) confirmed the anti-L1210 activity of dianhydrogalactitol and its superiority over DBD which has elicited only a moderate response against L1210. In addition, dianhydrogalactitol was markedly active against P388 and produced substantial activity against B16 melanoma (Table 7).

Horvath _et al_ (40) showed that when DBD was incubated in phosphate buffer, the major detectable product was dianhydrogalactitol; and Gati _et al_ (41) demonstrated the formation of dianhydrogalactitol in serum and ascitic fluid of rats bearing Yoshida ascites tumor following DBD treatment. Elson _et al_ (37) had earlier suggested that the cytostatic effects of dibromohexitols might be partially mediated by metabolism to corresponding epoxides. Thus, it is believed that dianhydrogalactitol is a major active metabolic product of DBD. The diepoxyhexitols are active alkylating agents, capable of cross-linking native DNA and reacting with bistone and non-histone protein(42, 43). In general, dianhydrogalactitol is the most effective of the diepoxyhexitols and corresponding halohexitols with respect to biochemical and biological activities.

4,4'-Propylenedi-(±)-2,6-piperazinedione (NSC 129943), ICRF 159. Fig. 6) is one of a number of bis-diketopiperazines which were submitted to NCI for further testing following initial observations of animal antitumor activity in the laboratories of the Imperial Cancer Research Fund, London (44). Figure 6 summarizes our own data showing the activity of ICRF 159 against L1210. An interesting characteristic of the compound is its demons-

TABLE 7 : NSC 132313, Dianhydrogalactitol. Activity against mouse tumors*

Tumor	Treatment Route-Schedule	OD (Mg/Kg)	Av. ILS (%)	Survivors	No. of Expts.
B16 Melanoma (IP)	IP-qd.; Day 1-9	2.0,4.0	66	0/16	2
L1210 Leukemia (IP)	IP-qd.; Day 1-9	2.0-5.0	91	2/86	11
	SC-qd.; Day 1-9	2.0-4.0	52	0/36	4
	PO-qd.; Day 1-9	4.0	54	0/30	3
	IP-q4d.; D1,5,9	4.0-8.0	109	5/52	6
	SC-q4d.; D1,5,9	8.0	83	0/10	1
	PO-q4d.; D1,5,9	8.0	66	0/20	2
L1210 Leukemia (SC)	IP-q4d.; D1,5,9	4.0	55	0/8	1
P388 Leukemia (IP)	IP-qd.; Day 1-9	2.0,4.0	181	0/12	2

*Data from various NCI screening laboratories.

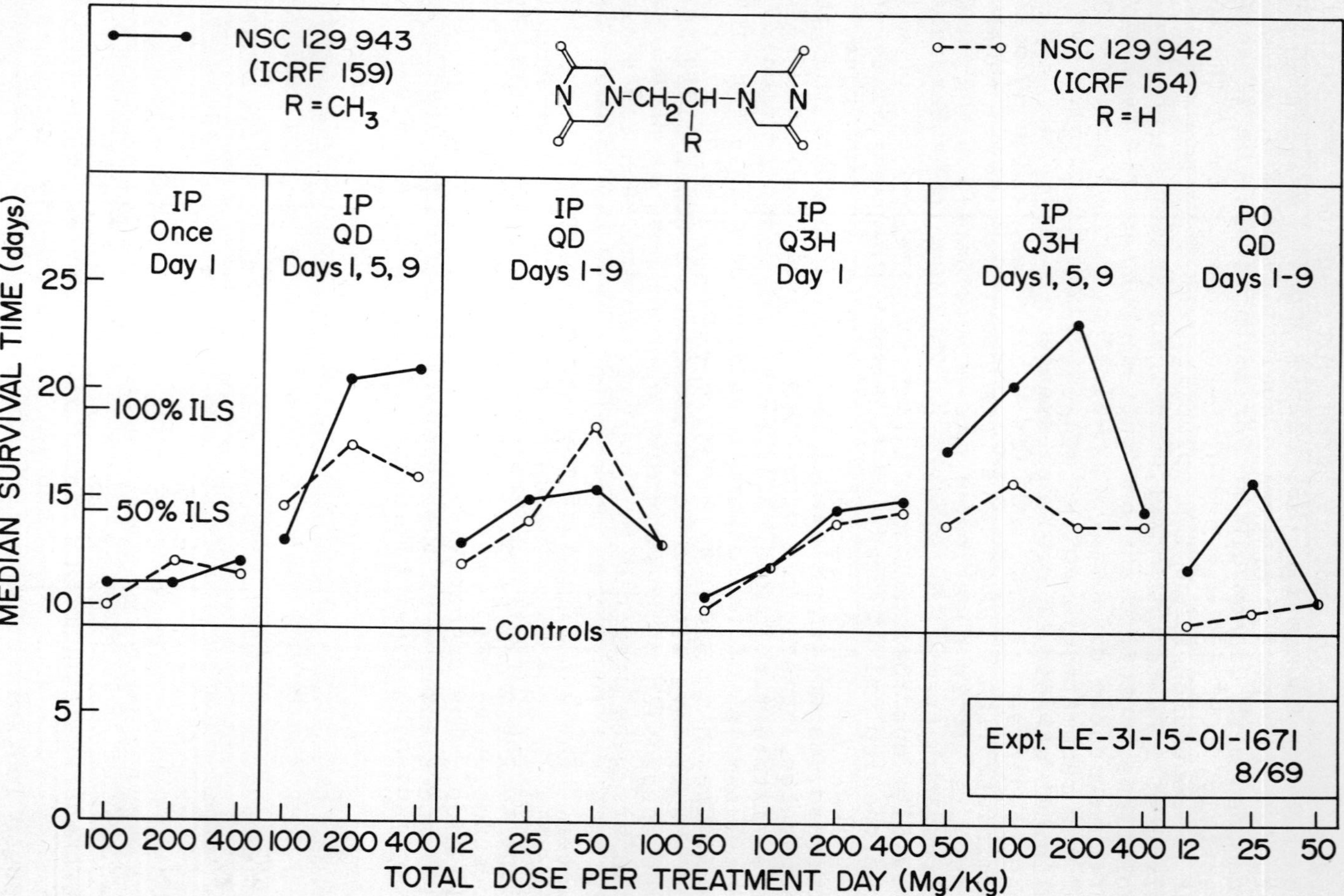

NSC 129 943 (ICRF 159) R = CH3
N-CH2-CH-N
R
NSC 129 942 (ICRF 154) R = H
IP Once Day 1
IP QD Days 1, 5, 9
IP QD Days 1-9
IP Q3H Day 1
IP Q3H Days 1, 5, 9
PO QD Days 1-9
MEDIAN SURVIVAL TIME (days)
0
5
10
15
20
25
100% ILS
50% ILS
Controls
Expt. LE-31-15-01-1671 8/69
100 200 400 100 200 400 12 25 50 100 50 100 200 400 50 100 200 400 12 25 50
TOTAL DOSE PER TREATMENT DAY (Mg/Kg)

trated ability to protect normal mice against the lethal toxicity of Daunomycin (NSC 82151) and its ability to provide therapeutic synergism against L1210 when combined with Daunomycin or Adriamycin (45). Up to very recently, ICRF 159 was administered to animals in the form of a suspension since the solubility of this racemic mixture, in water, 3 mg/ml, was insufficient to prepare solutions of sufficient concentration to permit delivery of therapeutic dosages. When given orally, a suspension of the racemate was active against L1210 (fig. 6). The clinical effects of oral preparations of ICRF 159 have been reported (46-48), and its toxicities following oral administration to dogs have been described (49). Thus, there is little question of its absorption from the gastro-intestinal tract. Nevertheless, in order to better relate toxicity and therapeutic efficacy to dose and to conduct pharmacological studies, we felt that the possibility of developing a soluble parenteral formulation should be persued, especially since we had been made aware that the separated isomers were considerably more water soluble than the mixture (Creighton, A.M., Personal Communication). Small samples of the separate isomers were received from A.M. Creighton and preliminary testing suggested solutions of the isomers were at least as active against L1210 as the suspension of the mixture. Larger amounts of the isomers were prepared in this program and each was shown to be about four times more soluble than the racemate in water. The activities of the separate isomers given parenterally in aqueous solution have been shown to be equivalent to the activity of the mixture, ICRF 159, given in suspension against L1210, B16 and the Lewis lung carcinoma in mice. The comparative activity of suspensions of ICRF 159 and solutions of the separate isomers (NSC 169779 and NSC 169780) against L1210 is summarized in Table 8.

←

LEGEND FOR FIGURE 6: Structure of ICRF 159, NSC 129943, and its effectiveness against mouse leukemia L1210. ICRF 159, a racemic mixture, was suspended in 0.5% carboxymethylcellulose. Data of I. Kline *et al*, Microbiological Associates, Inc (5).

TABLE 8

COMPARISON OF THE RACEMIC MIXTURE, ICRF-159, AND ITS SOLUBLE ISOMERS AGAINST IP IMPLANTED L1210 (10^5 CELLS/MOUSE)

Treatment Route-Schedule	Pct. Increase in Lifespan Over Controls at (Optimal Dose)* NSC-129943 ICRF-159	NSC-169779 (-) isomer	NSC-169780 (+) isomer
IP-qd.; D1-9	74(64)	75(32)	63(64)
IP-q4d.; D1,5,9	112(512)	94(1024)	87(1024)
SC-qd.; D1-9	77(32)	59(32)	61(64)
SC-q4d.; D1,5,9	110(512)	104(512)	139(1024)
PO-qd.; D1-9	45(16)	51(16)	85(64)
PO-q4d.; D1,5,9	115(1024)	107(1024)	137(1024)

*For each treatment regimen, each material was given over a series of dosages. Activities shown are the maximums observed. The optimal doses, mg/kg/injection, are shown in parentheses. Data of Barker *et al*., Battelle Memorial Institute, Columbus.

Summary. Pertinent animal antitumor data are presented for five drugs under study in the NCI pre-clinical drug development program. Three of the materials originated in projects sponsored by the program; Maytansine, NSC 153858, isolated from extracts of the Maytenus plant; the crystalline antibiotic, NSC 135758, isolated from fermentation broths of *Streptomyces griseoluteus*; and 5-methyl-tetrahydrohomofolic acid, synthesized on the basis of a biochemical pharmacological rationale. Dianhydrogalactitol, NSC 132313, was submitted to this program following its synthesis and initial animal testing in Hungary. The separated isomers, NSC 169779(-) and NSC 169780 (+) of the racemic mixture, ICRF 159 were originally submitted from Great Britain where ICRF 159 had first been tested. The drugs discussed are presented in order to emphasize our interest in identifying new drugs with potential anticancer activity by empirical screening and by rational drug design, and our interest in participating in the development of promising drugs found in other screening programs.

REFERENCES

1. Goldin, A. *et al* Cancer Chemotherapy Reports 50, 173, 1966.
2. Venditti, J.M. In *Pharmacological Basis of Cancer Chemotherapy*, p. 245, The Williams and Wilkins Co., Baltimore, 1975.
3. Venditti, J.M. Cancer Chemoth. Rep. Part 3, (2),1, 1972.
4. Venditti, J.M. & Abbott, B.J. Lloydia 30, 332, 1967.
5. Venditti, J.M. Cancer Chemoth. Rep. Part 3,2,35,1971.
6. Goldin, A. *et al*. In *Handbook of Experimental Pharmacology* 38/1. 411, Springer-Verlag, New York, 1974.
7. Schabel, F.M. Jr., Bioch. Pharmacol. 23 (Suppl. 2), 163, 1974.
8. Fugmann, R.A. *et al*. Cancer Chemoth. Rep. Part 2, 4(1), 25, 1974.
9. Martin, D.S. *et al*, Ibid, p. 13.
10. Wodinsky, I. *et al*. Ibid, p. 73.
11. Skipper, H.E. Ibid, p. 137.
12. Humphreys, S.R. & Karrer, K. Cancer Chemoth. Rep 54, 379, 1970.

13. Bono, V.H. Jr., Cancer Chemoth. Rep. Part 2, 4(1),131 1974.

14. Brockman, R.W. Ibid, p. 115.

15. Tobey, R.A. & Crissman, H.A. Cancer Research 35,448, 1975.

16. Tobey, R.A. & Crissman, H.A. Cancer Research 32, 2726 1972.

17. Kline, I. et al Cancer Chemother. Rep. 55, 9, 1971.

18. Venditti, J.M. et al. Cancer Chemother. Rep. 56, 483, 1972.

19. Schein, P. et al. Proc. American Assoc for Cancer Research 16, 122, 1975.

20. Geran, R.I. et al. Cancer Chemother. Rep. Part 3, 3(2), 7, 1972.

21. Kupchan, S.M. et al. J. Amer. Chem. Soc. 94, 1354, 1972.

22. Hartmann, G et al. Biochem. Biophys. Acta 145, 843, 1967.

23. Mizumo, S. et al. Biochem. Biophys. Acta 157, 322, 1968.

24. Yang, S.S. et al. J. Nat. Cancer Inst. 49, 7, 1972.

25. Kupchan, S.M. et al. J. Amer. Chem. Soc. 96, 3706, 1974.

26. Wolpert-DeFilippes, M.K. et al. Bioch. Pharmacol. 24, 751, 1975.

27. O'Connor, T.E. et al. Proc. of the Amer. Assoc. for Cancer Research 16. 29, 1975.

28. Goldin, A. & Venditti, J.M. Cancer Chemother. Rep. 17, 145, 1962.

29. Remillard, S. et al Science (in press).

30. Gitterman et al. J. Antibiotics (Tokyo) 23, 305, 1970.

31. Mead, J.A.R. In Pharmacological Basis of Cancer Chemotherapy, p. 197, Williams and Wilkins Co., Baltimore, 1975.

32. Misra, D.K. et al. Nature 189, 39, 1961.

33. Mead, J.A.R. et al. Cancer Research 26, 2374, 1966.

34. Mishra, L.C. & Mead, J.A.R. Biochem. Pharmacol. 21, 579, 1972.

35. Knott, R. & Taunton-Rigby, A. Abs. 162nd National Meeting, ACS, Washington, D.C., Medicinal Chemistry, No. 27, 1971.

36. Institoris, L. et al. Neoplasma 17, 15, 1970.

37. Elson, L.A. et al. Europ. J. Cancer 4, 617, 1968.

38. Nemeth, L. et al. Cancer Chemother Reports 56, 593, 1972.

39. Kellner, B. et al. In Advances in Antimicrobial and Antineoplastic Chemotherapy, Vol II, p. 39, University Park Press, Baltimore, 1972.

40. Horvath, I.P. et al. Ibid, p. 27.

41. Gati, E. et al. Ibid, p. 33

42. Institoris, E. et al. Ibid, p. 31.

43. Otvos, L. et al.Magy Kem Foly 77, 646, 1971 (abstracted in Chem. Abs. 76. 109327g, 1972).

44. Creighton, A.M. et al. Nature 222, 384, 1969.

45. Woodman, R.J. et al. Cancer Chemother. Rep. (in press)

46. Hellmann, K. et al. Brit. Med. J. I, 822, 1969.

47. Hellmann, K. et al. In Advances in the Treatment of Acute (Blastic) Leukemias, p. 52, Springer-Verlag New York, 1970.

48. Bellet, R.E. et al. Cancer Chemother Rep. 57, 185, 1973.

49. Gralla, E.J. et al. Cancer Chemother Rep. Part 3, 5 1, 1974.

PLATINUM COMPLEXES AS ANTI-CANCER DRUGS

M.J. Cleare

Johnson Matthey and Co. Ltd.

Research Laboratories, Wembley, Middlesex, U.K.

In 1969 Rosenberg and Van Camp announced the discovery of potent antitumour activity in four platinum coordination compounds (1). Perhaps not surprisingly, prior to this very few of the hundreds of thousands of compounds screened for antitumour activity were metal-based or even inorganic in nature. The major involvement of metals had concerned their relative concentrations in cancerous and noncancerous tissues. The platinum discovery came about somewhat serendipitously whilst the investigators were studying the effects of an electric field on the growth processes in bacteria (2). Extensive experimentation showed that the resulting filamentation effect (continued growth without cell division) was due to a platinum compound, <u>cis</u>-($Pt(NH_3)_2Cl_4$), which was formed by reaction of the Pt electrodes with the nutrient medium under the influence of the electric current. Testing of synthesised compounds showed that only the <u>cis</u> geometric isomer was active and this condition remained true when these compounds and their Pt(II) analogues were tested against transplanted tumours in mice; initially S 180 in ICR mice and confirmed by the NCI for L 1210 in DBA mice (1). Since then the study of Pt and other heavy metal complexes in this context has greatly increased, particularly as coordination chemists saw a useful application of their talents. The work can be very roughly divided into the following four areas and in the brief time available, a short summary of progress in each has been attempted.

(1) Synthesis of Pt complexes to determine structure-activity relationships.

(2) Animal and clinical testing of the initially most active compound, cis($Pt(NH_3)_2Cl_2$).

(3) Research into the mechanism of action.

(4) Testing of other metal complexes-new areas of interest

1. Synthesis of Pt complexes to determine structure-activity relationships.

A wide variety of Pt complexes has been tested and at present only complexes of the type cis-($Pt(II)A_2X_2$) (where A_2 = one bidentate or two monodentate amine ligands and X_2= one bidentate or two monodentate anionic ligands) show activity with exception of the uncharacterised Pt blues (see below)(3). Few firm guidelines are available for compounds of this type to be active but in general:

a) The complex should be neutral. Charged complexes which satisfy the other criteria do not show appreciable activity. This may be a membrance transfer effect as Pt (II) substitution rates are generally independent of charge.

b) They should contain a pair of cis leaving groups (X) usually of intermediate lability (e.g. Cl, Br) although some bidentate O-donor ligands (carboxylates) are also effective. Strongly bound groups (e.g. NO_2-,SCN-) give compounds which pass through unchanged, while those with readily replaced legands (e.g. H_2O, NO_3-) are highly toxic. In vivo biochemical activation of the chelated carboxylates (e.g. malonate) has been postulated (3).

c) The other ligands (A) play an important part; there appears to be a great preference for inert amine systems. The nature of the A ligand has a secondary effect on the reaction kinetics (barring extreme steric hindrance) but has an important bearing on the anti-tumour property (3,4) Tables 1 and 2 show two series of results (amoung many) against the particularly Pt sensitivie ADJ/PC6A tumour (4,5).

d) Although all the antitumour compounds also show bacterial activity (filamentation), the reverse is not true. It has been claimed that all compounds which induce lysis in lysogenic bacteria are antitumour active (6).

2. Animal and clinical testing of the initially most active compound, cis ($Pt(NH_3)_2Cl_2$).

Cis-($Pt(NH_3)_2Cl_2$) (cis Pt II) has been tested against a large number of experimental tumours and has a wide spectrum of activity. Although most tests were on transplanted systems, activity has also been shown against virally and chemically induced tumours (7). This led to a full toxicological study by the NCI in animals up to dogs and monkeys, followed by clinical trials in man (8), which are now well into the Phase II stage. The major toxic effects encountered in man are:

a) Nephrotoxicity - largely tubular damage and this is the dose limiting factor.
b) Myelosuppression (hematologic toxicity) - leukopaenia, thrombocytopenia and occasionally a fall in the haemoglobin count.
c) Ototoxicity - tinnitus and loss in high frequency hearing - not usually noticed but probably irreversible.
d) Gastroenteric toxicity manifested in nausea and difficult to control vomiting plus anorexia. (dose dependent above 37.5 mg/m^2).

The compound has been given at single doses up to 100 mg/m^2 but doses at 15-25 mg/m^2 for several days every month are preferred. This greatly reduces renal toxicity.

The drug has shown some effect on a variety of tumours but the most susceptible major group at present appears to be genitourinary particularly testicular and ovarian tumours. Combination therapy is beginning to show promise in several different systems.

3. Mechanism of Action

This area of study is large and very difficult to summarise especially as itis rife with speculation. Tissue culture studies have shown selective and persistent inhibition of DNA synthesis in comparison to that of RNA and proteins, using cis Pt (II) at 5 μM or less, which is approximately equivalent to that found in tumour tissue (9,10). The level of inhibition is dose dependent and reaches a nadir some 4-6 hours after removal of the drug; there is not a high cell kill at these levels. Active Pt complexes show similar effects while inactive complexes show nothing comparable at these concentrations (9). Chemical Pt complexes are known to interact quite strongly at the N7 of guanine and adenine. The activity of the cis and not the trans isomers suggests a chelation interation (3). A certain parrellism exists between Pt drugs and alkylating agents, (Table 3) which are known to react at the N7 of guanine, but this is not complete as synergism has been indicated in combination therapy and Pt can affect alkylating agent resistant tumours (11). Crosslinking has been demonstrated for Pt drugs (12) but geometric considerations rule out N7 guanine bridging as the Cl's

TABLE 1

ADJ/PC6 Plasma Cell Tumour[4] A	Solvent	Dose Range mg/kg	Dose Response	LD_{50}	ID_{90}	T.I.
NH_3	A	0.1–40	+	13.0	1.6	8.1
CH_3NH_2	A		−	18.5	18.5	1.0
$ClC_2H_4NH_2$	A		+	45.0	17.5	2.6
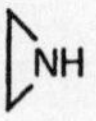 NH	A	2.5–160	+	56.5	2.6	21.7
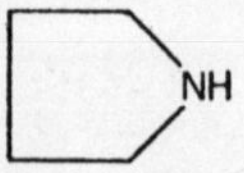 NH	A	3–200	+	141	10.8	13.1
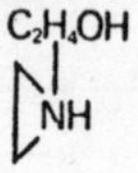 C_2H_4OH NH	A		−	90	>90	< 1.0
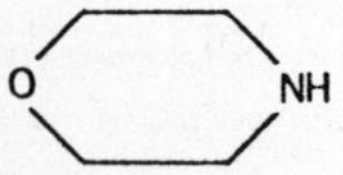 O NH	A		−	18	>18	<1.0
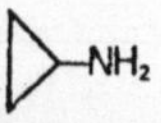 $-NH_2$	A	1–80	+	56.5	2.3	24.6
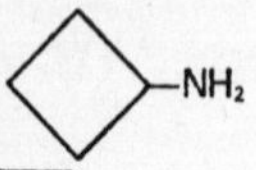 $-NH_2$	A	6–750	+	67	<6	>11.1
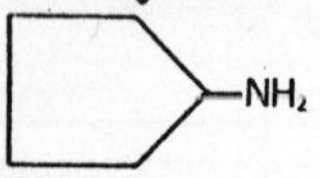 $-NH_2$	A	1–3200	+	480	2.4	200
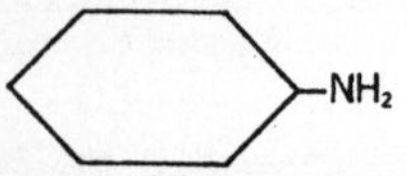 $-NH_2$	A	1–3200	+	>3200	12	>267
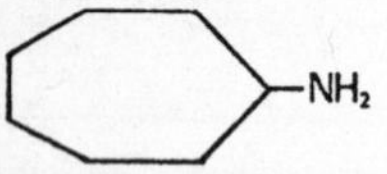 $-NH_2$	A	5–625	+	>625	18	>35

are only 3.3-3.4 Å apart. There issome evidence that the amount of crosslinking is insufficient to account for the total cytotoxic effect and as suggested by Harder, intra-strand links may be important (13). There is evidence that these are the major toxic cytotoxic lesion for bacteriophage (14). Studies on DNA in vivo to determine the Pt binding sites (as for alkylating agents) are highly desirable. It is most unlikely that all actions of heavy metal drugs will be at the DNA level, they will also react with RNA and particularly proteins.

TABLE 2

BRANCHED CHAIN ALKYLAMINE COMPLEXES

COMPLEX (<u>cis</u> - [PtA_2Cl_2]) A =	ACTIVITY	ID_{90}	LD_{50}	T.I.
		<............ mg/kg)		
(C)(C)C - NH_2 (isopropyl-)	+	0.90	33.5	37.1
(C)(C)C - C - NH_2 (isobutyl-)	+	6.2	83	13.4
(C)(C)C - C - C - NH_2 (isoamyl -)	+	5.8	1150	198
C - C - C - C - C(C)(NH_2) (2-aminohexane -)	+	27.5	730	26.5

TABLE 3

PARALLELISMS OF ALKYLATING AGENTS AND Cis-Pt(II)$(NH_3)_2Cl_2$

1. Two chloride leaving groups
2. Grian cell formation
3. Persistent Inhibition of cell division
4. Selective inhibition of DNA synthesis
5. Filamentation in bacteria
6. Induction in lysogenic bacteria
7. Enhanced DNASE and DNA polymerase activities in treated cells
8. Cross links double stranded DNA

TABLE 4

SOME REPRESENTATIVE TESTING RESULTS FOR PLATINUM BLUES - S 180 ASCITES[b]

COMPOUND	SOLVENT	DOSE RANGE	TOXIC LEVEL	BEST % ILS	DOSE	CURES[+] (out of 6)
Cis-$[Pt(NH_3)_2Cl_2]$	S	7	10	49	7	1
CLASS I (ammine-pyrimidine/amide) BLUE						
URACIL	W	50–400	400	91	200	5
THYMINE	W	150–600	450	72	300	2
5,6-DIHYDROURACIL	W	20–800	400	92	200	4
6-METHYLURACIL	S	200–800	> 800	87	600	3
5,6-DIMETHYL URACIL	W	50–400	> 400	100	400	5
1-METHYLTHYMINE	S	50–400	200	94	100	3
ACETAMIDE	S	25–200	25	-94	25	0
BENZAMIDE	S[+]	50–400	400	23	400	0

[+] Slurry   [+] SWISS MICE

W = Water   S = Saline

[b] Rosenberg et al, Cancer Chemo. Reps. Part 1, 59, 287 (1975).

CONCLUSION

4. New areas of interest centre round:
   (a) The search for more water soluble Pt drugs
   (b) Investigations on other heavy metal systems.

(a) One of the drawbacks of many of the active compounds discovered since cis PtII is their extremely low aqueous solubility. Indeed cis PtII in saline is only usable at 1 mg/ml. The most interesting development here concerns the Pt blues which are formed from the reaction of cis($Pt(NH_3)_2(H_2O)_2)^{2+}$ with pyrimidines and substituted pyrimidines (15). The structure of these compounds is not yet understood but there is a general agreeement that they are polymeric cationic species with platinum in a mixed or more likely non-integral oxidation state (16,17). They are highly water soluble and show activity comparable or better than cis Pt(II)against several test tumours (Table 4). Surprisingly enough, they are not very active against the Pt-sensitive ADJ/PC6 tumours. Microscopic histopathologic studies show much less kidney damage than with cis Pt (II) (15). They are undergoing intensive study with with respect to toxicology and structural analysis. They are also excellent electron microscopy stains as they have a high affinity for nucleic acids. Indeed there is some evidence that they can identify tumourigenic cells (18). Another development involves the use of Pt(IV) analogues of active species. Pt(IV) compounds are believed, but not proven, to undergo reduction to Pt(II) in vivo. The use of trans-dihydroxo Pt (IV) derivatives increases the aqueous solubility but presumably leads to the PtII drug in vivo. The best example at present is cis(Pt (isopropylamine)$_2Cl_2$) which is very active against the L1210 (NCI) but has a low solubility. (Pt(IV)(isoprop)$_2Cl_2(OH)_2$) is soluble to the extent of 18 mg/ml and more active than cis Pt(II) against the ADJ/PC6A. It is about to be tested against the L1210.

(b) The obvious analogue Pd(II) shows no activity even when exactly analogous complexes to active Pt(II) ones are used (3). However, when the Pt(II) criteria were applied to Rh(III) the corresponding complex ($Rh(NH_3)_3Cl_3$) was found to be active against several systems (19) although to a considerably lesser extent than Cis Pt (II), except in the case of the Walker 256 carcinosarcoma.

Rh acetate has been used in combination with arabinosylcytosine and it is thought to act by inhibiting the deamination of this fraudulent nucleoside (20).

REFERENCES

1. B. Rosenberg, L. Van Camp, J.E. Trosko and V.H. Mansour. Nature (London), 222, (1969) 385.

2. B. Rosenberg, L. Van Camp and T. Krigas, Nature (London), 205, (1965), 698.

3. M.J. Cleare and J.D. Hoeschele, Bioinorg, Chem., 2 (1973), 187.

4. T.A. Connors, M. Jones, W.C.J. Ross, P.D. Braddock, A.R. Khokhar and M.L. Tobe. Chem.-Biol. Interactions, 5 (1972) 415.

5. T.A. Connors, M. Jones, P.D. Braddock, A.R. Khokhar and M.L. Tobe. Chem.-Biol. Interactions, in press.

6. S. Reslova. Chem.-Biol. Interactions, 4(1971, 66.

7. B. Rosenberg, Naturwissenschaften, 60(1973) 399.

8. U. Schaeppi, I.A. Heyman, R.W. Fleischman, H. Rosenkrautz, V. Ilievski, R. Phelan, D.A. Cooney and R.D. Davis. Toxicol and App. Pharmacol. 25 (1973) 230.

9. H.C. Harder and B. Rosenberg. Int. J. Cancer, 6 (1970) 207.

10. J.A. Howle and G.R. Gale, Biochem. Pharmacol., 19 (1970) 2757.

11. E. Wiltshaw and T. Kroner, in press.

12. J.J. Roberts and J.M. Pascoe. Nature (London) 235 (1972) 282.

13. H.C. Jarder, Ph.D. Thesis, Michigan State University 1970.

14. E.V. Shooter, R. Howse, R.K. Merrifield and A.B. Robins. Chem.-Biol. Interactions, 5 (1972) 289.

15. J.P. Davidson, P.J. Faber, R.G. Fischer jr., S. Mansy, H.J. Reresie, B. Rosenberg and L. Van Camp. Cancer Chemotherapy Reports, 59 (1975) 287.

16. D.R. Hepburn and M.J. Cleare, unpublished results.

17. B. Rosenberg, personal communication.

18. S.K. Aggarwal, R.W. Wagner, P.K. McAllister and B. Rosenberg. Proc. Nat. Acad. Sci 72 (1975) 928.

19. M.J. Cleare, J.D. Hoeschele, T.A. Connors, B. Rosenberg and L. Van Camp, Recent Results in Cancer Reserach 48 (1974) 12.

20. S.H. Lee, D.L. Cjao, J.L. Bear and A.P. Kimball. Cancer Chemotherapy Reports 59 (1975) 661.

STREOPTOZOTOCIN, CHLOROZOTOCIN AND RELATED NITROSOUREA ANTITUMOUR AGENTS

Phillip S. Schein, Tom Anderson, Mary G. McMenamin and Joan Bull
Division of Medical Oncology, Georgetown University School of Medicine, Washington, D.C., USA 20007
and Medicine Branch, National Cancer Institute, Bethesda, Maryland, U.S.A. 20014

In 1959, 1-methyl-1-nitroso-3-nitroguanidine (MNNG) was found to increase the life span of mice bearing leukaemia L1210 (1). While MNNG did not have sufficient activity to warrant extensive clinical testing, the demonstration of antitumour effect gave impetus for further evaluation of the N-nitroso class of compounds as potential antineoplastic agents. In 1961 1-methyl-1-nitrosourea (MNU) was reported to be not only more effective against intraperitoneally implanted L1210 than MNNG, but also was capable of penetrating the blood-brain barrier; MNU produced limited but reproducible antitumour activity in mice with intracerebral leukaemic cells (1). Since that time over 300 alkylnitrosourea compounds have been screened for antitumour activity, the majority of the synthetic work having been undertaken by Montgomery, Johnston and co-workers at the Southern Research Institute (3).

Major emphasis has been placed on halogenated ethyl derivatives after BCNU (1,3-bis(2-chloroethyl)-1-nitrosourea) was shown to have curative antitumour activity in mice implanted either intraperitoneally or intracranially with L1210 (2). The chloroethylnitrosoureas as a group, BCNU, CCNU, and methyl CCNU, have been established as an important class of clinical antitumour agents with activity having now been demonstrated against lymphomas, small cell carcinomas of the lung, malignant melanomas, intracerebral gliomas, and gastrointestinal cancer when combined with 5-fluorouracil (3-5). However, these agents produce profound and delayed bone marrow toxicity which can significantly limit the ability of patients to receive other forms of myelosuppresive therapy during the prolonged period of white blood cell and platelet depression. In addition, with repeated courses of treatment, the chloroethly nitrosoureas can produce cumulative bone marrow injury resulting in a chronic state of myelosuppression (4-5).

Concurrent with this work on chloroethyl derivatives there have been extensive laboratory and clinical investigations of the naturally occurring methlynitrosourea streptozotocin, a fermentation product of Streptomyces acromogenes. While streptozotocin has not proved as clinically useful as the chloroethly derivatives, this compound has been demonstrated to have activity against islet cell carcinomas, malignant carcinoid tumours, soft tissue sarcomas and advanced stages of Hodgkin's disease (6). Equally important has been the pharmacologic information derived from the studies of streptozotocin which may have a significant impact upon future developments for the alkylnitrosourea class of compounds as a group.

Chemically, streptozotocin is composed of 1-methyl-1-nitrosourea attached to a glucosamine carrier (7). The compound has been demonstrated to produce two unique pharmacologic actions in experimental systems. The first is the ability to selectively destroy the pancreatic beta cell of the islet of Langerhans in animals, which results in a permanent diabetic state. Studies of the biochemical basis of this diabetogenic activity have demonstrated it to be mediated through a rapid reduction in pyridine nucleotide concentrations, an observation initially demonstrated in liver and subsequently confirmed in isolated pancreatic islets (8-10). Of interest was the finding that pharmacologic doses of nicotinamide was quite specific for this effect. We believe that streptozotocin's activity against human malignant insulinoma is mediated through the mechanism of NAD depression. We subsequently demonstrated that all compounds which possessed an N-nitroso methyl or ethyl end group could depress liver NAD concentrations, the methyl compounds being ten-fold more active based upon molar dose (11). This has been confirmed in our recent studies of an ethyl derivative of streptozotocin. DENU is diabetogenic, but a ten-fold increase in molar dose is required for biologic activity comparable to that of the methylnitrosourea streptozotocin (12). Placement of a halide on the alkyl end group of all compounds tested completely removed the ability to depress liver and islet NAD concentrations and thus the potential for diabetes (11). Thus, the chlorethyl nitrosoureas, BCNU, CCNU, and the newly synthesized glucose containing compound chlorozotocin do not depress liver NAD and are not diabetogenic.

We had originally considered MNU to be non-diabetogenic since no increase in blood glucose was observed at doses that produced lethal bone marrow toxicity in mice. However, at supra-lethal doses diabetes could be produced as documented by disruption of beta cell morphology and measurements of plasma glucose; a four-fold increase in molar dose compared to streptozotocin was required for production of comparable degrees of diabetes and depression of islet NAD (13). This has subsequently been correlated with the relative uptake of the two compounds into the pancreatic islets. Whereas the exocrine portion of the gland preferentially took up MNU (ratio of 2:1 compared with streptozotocin), the islets preferentially took up streptozotocin compared to MNU, 4:1. Based upon these observations we feel that the glucose carrier on the streptozotocin molecule facilitates transport of the active cytotoxic group, MNU, into the islet and thus allows for the selective destruction of the beta cell.

The second unique pharmacologic property of streptozotocin is the compound's relative lack of myelosuppressive activity, in contrast to the cytotoxic group, MNU, which is significantly bone marrow toxic in animals (11). We have been able to use streptozotocin effectively in patients with severely depressed bone marrow function and have observed a complete return of white blood cell counts to normal in the face of continued treatment with this agent (6). It appears that nitrosourea myelosuppression is reduced by the attachment of the cytotoxic group to the carbon-2 position of glucose.

To further evaluate the influence of the glucose carrier on chloroethyl nitrosourea bone marrow toxicity, two new compounds, 2-(3-(2-chloroethyl)-3-nitrosoureido)-2-deoxy-D-glucopyranose, chlorozotocin, and the tetra-acetate form of the same agent were synthesized for our studies by Dr. John Montgomery and co-workers. The biological and chemical properties of these two compounds were compared to those of BCNU and CCNU (14,15).

To evaluate the relative bone marrow toxicity, groups of ten normal BDF_1 mice received single intraperitoneal doses of chlorozotocin, ranging from 10-50 mg/kg. Serial peripheral white blood cell (WBC) counts were performed over a 30-day period of observation. The results were compared with WBC counts from mice that had received single intraperitoneal doses of BCNU, 20 or 30 mg/kg (15). The nadir of WBC depression occurred three days after administration for both drugs.

Chlorozotocin, administered at a maximum nonlethal dose, 15 mg/kg, produced an 18% reduction in mean WBC count. This degree of WBC depression was not significantly different from the control. A 10% lethal dose, 20 mg/kg, produced a 28% decrease in WBC count with no specific alteration in neutrophil lymphocyte ratio. Administration of a 100% lethal dose, 50 mg/kg, decreased the WBC count by 76%, with a preferential reduction in circulating lymphocytes. Histological examination of the bone marrows of these animals demonstrated only a moderate reduction in the granulocytic series, whereas there was a major decrease in size of splenic lymphoid follicles. With the 50 mg/kg dose all animals died between the fourth and sixth day following injection.

BCNU, administered at a maximum non-lethal dose of 20 mg/kg, produced a 40% reduction in WBC count, which was significantly different from control ($P < 0.05$). In contrast to chlorozotocin, WBC differential counts demonstrated a preferential reduction in circulating neutrophils. A 20% lethal dose of BCNU, 30 mg/kg, caused a reduction in WBC count comparable to a 100% lethal dose of chlorozotocin. The bone marrows of mice sacrificed at day 3 post-injection demonstrated a generalized hypoplastic state, whereas the splenic lymph follicles were only moderately reduced in size compared to controls. Animals died between 21 and 30 days after treatment at this dose of BCNU, in contrast to the actue mortality observed with chlorozotocin at lethal dose levels. This relative bone marrow sparing property of chlorozotocin has been confirmed by Dr. Leon Schmitt and co-workers at the Southern Research Institute.

Relative antitumour activity was evaluated in mice implanted intraperitoneally with 10^5 L1210 leukaemic cells. The animals received graded single intraperitoneal doses of chlorozotocin or BCNU after two or six days of tumour growth. The maximally effective dose of chlorozotocin against day two tumour was 15 mg/kg i.p., which produced a 70% increase in life-span compared to untreated controls; 60% of the mice survived for 90 days. This dose level was not myelosuppressive in normal mice. The maximally effective dose for BCNU against the day 2 tumour was 30 mg/kg. This dose resulted in a 632% increase in life-span compared to untreated controls, with seven of nine animals alive after 90 days of observation. This dose of BCNU in normal mice had produced a 72% reduction in normal circulating white blood cells.

In animals treated on day six of tumour growth chlorozotocin, 20 mg/kg, resulted in a 401% increase in life-span, with 30% of the animals surviving for 90 days. With BCNU, mice demonstrated a 493% maximum increase in life-span, with 50% of animals surviving for 90 days. Thus the antitumour activities of chlorozotocin and BCNU in the L1210 leukaemic system are almost identical, both agents demonstrating curative activity in both the early and late stages of tumour growth.

As a correlate of the relative bone marrow toxicity and antitumour activity of chlorozotocin and BCNU, measurements of DNA synthesis were carried out using mice with four days of L1210 tumour growth (15). Chlorozotocin, 15 mg/kg, or BCNU, 30 mg/kg, were administered intraperitoneally and one hour prior to sacrifice the mice were given 100 μCi of ^{3}H-thymidine intraperitoneally. The ascites tumour cells were aspirated from the peritoneal cavity and the normal bone marrow expressed with phosphate buffered saline. DNA was extracted and counted for radioactivity, results being expressed as dpm/μg DNA.

Chlorozotocin, 15 mg/kg, produced a 96% inhibition of L1210 DNA synthesis within 24 hours of administration, as measured by ^{3}H-thymidine incorporation into DNA. BCNU, 30 mg/kg, resulted in an 85% inhibition at the same time period. Both drugs produced a 94% inhibition in DNA synthesis by 48 hour post-treatment.

Chlorozotocin did not significantly reduce DNA synthesis of bone marrow. BCNU, however, did reduce the incorporation of thymidine into DNA to 37% of control by 24 hour post-treatment. This degree of inhibition was significant ($P < 0.01$). With both drugs, a rebound in DNA synthesis above the control level was observed by 48 hours after administration.

We have now extended this observation to normal human bone marrow, comparing the _in vitro_ effect of chlorozotocin and BCNU on DNA synthesis to determine whether the differential effect noted in animals would be reproduced in a human system (11). Four millilitres of bone marrow were obtained from iliac crest aspirates of normal volunteers, incubated with graded concentrations of the two drugs and then pulsed with ^{3}H-thymidine. The time relationship of DNA synthesized at 2, 8 and 24 hours after expsoure to a 10^{-3}M and 10^{-4}M concentration of chlorozotocin and BCNU, 10^{-3}M, produced a 94% reduction in synthesis by 24 hours. In contrast, chlorozotocin at a comparable concentration produced only a 30% maximum reduction in uptake of ^{3}H-thymidine into bone marrow DNA.

Attempts are now being made to better understand the biochemical mechanisms which allow for the differences between chlorozotocin and the remaining chlorethyl nitrosoureas. The aqueous decomposition of BCNU and CCNU have been studied. In addition to the formation of an isocyanate, there is also decomposition to alkylating chloroethyl carbonium intermediates (16,17). Wheeler has subjected 17 haloethyl nitrosoureas to a computer analysis to estimate the relative role of carbamoylating and alkylating activities by the isocyante group in determining the toxicity and the antitumour activity against L1210 leukaemia in mice. Alkylating activity was found to correlate closely with the relative antitumour activity, whereas carbamoylating activity was suggested as the principal contributing mechanism for lethal toxicity (18).

We have attempted to correlate the differences of chlorozotocin and BCNU on bone marrow DNA synthesis with their relative alkylating and carbamoylating activities. Measurement of alkylating activity with 4-(para-nitrobenzyl) pyridine was performed by the method proposed by Wheeler using a temperature of 37°C at pH 6.0 (18). Nitrogen mustard at a comparable concentration was used as a standard for comparison. Chlorozotocin and BCNU demonstrated equal alkylating activity. Under the conditions of 100°C incubation BCNU produced 5 times more alkylating activity, probably due to the release of chloroethylamine from the second mustard arm of this compound. We consider the method of Wheeler more valid because of the more physiologic nature of the conditions of the incubation. This correlates with the findings in L1210 leukaemia where the therapeutic results obtained with chlorozotocin and BCNU are comparable.

Carbamoylating activity was estimated by incubation of the test nitrosourea with ^{14}C-lysine. Separation of parent lysine from the carbamoylated product was accomplished by paper electrophoresis. With chlorozotocin only 1% of total lysine counts were present as carbamoylated product in contrast to 82% for BCNU. Thus, these studies support Wheeler's theory that carbamoylating activity correlates closely with toxicity, as estimated by degree of inhibition of bone marrow DNA synthesis and myelosuppression. The mechanism for the reduced carbamoylating activity of chlorozotocin is not as yet established. Structural modeling suggests that it can result from an internal detoxification by combination of the isocyanate with the carbon-4 hydroxyl of the glucose ring. Studies to identify the resulting two-ring structure are now in progress.

In summary, structure-activity studies of nitrosourea pharmacology have resulted in the synthesis of a new water-soluble agent, chlorozotocin, which has significant antitumour activity against the L1210 leukaemia system, and produces only a minor degree of inhibition of mouse and human bone marrow DNA synthesis compared to BCNU. It is important to emphasize that the bone marrow sparing feature of chlorozotocin is relative and that when the drug is administered at lethal dose levels in mice, myelosuppression is observed.

The potential importance of these studies is the identification of a new, active nitrosourea antitumour agent with modified bone marrow toxicity. If glucose modification of nitrosourea bone marrow toxicity can be confirmed in man without significant loss of antitumour activity the use of such a compound could facilitate treatment of patients with neoplastic disease who have pre-existing abnormal bone marrow function or could allow for the more effective use of a nitrosourea agent in combination with anticancer agents possessing more potent myelosuppressive properties.

REFERENCES

1. Skipper, H.E., Schabel, F.M.,Jr., Trader, M.W. et al. (1961). Experimental evaluation of potential anticancer agent. VI. Anatomical distribution of leukaemic cells and failure of chemotherapy. Cancer Res., 21, 1154-1164.
2. Skipper, H.E., Schabel, F.M., Jr., and Wilcox, W.S. (1964). Experimental evaluation of potential anticancer agents. XII. On the criteria and kinetics associated with "curability" of

experimental leukemia. Canc. Chemotherapy Rep., 35, 1-111.
3. Carter, S.K. (1973). An overview of the status of the nitrosoureas in other tumors. Cancer Chemotherapy Rep., 4, 35-46.
4. Walker, M.D. (1973). Nitrosoureas in central nervous system tumors. Cancer Chemotherapy Rep., 4, 21-26.
5. Moertel, C.G. (1973). Therapy of advanced gastrointestinal cancer with the nitrosoureas. C ncer Chemotherapy Rep., 4, 27-34.
6. Schein, P.S., O'Connell, M.J., Blom, J. et al. (1974). Clinical antitumor activity and toxicity of streptozotocin (NSC 85998). Cancer, 34, 993-1000.
7. Herr, R.R., Jahnke, H.K. and Argoudelis, A.D. (1967). The structure of streptozotocin. J. Am. Chem. Soc., 89, 4808-4809.
8. Schein, P.S., Cooney, D.A. and Vernon, M.L. (1967). The use of nicothamide to midify the toxicity of streptozotocin diabetes without loss of antitumor activity. Cancer Res., 27, 2324-2332.
9. Schein, P.S. and Loftus, S. (1968). Streptozotocin: depression of mouse liver pyridine nucleotides. Cancer Res., 28, 1501-1506.
10. Schein, P.S., Cooney, D.A., McMenamin, M.G. and Anderson, T. (1973). Streptozotocin diabetes: further studies on the mechanisms of depression of nicotinamide adenine dinucleotide concentrations in mouse pancreatic islets and liver. Biochem. Pharmacol, 22, 2625-2631.
11. Schein, P.S. (1969). 1-Methyl-1-nitrosourea and dialkylnitrosamine depression of nicotinamide adenine dinucleotide. Cancer Res., 29, 1226-1232.
12. Anderson, T., McMenamin, M.G. and Schein, P.S. (1975). Diabetogenic activity of deoxy-2-[(ethylnitrosoamino) carbonyl amino]-D-glucopyranose. Biochem. Pharmacol. 24, 746-747.
13. Anderson, T., Schein, P.S., McMenamin, M.G. and Cooney, D.A. (1974). Streptozotocin diabetes: correlation with extent of depression of pancreatic islet nicotenamide adenine dinucleotide. J. Clin. Invest., 54, 672-677.
14. Schein, P.S., McMenamin, M. and Anderson, T. (1973). 3-Tetraacetyl glucopyranose-2-yl)-1-(2-chlorethyl)-1-nitrosourea, an antitumor agent with modified bone marrow toxicity. Cancer Res., 33, 2005-2009.
15. Anderson, T., McMenamin, M.G. and Schein, P.S. (1975). Chlorozotocin, 2-(3-(2-chlorethyl)-3-nitrosoureido)-D-glucopyranose, an antitumor agent with modified bone marrow toxicity. Cancer Res., 35, 761-765.
16. Montgomery, J.A., James, R., McCaleb, G.S. and Johnston, T.P. (1967). The modes of decomposition of 1,3-bis(2-chloroethyl-1-nitrosourea and related compounds. J. Med. Chem. 10,668-674.

17. Cowens, W., Brundratt, R. and Colvin, M. (1975). Mechanism of action of bischloroethyl nitrosourea. Proc. Am. Assoc. Cancer Res., 66, 100.

18. Wheeler, G.P., Bowdon, B.J., Grimsley, J.A. and Lloyd, H.H. (1974). Interrelationships of some chemical, physiochemical, and biological activities of several 1-(2-haloethyl)-1-nitrosoureas. Cancer Res., 34, 194-200.

19. Schein, P.S., Bull, J., McMenamin, M.G. and Macdonald, J.S. (1975). DNA synthesis by human bone after incubation with BCNU or chlorozotocin (DCNU, NSC-178248). Proc. Am. Assoc. Cancer Res., 66, 122.

ANALOGUES AND METABOLITES OF CYCLOPHOSPHAMIDE

K. Norpoth

Institute for Pneumoconiosis Research and Occupational Medicine,

University of Muenster (German Federal Republic)

In 1969 I proposed a mechanism of biological Cyclophosphamide (CYM) activation (18) which is shown by figure 1. This pathway was concluded from circumstantial evidence that 4-carboxy-CYM is the main CYM metabolite and the C-4 atom of the molecule ring is the preferential site of biological oxidation. I assumed that one of the metabolites should account for the tumour specific activity of the drug. This we could rule out concerning 4-carboxy-CYM although this compound has been identified as the main metabolite by Struck and co-workers in addition to 4-keto-CYM, a non toxic minor metabolite (27).

The latter two compounds therefore must be regarded as detoxication products. On the other hand the metabolic pathway of CYM, shown by the diagram became more evident when Hill and co-workers and Struck found an aldehyde as the primary product of CYM biotransformation (13, 28) and Alarcon and Meienhofer could show that acreolein arises from the microsomal oxidation of CYM (1). Now the metabolism of the drug became more intelligible and could be described in a more detailed way as shown by Figure 2. The hope of finding better drugs for cancer chemotherapy by clarifying the metabolism of CYM was then based on the required synthesis of 4-OH-CYM and the so called "Aldophosphamide". In 1973 Takamizawa and co-workers reported the successful synthesis of 4-OH-CYM, a rather unstable compound, and simultaneously they described the synthesis of 4-hydroperoxy-CYM which can be regarded as a stable preactivated derivative of CYM (29). This was a break-through in the field of CYM research because 4-OH-peroxy-CYM and later on also its dimer (30) which has also been found by Benckhuysen and co-workers as a product of CYM oxidation in the Fenton reaction (6)

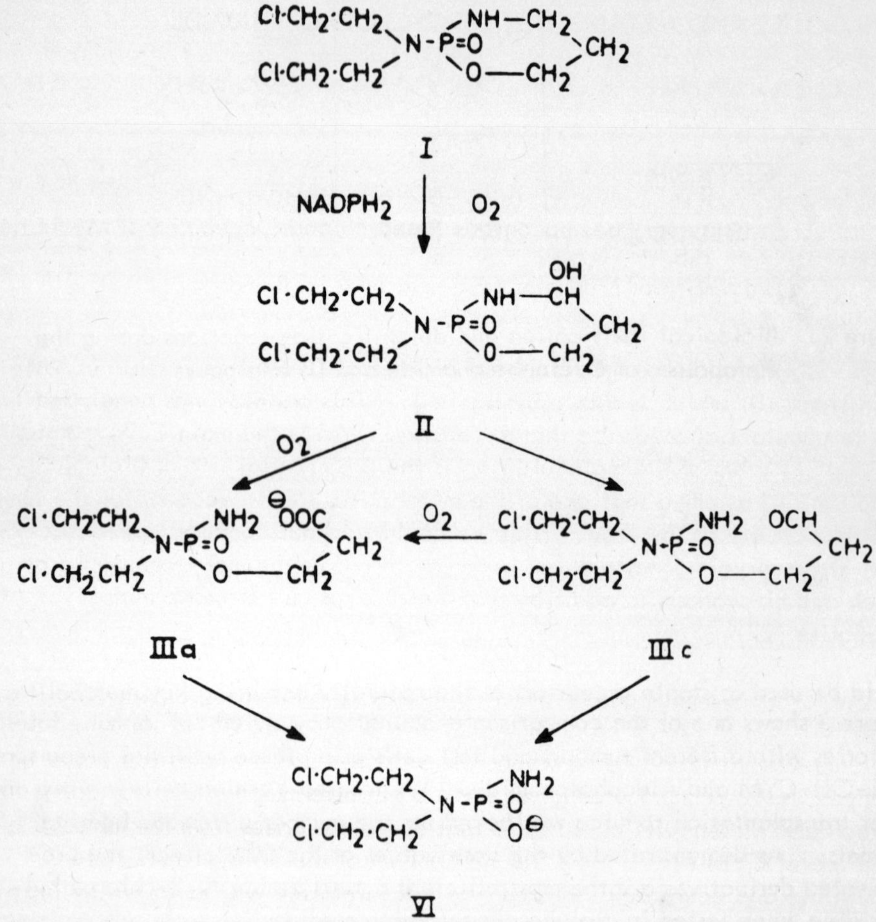

I

$NADPH_2$ O_2

II

O_2

IIIa O_2 IIIc

VI

Figure 1. Metabolic pathway of Cyclophosphamide proposed in 1969 (18).

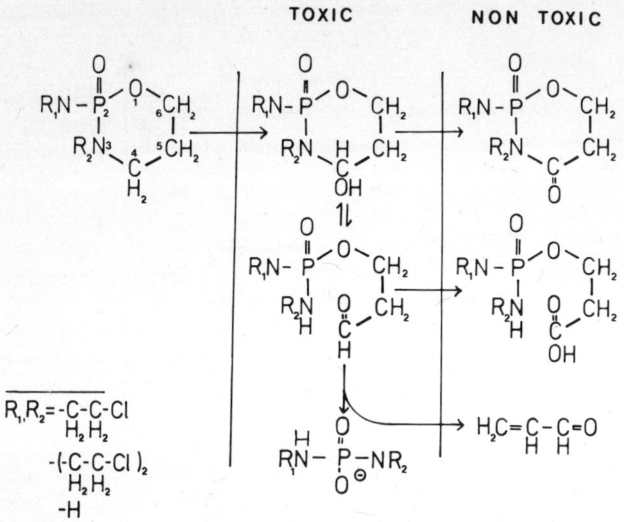

Figure 2. Biological toxification and detoxification reactions during the metabolism of Cyclophosphamide and its analogues

could be used as stable precursors of the naturally occurring key metabolites. Figure 3 shows one of the comparison examinations carried out in many laboratories with different tumours and test cells using these artificial precursors of 4-OH-CYM and Aldophosphamide. We treated Yoshida cells in vitro and after transplantation to mice we looked for the number of tumour-bearing animals. As demonstrated by the dose values of the 50% effect, the preactivated derivatives are the most efficient agents beside N-2-chloroethyl-aziridine when tested in a glucose-containing medium.

The OH-Peroxy-CYM dimer on the other hand did not show increased toxicity in the presence of glucose. We must realise regarding the molar ED_{50} value that this compound contains two molecules of preactivated CYM metabolites. Referred to those metabolites the lowest value we have ever found must therefore be specified as 12 n moles/ml. Acrolein has only been tested up to 180 n moles/ml. It may not be considered as completely inactive. Phosphoramide mustard, tested as free acid, has shown no

	Inhibitor	Variations of the Medium Phos - phatebuffer, pH 7.2)	ED_{50} nmol/ml	Number of Animals
Cl, NH, Cl	Bis-(2-chlo-roethyl)-aminhydro-chloride	——	137	53
Cl, N	N-(2-chlo-roethyl)-aziridine	——	105	50
Cl, N	N-(2-chlo-roethyl)-aziridine	100 mg % Glucose	37	59
Cl, Cl, NH_2, COOH, N-P=O, O	4-Carboxy-cyclophos-phamide	——	> 200	60
Cl, Cl, NH_2, N-P=O, OH	N,N-Bis(2-chloroethyl)-phosphorodi-amidic acid	——	152	32
Cl, Cl, NH, O-OH, N-P=O, O	Hydroper-oxycyclo-phosphamide	——	47	39
[Cl, Cl, NH, O, N-P=O, O]$_2$	Peroxy-cyclophos-phamide	——	6	60
$H_2C = CH-C(=O)H$	Acrolein	——	> 180	70

Figure 3. ED_{50} values of some Cyclophosphamide derivatives as measured with Yoshida ascites cells transplanted to mice after in vitro treatment (23).

significantly higher toxicity compared with Nor-nitrogen-mustard. This is in contrast to the findings of some other authors who used other test tumours but in better accordance with data presented by Brock (7) who used the same tumour. The difference, however, may not only be due to the different test tumours but perhaps also to different properties of the free acid and the cyclohexylammonium salt. Nevertheless it seems to be ascertained that Phosphoramide mustard as the ultimate alkylating agent does not exhibit the same tumour toxic activity as do the precursors and that this compound must be liberated within the cancer cell.

Increasing knowledge of the selectivity of preactivated derivatives of CYM has established a surprising result. Until now nobody has found a selectivity comparable to CYM itself neither with 4-hydroxy-CYM nor with any of its artificial precursors. This may be due to the fact that the pharmakokinetics of preactivated CYMs differ completely depending on whether these compounds are liberated during the course of CYM biotransformation or are administered directly. It must be emphasized in this connection that the design of new preactivated CYMs provides a new approach to the problem of selectivity. Recently it has been shown by Peter and Hohorst that S-alkyl-4-mercapto derivatives of CYM can be regarded as a new class of preactivated oxazaphosphorine mustards (24). Cox and co-workers described some correlations between the cytotoxic effects of ring deuterated CYM's and the spontaneous degradation kinetics of its oxidation products (11). Furthermore the successful synthesis of a preactivated analogue of CYM - the 4-OH-peroxy-Ifosfamide - has been reported by Takamizawa and co-workers (31). I would like to mention that some of the precursors have become useful tools in the field of clinical predictive tests of tumour sensitivities.

Considering the hope to improve the chemotherapeutic effect of CYM by changing the regimens of the treatment with stable preactivated derivatives and by designing new precursors of Aldophosphamide and its analogues I would like to move on to the question of whether a single principle actually may account for the cytotoxic effects of CYM or whether these effects may rather be due to different events during CYM treatment. In this connection I should like to comment on experiments we have carried out in order to clarify whether the cell toxicity of rat urine after CYM treatment can be explained by the action of a single metabolite. For this reason we infused intravenously to narcotised rats 1 ml of a sodium chloride solution containing 10% glucose one hour after i.p. administration of 500 mg/kg CYM. The urine immediately excreted and trapped at 0°C contains large amounts of Nitro-benzyl-pyridine reactive metabolites and shows a high cytotoxic activity. The NBP-activity we found remains unchanged at 37°C for over two hours even in the presence of rat serum (figure 4a) and in phosphate buffer (pH 7.2) alone (figure 4b). In contrast the cytotoxic activity

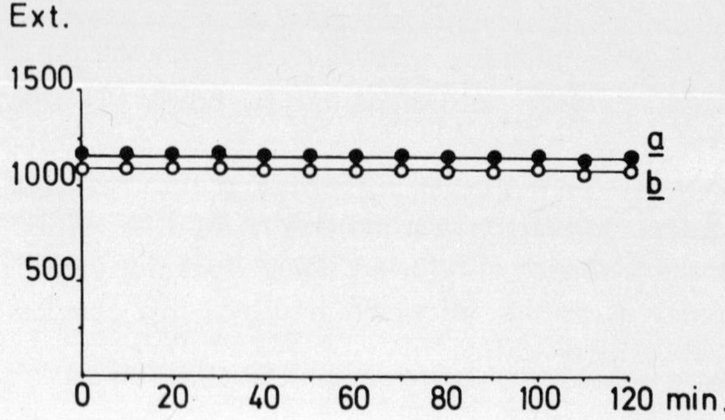

Figure 4. NBP-activity of rat urine obtained after treatment with 500 mg/kg Cyclophosphamide and incubated in 0.1M phosphate buffer pH 7.2 (b) and in rat serum containing phosphate buffer (a) at 37°C.

measured with Yoshida cells decreased very rapidly at 37°C in phosphate buffer solution. This is demonstrated by figure 5. It is well known by findings of Hohorst and co-workers that 4-OH-CYM and Aldophosphamide, respectively, can be detoxicated by thiol group containing compounds (15). Thus the rapid decrease of cytotoxicity may be due to the presence of some mercapto compounds in the urine obtained artificially. Therefore we measured the amounts of acrolein releasing compounds in the rat urine after treatment with CYM and its analogue Ifosfamide. As shown by table 1 we obtained no reasonable results when referring the concentration values to the cytotoxic activities. Looking only to the table on the right hand we must remember that the lowest ED_{50} value we have ever found with preactivated CYM's was 12 n moles/ml. That means that the activity of the urine relative to the concentrations of acrolein releasing metabolites was at least ten times higher than expected. Another point is that we have found a very striking glucose effect of the urine metabolites which has never been found with preactivated CYMs. Thus the cytotoxic activity cannot be explained by the effect of the primary CYM metabolites alone.

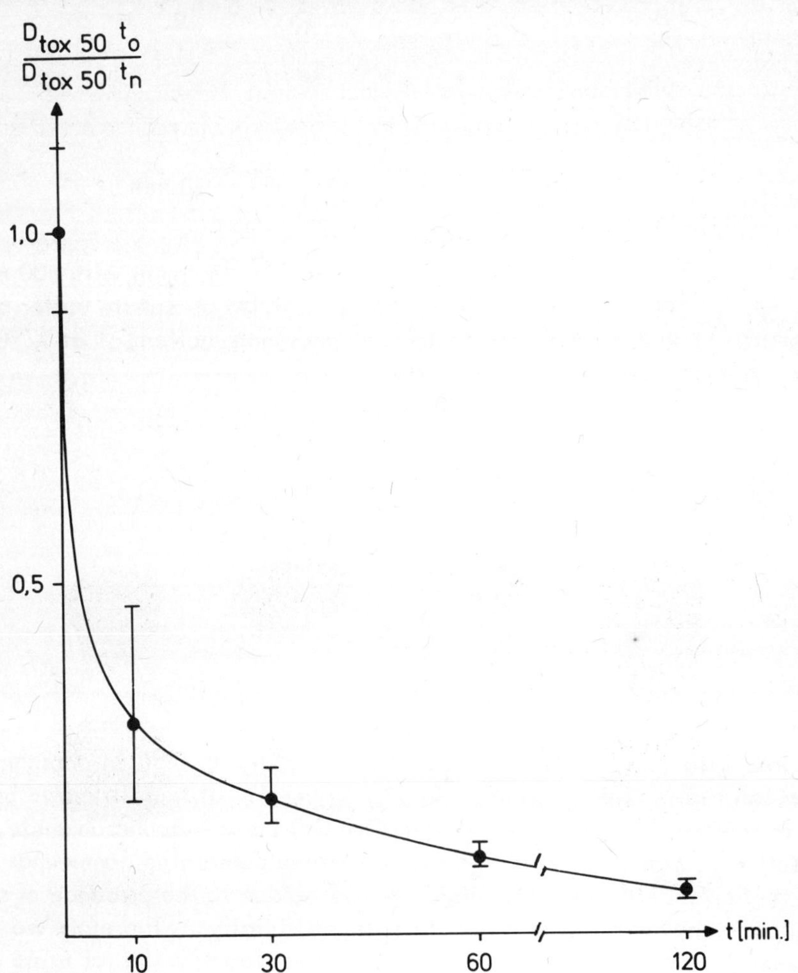

Figure 5. Decrease of the cytotoxic activity of rat urine collected after treatment with 500 mg/kg Cyclophosphamide and tested with Yoshida cells in vitro. Preincubation in phosphate buffer, pH 7.2 at 37°C for 10–20 minutes (Abscissa).

Table 1

INHIBITED TRANSPLANTABILITY OF YOSHIDA-CELLS TO MICE BY URINE METABOLITES OF CYCLOPHOSPHAMIDE AND ISOFOSFAMIDE

	A: ED_{50}-values calculated from NBP-reaction measurements of the total alkylating activity		B: ED_{50}-values calculated from estimations of the total amount of acrolein releasing metabolites	
	Cyclophos-phamide	Ifosfamide	Cyclophos-phamide	Ifosfamide
N	155	40	155	40
$\bar{x}$ [nMol/ml]	15,7	71,4	1,1	8,7
s [nMol/ml]	13,9-17,5	23,6-85,7	0,98-1,2	7,3-10,5

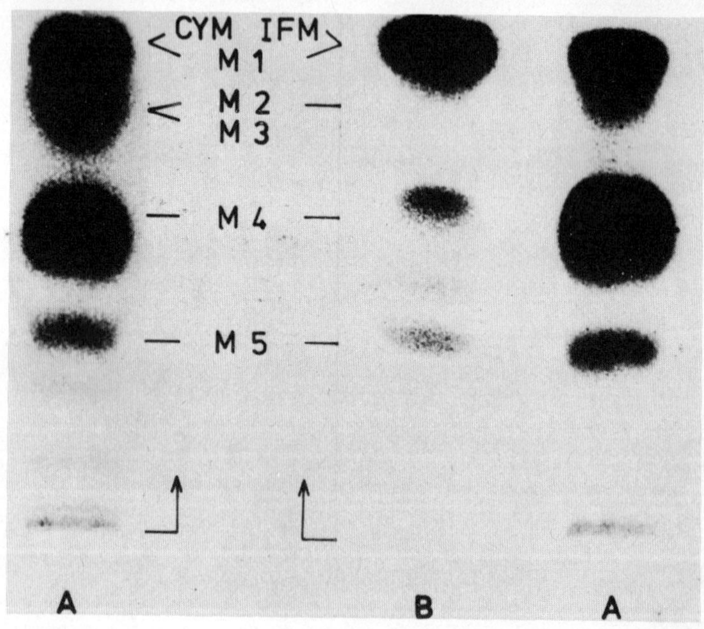

Figure 6. DC-chromatograms of CYclophosphamide and its urine metabolites (A) and Ifosfamide and its metabolites (B) obtained after PBH-Spray (see 19).

The second topic I would like to discuss is the selectivity of Ifosfamide, an analogue of CYM with preferential activity against some solid tumours. As we showed using Walker carcinosarcomas grown in the embryonated egg, the embryotoxic effect of Ifosfamide is significantly lower compared with the effect of CYM whereas both compounds have nearly the same tumourtoxic activity (22). This is in accordance with the findings of Brock, Ardenne and co-workers and Druckrey who found that the therapeutic usefulness of Ifosfamide exceeds that of CYM in the case of certain solid and even CYM resistent test tumours (4,8,12). Concerning the metabolism of Ifosfamide these results are not easy to understand since Hill and co-workers (13) and Alarcon and co-workers (2) could show that the microsomal turnover of Ifosfamide to acrolein releasing metabolites proceeds much more slowly than the turnover of CYM.

Moreover investigations on the urine metabolites of Ifosfamide in man carried out in our laboratory have established the role of another metabolic pathway which we call side chain oxidation (21). Figure 6 shows a TLC-chromatogram of CYM and Ifosfamide and its alkylating urine metabolites

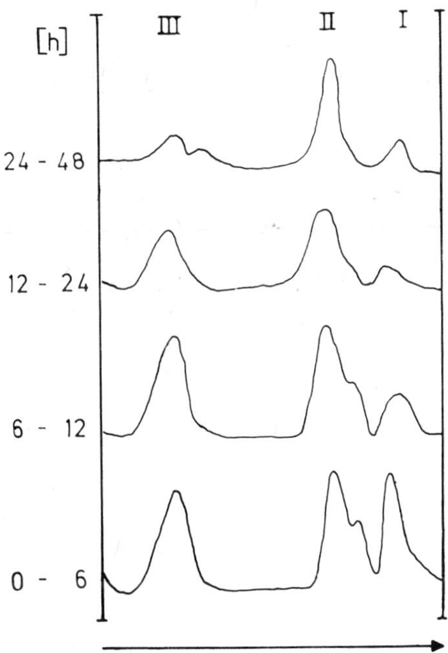

Figure 7. TLC-spectrograms of PBH-reactive urine components found after Ifosfamide treatment (5g). Explanation see text.

Table 2. Mean values (X) and standard derivations (S) of the excreted amounts of Ifosfamide and three metabolites (% of the given dose) calculated from 19 measurements.

URINE EXCRETION				
	n	$\bar{x}$	s	s[%$\bar{x}$]
IFOSFAMIDE	19	17,6	±12,3	±70
4-CARBOXY-IFOSFAMIDE	16	22,3	±12,7	±57
DECHLORO-ETHYL-IFOS-FAMIDE I + II	17	17,6	±11,6	±66
TOTAL	19	52,6	±24,1	±46

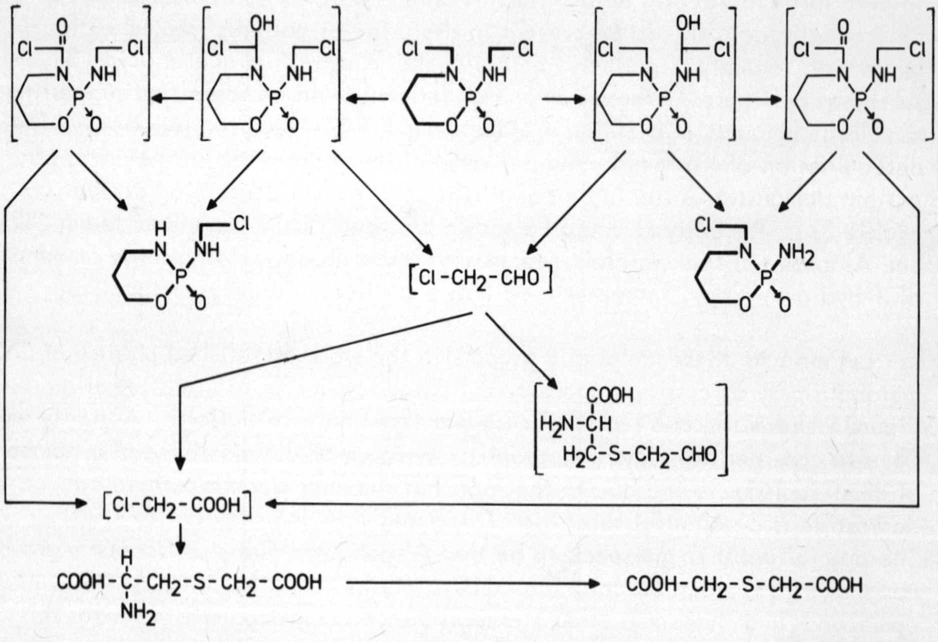

Figure 8. Metabolism of Ifosfamide by side chain oxidation. The compounds in brackets were not isolated.

coloured with pyridinealdehyde - benzothiazolylhydrazone after Sawicki and co-workers (25, 26). The stable spots obtained allow the quantitative spectroscopic determination of PBH-reactive compounds in the urine of patients treated with high doses of Ifosfamide (19,20,21). Figure 7 shows TLC-spectrograms obtained from 0.02 samples of urine collected at different intervals after the beginning of the treatment. In the first position unchanged Ifosfamide appears. In the second position two metabolites follow whose structure we could clarify by elemental analysis and mass spectrometry (21). These derivatives are two different dechloroethylated metabolites of low toxicity arising from side chain oxidation. In the third position 4-carboxy-Ifosfamide appears which is often the main urine metabolite. Table 2 shows the mean values of 19 urine analyses in the cases of 11 patients. The main metabolite was 4-carboxy-Ifosfamide amounting to about 22% of the given dose. Unchanged Ifosfamide as well as the two dechloroethylated derivatives were excreted to about 18% each.

Since we can conclude that side chain oxidation of Ifosfamide is not a minor metabolic pathway as assumed in the case of CYM (5, 9, 10) considerations about the structure of the phosphorous free splitting product became more important. Whitehouse and co-workers assumed that it should be chloroacetaldehyde (32), a toxic alkylating agent which may be rapidly converted in vivo into chloracetic acid. In this case the well known metabolites of chloroacetic acid should be present in the urine of patients treated with Ifosfamide, namely S-carboxy-methyl cysteine and thiodiacetic acid (33,34). As shown by figure 8, these compounds indeed could be identified suggesting that large amounts of cysteine are consumed for detoxication reactions. The determination of Ifosfamide and a number of its metabolites in the urine of a patient demonstrates the large quantities of sulfurous-containing derivatives (Table 3). Recently it could be shown by Kaye (16), Kaye and Joung (17) and Alarcon (3) that acrolein reacts with glutathione yielding large amounts of 3-hydroxy-propylmercapturic acid as a further main urine metabolite.

Let me add these metabolic aspects to the well-established picture of CYM metabolism by discussing a more complicated scheme of biotransformation. Figure 9 shows the two routes of ring and side chain oxidation. Actually we have to consider many more metabolites because of the existence of a number of diastereoisomers and due to the fact that the monodechloroethylated derivative is a potential substrate of ring and side chain oxidation itself. The crucial point to me seems to be that Aldophosphamide, as Hohorst's group has shown (15), can be detoxicated by cysteine and other thiol group containing compounds and that some other metabolites are competing substrates for this spontaneous reaction, at least acrolein, chloroacetic acid and perhaps chloroacetaldehyde. Thus the detoxicating capacity of the cancer cell may be lowered by each agent which can react with protective thiol groups until the cell becomes defenceless against the impact of the crucial alkylating reaction.

Table 3. Urine excretion of Ifosfamide and some of its metabolites in the case of a patient treated with the drug and with the diuretic agent 4-Chlor-N-(2-furfurylmethyl)-5-sulfamoyl-anthranilic acid (Lasix[R])

	IFOSFAMIDE [mMol]	CARBOXY-IFOSFAMIDE [mMol]	DECHLORO-ETHYLIFOSFAMIDE I [mMol]	DECHLORO-ETHYLIFOSFAMIDE II [mMol]	S-CARBOXY-METHYL-CYSTEINE [mMol]	THIODIACETIC ACID [mMol]	ACROLEIN RELEASING METABOLITES [μMol]
6 h	0.106	0.28	0.11	0.62	—	0.02	0.6
12 h	0.019	trace	0.87	0.95	1.5	0.13	1.2
24 h	—	—	0.45	1.31	0.9	0.45	0.9
48 h	—	—	—	—	>0.05	0.30	1.0
72 h	—	—	—	—	trace	0.17	0.8
TOTAL	0.125	0.28	1.43	2.88	2.4	1.07	4.5

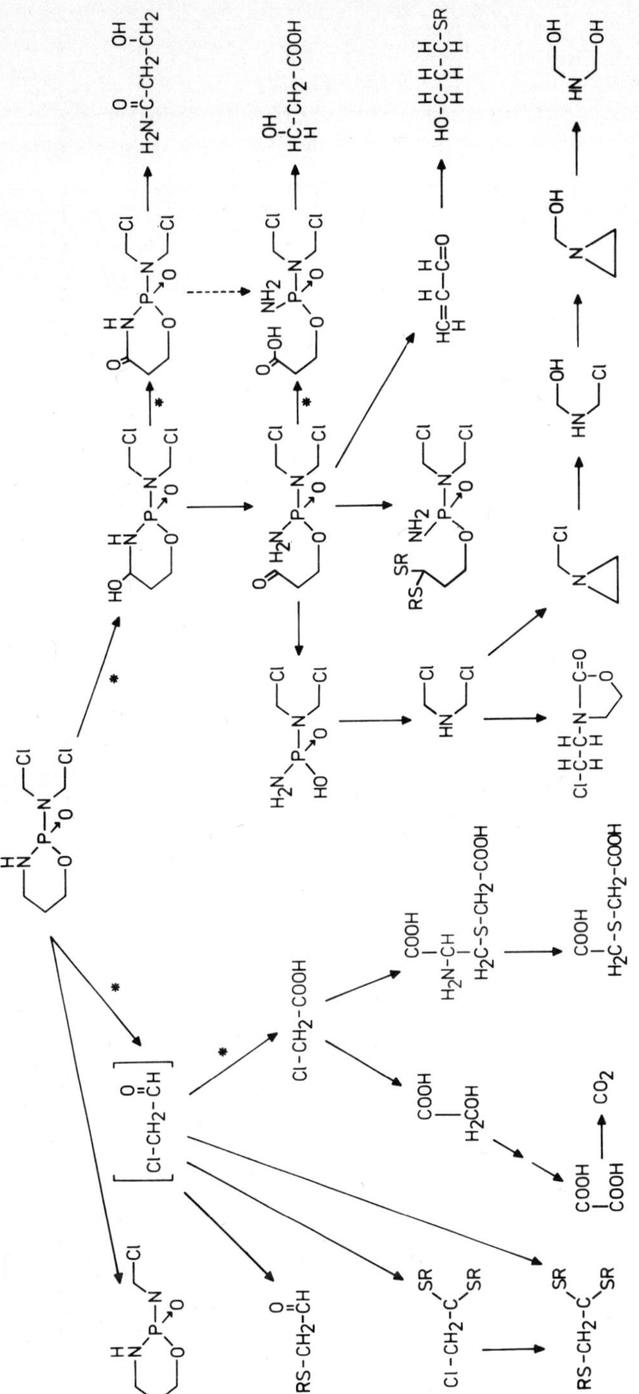

Figure 9. Metabolites of Cyclophosphamides which have been found or which can be assumed after identification of the biological precursors.

Another concept of selectivity which stresses the differences between cancer cells and normal cells concerning the O_2 dependent detoxication reactions is still under discussion. Both hypotheses may be verified or refuted in the near future because the use of inhibitors and competing substrates of detoxication reactions as well as the design of new CYM analogues provides some new approaches to the problem of selectivity. At that stage it should become fairly clear whether a new regimen of Cyclophosphamide and Ifosfamide treatment or the replacement of these drugs by new analogues or preactivated derivatives, respectively, is the best way towards a more effect use of oxazaphosphorine anticancer agents. Whatever the answer may be, it will indeed mark another important step forward in cancer chemotherapy.

REFERENCES

1. Alarcon, R.A. and Meienhofer, J. (1971). Nature, New Biology, 233, 250-252.
2. Alarcon, R.A., Meienhofer, J. and Atherton, E. (1972). Cancer Research, 32, 2519-2523.
3. Alarcon, R.A. Symposium on Metabolism and Mechanism of Action of Cyclophosphamide, London July 10th-12th, 1975. (In press)
4. Ardenne, M. von, Reitnauer, P.G. and Rohde, K. (1971). Arch. Geschwulstforsch, 38, 15-26.
5. Bakke, J.E., Feil, V.J., Fjeilstul, C.E. and Thacker, E.J. (1972). J.Agr.Food Chem., 20, 384.
6. Benckhuysen, C., Van Der Steen, J. and Spanjersberg, E.J. Symposium on Metabolism and Mechanism of Action of Cyclophosphamide, London, July 10th-12th 1975 (In press).
7. Brock, N. Symposium on Metabolism and Mechanism of Action of Cyclophosphamide, London, July 10th-12th 1975 (In press)
8. Brock, N. (1972). Czechoslowak Medical Press, Vol. II, Avicenum, Prague, p. 749-756.
9. Connors, T.A., Cox, P.J., Farmer, P.B., Foster, A.B., Jarman, M. and Macleod, J.K. (1974). Biomedical Mass Spectrometry, 1, 130-136.
10. Connors, T.A., Farmer, P.B., Foster, A.B. and Jarman, M. (1974). Biochem. Pharmacol., 23, 115-129.
11. Cox, P.J., Farmer, P.B., Foster, A.B., Gilby, E.D. and Jarman, M. Symposium on Metabolism and Mechanism of Action of Cyclophosphamide. London, July 10th-12th, 1975 (In press).
12. Druckrey, H. (1970). J. Kanser (Ankara), 1, 131-149.
13. Hill, D.L., Laster, W.R., Jr. and Struck, R.F. (1972). Cancer Research, 32, 658-665.

14. Hill, D.L., Laster, W.R., Jr., Kirk, M.C., El D reer, S. and Struck, R.F. (1973). Cancer Research, 33, 1016-1022.
15. Hohorst, H.J. (1973). Paper held at the second meeting of the European Association for Cancer Research, Heidleberg, October 2-5th.
16. Kaye, C.M. (1973). Biochem. J., 134, 1093-1101.
17. Kaye, C.M. and Joung, (1974). Biochem. Soc. Trans. 2, 308.
18. Norpoth, K. (1969). Habilitationsschrift, Munster.
19. Norpoth, K., Addicks, H.W. and Witting, U. (1973). Arzneim. Forsch. (Drug Res.), 23, 1529-1535.
20. Norpoth, K., Wust, G. and Witting, U. (1972). Verhandlungen der Deutschen Gesellschaft fur Innere Medizin, 78, 1561-1564.
21. Norpoth, K. Symposium on Metabolism and Mechanism of Action of Cyclophosphamide, London, July 10-12th, 1975.
22. Norpoth, K., Witting, U. and Rauen, H.M. (1974). Arzneim. Forsch. (Drug Res.), 24, 86-89.
23. Norpoth, K. and Witting, U. Unpublished results.
24. Peter, G. and Hohorst, H.J. Symposium on Metabolism and Mechanism of Action of Cyclophosphamide. London, July 10-12th, 1975. (In press).
25. Sawicki, E., Bender, D.F., Hanser, T.R., Wilson, R.M. and Meeker, J.E. (1963). Anal. Chem., 35, 1479-1486.
26. Sawicki, E. and Sawicki, C.R. (1969). Ann. N.Y. Acad. Sci., 163, 895-920.
27. Struck, R.F., Kirk, M.C., Mellet, L.B., El Dareer, S. and Hill, D.L. (1971). Molecular Pharmacology, 7, 519-529.
28. Struck, R.F. (1974). Cancer Research, 34, 2933-2935.
29. Takamizawa, A., Matsumoto, S., Iwata, T., Katagiri, K., Tochino, Y. and Yamaguchi, K. (1973). J. Am. Chem. Soc, 95, 985-986.
30. Takamizawa, A., Matsumoto, S. and Iwata, T. (1974). Tetrahedron Letters, 6, 517-520.
31. Takamizawa, A., Iwata, T., Matsumoto, S., Yamagucki, K., Shiratory, O., Harada, M. and Tochino, Y. Symposium on Metabolism and Mechanism of Action of Cyclophosphamide. London, July 10-12th, 1975. (In press).
32. Whitehouse, M.W., Beck, F.J. and Kacena, A. (1974). Agents and Action, 4, 1.
33. Yllner, S. (1971). Acta pharmacol. et toxicol., 30, 69-80.
34. Yllner, S. (1971). Acta pharmacol. et toxicol., 30, 257-265.

ICRF 159 AND OTHER BISDIOXOPIPERAZINES

K. Hellmann

Cancer Chemotherapy Department

Imperial Cancer Research Fund, London, U.K.

ICRF 159 (($\pm$)1,2-bis(3,5-dioxopiperazin-1-yl)propane) and a number of other bisdioxopiperazines are potent antimetastatic compounds which inhibit the development of metastases from primary implants of the syngeneic Lewis lung carcinoma (3LL) in C_{57} BL mice (Hellmann & Burrage 1969; Salsbury, Burrage and Hellmann 1970). This effect is produced without evident influence on the growth rate of the primary tumour and thereby shows that it is possible to delete selectively one malignant characteristic of a tumour without influencing another. While this antimetastatic effect is not apparently unique amongst anticancer agents it seems to be the exception.

ICRF 159 and a number of closely related bisdioxopiperazines also have a modest antimitotic activity. The antimitotic activity however in contrast to the antimetastatic activity is not selective and normal as well as malignant replicating cells are inhibited with equal facility (Creighton, Hellmann and Whitecross 1969). The non-selective nature of the antimitotic activity gives rise to a predictable clinical toxicity pattern. In rodents as well as man, ICRF 159 is active when given by mouth, and in mice the drug is active by all routes against a variety of transplantable tumours. It is even active against leuk aemias implanted intracerebrally.

Examination of a series of some 40 related compounds and analogues of ICRF 159 made by the customary chemical exploration of a series around an active compound - ICRF 154 (1,2-bis(3,5-dioxopiperazin-1-yl)ethane) the parent compound of the series - has shown that the structure of active *bis*dioxopiperazines is confined to those with no more and no less than two carbon atoms in the central bridge and no substitution in either of the rings. Openin of either (or both) of the rings leads to total loss of activity. The (+) isomer (ICRF 187) and the (-) isomer (ICRF 186) of ICRF 159 are each as active as the racemic ICRF 159. The toxicity of these isomers is also not different from ICRF 159 and there seemed to be no improvement in the therapeutic index by use of the optical isomer over that of ICRF 159 itself. ICRF 159 has been useful as a probe for the discovery of new approaches to cancer chemotherapy. These approaches have centered around the antimetastatic action. The mechanism of this action has been traced to the ability of the compound to prevent release from the primary tumour of 3LL cells into the bloodstream; itself a somewhat improbable goal, but now clearly shown to be realizable (Salsbury, Burrage and Hellmann 1970 and 1974). Even tumours which do not normall produce metastasis (Sarcoma S 180) but shed cells into circulation, can also be effectively prevented from releasing their malignant cells into the circulation.

The observations correlate best - though it is not completely certain whether the events are causally related with the finding that under influence of ICRF 159 there is a normalization of the developing tumour neovasculature (James and Salsbury 1974); the angiometamorphic effect. It seems most probable however, that this effect is responsible for preventing cell release from primary tumours. Although these changes are brought about without interfering with the usual growth rate of the primary tumour, the normalized vasculature may be due to changes in the respiratory activity in the malignant cells as a result of treatment by ICRF 159, thereby reducing their demand for oxygen and permitting more time for a more orderly neovascular development.

It seemed possible, that a normalized tumour vasculature would result in an improvement in the usual poor blood supply which obtains in most tumours. It also presented the possibility that the hypoxia generally present, particularly in the more central regions of tumours, might be reduced and that thereby, radiation might become more effective. This combination is being examined clinically, but it is clear from animal experiments that the growth inhibitory effect of radiation can be considerably enhanced by the simultaneous administration of doses of ICRF 159, which themselves are ineffective in inhibiting tumour growth.

Contrary to the findings with many other antitumour agents and in particular all the antimetabolites and alkylating agents, the point in the cell generation cycle at which the active *bis*dioxopiperazines block, is not as was proposed by Creighton and Birnie (1970) the DNA synthesis phase (S phase) but the late G_2 or possibly G_2/M phase (Hellmann & Field 1970, Sharpe, Hellmann and Field 1970, Hellmann, West and Hallowes 1974). This is a point where cells become very radiosensitive and may be an added (or even the main) reason why radiation is potentiated by ICRF 159 (Hellmann & Murkin 1974; Ryall et al 1974).

The mechanism of action of the *bis*dioxopiperazines is at present quite unknown. They are closely related to EDTA and ICRF 154 and ICRF 159 are able to act as *in vitro* and *in vivo* chelating agents but so are closely related compounds that are totally devoid of antitumour activity.

The poor selectivity of the active compounds inevitably results in poor antitumour performance when the compounds are used alone. A response rate of probably less than 10% is all that can be anticipated in man and is all that has been found when ICRF 159 is used as a single agent. In the acute leukaemias, ICRF 159 alone can sometimes produce complete or partial short-lived remissions though it seems clear that its use in combination with other drugs or with other modalities of treatment is to be preferred. There are also more specific reasons than poor selectivity for the use of this compound in combination treatment, since it has been shown clearly that the drug potentiates most of the currently available antitumour compounds while with some of them it simultaneously reduces their toxicity (Goldin, Venditti and Mantel 1975; Wampler 1974). The combination with adriamycin and daunomycin has been shown to reduce the cardiotoxicity of these drugs (Mhatre and Herrman 1972;, Woodman, Kline and Venditti 1972). This would be a fairly important contribution to cancer chemotherapy since it seems to be the usual rule that reduction of toxicity leads to reduction of activity.

Clinical trials in patients with a variety of soft tissue sarcomas treated with a combination of radiotherapy and ICRF 159 have now shown that the disease progression free interval is significantly greater in those patients treated with the combination than in similar patients treated only with radiotherapy. A similar trend is emerging from a trial in carcinoma of the bronchus using the same combination compared with radiotherapy alone.

1. Hellmann, K. & Burrage, Karen. Nature 224, 273-275 (1969).

2. Salsbury, A.J., Burrage, Karen and Hellmann, K. (1970) British Medical Journal, 4, 344-346.

3. Creighton, A.M., Hellmann, K. & Whitecross, Susan (1969) Nature, 222, 384-385.

4. Salsbury, A.J., Burrage, Karen, & Hellmann, K. (1974). Cancer Research, 34, 843-849.

5. James, Sandra E. & Salsbury, A.J. (1974) Cancer Research, 34, 839-842.

6. Creighton, A.M. & Birnie, G.D. (1970) International Journal of Cancer, 5, 47-54.

7. Hellmann, K. & Field, E.O. (1970) J. Nat. Cancer Inst. 44, 539-543.

8. Sharpe, Heather B.A., Field, E.O. & Hellmann, K. (1970) Nature, 226, 524-526.

9. Hallowes, R.C., West, D.G. & Hellmann, K. (1974) Nature, 247, 487-490.

10. Goldin, A., Venditti, J. & Mantel, N. (1975). in Antineoplastic and immunosuppressive agents Vol 1. Eds. A.C. Sartorelli & D.G. Johns, Springer, New York.

11. Wampler, G.L. (1973). Minutes of ICRF 159 meeting, National Cancer Institute, Bethesda, U.S.A. Ed. Wasserman, T.H.

12. Woodman, R.J., Kline, I. & Venditti, J.M. (1972). Proc. Amer. Ass. Cancer Res. 13, 31.

BIOLOGICAL BASIS OF RADIOSENSITIZATION BY HYPOXIC-CELL RADIOSENSITIZERS

G.E.ADAMS, J.DENEKAMP & J.F.FOWLER

Gray Laboratory of the Cancer Research Campaign

Mount Vernon Hospital, Northwood, HA6 2RN, England

ABSTRACT

Radiosensitizing drugs can only be clinically useful if they give a greater increase in sensitivity to radiation in the tumour than in normal tissues. This differential may be based on differences in the proliferation characteristics or on other known differences between normal and tumour cells, such as their oxygen status. The degree of oxygenation profoundly influences the radiosensitivity of all cells: hypoxic cells occur in most animal tumours and can be more effectively killed if their hypoxic protection is overcome e.g. with hyperbaric oxygen, high LET radiation or with electron affinic chemical radiosensitizers. This latter group of drugs includes nitroimidazoles which have recently been shown to mimic oxygen in its sensitizing ability. The drugs can diffuse to hypoxic tumour cells because, unlike oxygen, they are not rapidly metabolised by respiring cells.

Experiments in vitro and in vivo have shown that large sensitization occurs only in cells which lack oxygen. No sensitization is observed in well oxygenated cells or tissues. At least 10 different types of animal tumours have shown greatly increased sensitivity to single doses of X-radiation in the presence of the drug Ro-07-0582. Several tumours have also been tested with fractionated doses of radiation and drug and a therapeutic advantage was still observed.

Preliminary clinical studies with metronidazole and with Ro-07-0582 have been carried out. Significant radiosensitization of human tumours with no extra damage to normal tissues has been demonstrated with Ro-07-0582.

INTRODUCTION

Several different classes of radiosensitizing drug have been described (Adams,1970; Bridges,1969; Emmerson,1972). However, if radiation sensitizers are to be of any practical clinical value, they must cause more damage to tumours than to normal tissues. This is not the case with the DNA-intercalating radio-sensitizers such as BUdR and FUdR and their use has decreased.

The largest difference in radiosensitivity known between tumours and normal tissues is due to the radioresistance of hypoxic cells in tumours. X-ray doses have to be about three times higher to kill a given proportion of hypoxic cells than of well-oxygenated cells. The presence of hypoxic cells has been demonstrated repeatedly in animal tumours and results in a resistance to radiation which makes cure with single doses of X-rays difficult or impossible. Clinical trials indicate that hypoxic cells also limit the radiocurability of some human tumours, including carcinoma of the cervix uteri and of the head and neck (Henk et al.,1975; Catterall et al.,1975). This disadvantage of hypoxic cells is reduced in tumours which can reoxygenate their hypoxic cells during fractionated radiotherapy, for example by shrinkage. It is probably reoxygenation during the course of radiation therapy which enables cures to be achieved at present.

Methods suggested to overcome the problem of hypoxic cells in tumours include treatment in high pressure oxygen chambers (HPO) and radiotherapy with beams of high-energy nuclei (neutrons or negative pi mesons) as outlined in Figure 1. Recently a third method has become available: the application of chemical radiosensitizers which are active against hypoxic cells only. Sensitizers of this type are electron-affinic compounds which mimic the radiosensitizing effect of oxygen. A vital point is that they are not used up in the metabolism of the cells through which they diffuse, so that they can penetrate further from the capillary vessels than oxygen does and so can reach the hypoxic cells in tumours.

ELECTRON-AFFINIC RADIOSENSITIZERS

In 1963, Adams and Dewey proposed that a relationship existed between the ability of a few chemical compounds to sensitize hypoxic bacterial cells and the electron-affinity of these compounds. Subsequent work with bacterial systems (Ashwood-Smith et al.,1967; Adams and Cooke,1969) and later with mammalian cells in vitro, led to the characterization of a large number of radiosensitizers. The electron-affinity hypothesis was verified in the main, and this aided the search for more active compounds. A report of the radiosensitizing properties of several nitrofurans, including some known urinary antibiotics, on hypoxic mammalian cells in vitro was significant because toxicological and pharmacological information was available for these compounds (Chapman et al.,1972). However, subsequent attempts to demonstrate appreciable sensitization in vivo with these compounds have been disappointing, in some cases because the metabolic half-life was only a few minutes.

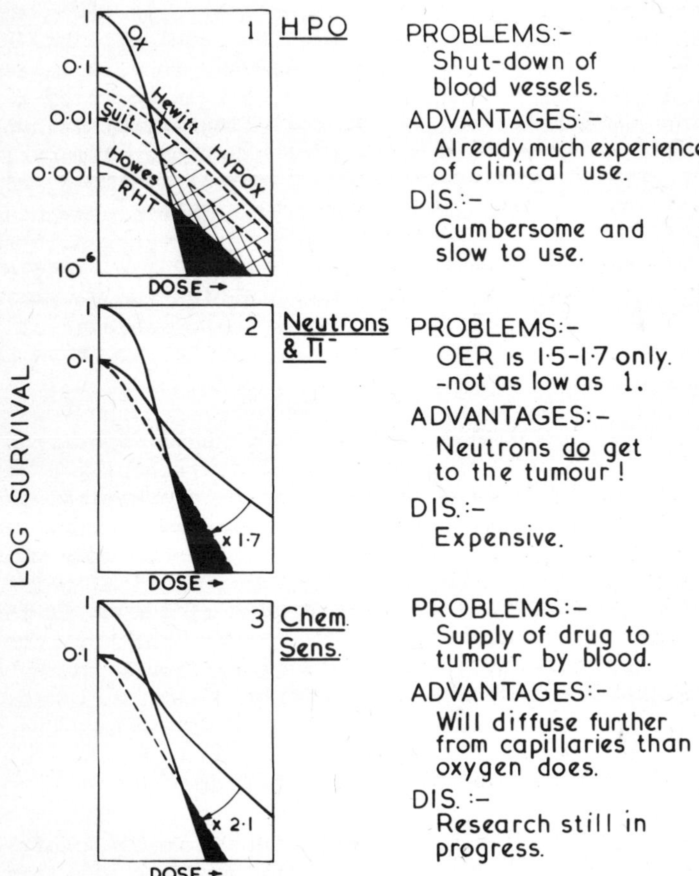

Figure 1. The black areas represent the number of hypoxic cells surviving, i.e. the size of the problem remaining, after a single dose of X-rays with each of the three main methods of overcoming this problem. 1 - High Pressure Oxygen tanks. 2 - Nuclear physics beams of neutrons or negative pions. 3 - Chemical sensitizers of the electron-affinic type.

Another significant step forward occurred with the successful demonstration of the radiosensitization, in vivo, of epidermal cells in mice that were made artifically hypoxic by breathing nitrogen for 35 seconds (Denekamp and Michael, 1972). The first compound used was NDPP, a soluble derivative of paranitroacetophenone which was known to be an active sensitizer in vitro (Adams, Asquith, Watts and Smithen, 1972). A small degree of radiosensitization was also observed in mouse ascites tumour cells irradiated in vivo (Berry and Asquith, 1974) and in solid tumours in mice (Sheldon and Smith, 1975). However, encouraging as these results were, the chemical instability of NDPP and its high attachment to serum proteins ultimately limited its usefulness (Whitmore, 1975).

Further searches for other drugs already in clinical use and possessing a chemical structure associated with electron-affinity led to the discovery in 1973 of the radiosensitizing action of metronidazole* (Foster and Willson, 1973; Chapman, Reuvers and Borsa, 1973; Asquith, Foster, Willson, Ings and McFadzean, 1974). Although this sensitizer is only moderately active on a concentration basis, experiments in various types of systems in vivo, including solid tumours in mice, gave promising results. This was due to its low toxicity, wide distribution in tissues and, very importantly, its long metabolic half-life, all of which are properties necessary for a clinically useful hypoxic cell radiosensitizer.

Several other compounds related to metronidazole, a 5-substituted nitroimidazole, were investigated in attempts to find more active compounds. On theoretical grounds related to the effect of chemical structure on the electron-affinity of the nitroimidazoles, it was anticipated that the 2-substituted nitro compounds might be more effective than the 5-nitro derivatives. Recently, one such compound has been shown to be even more effective than metronidazole (Asquith, Watts, Patel, Smithen and Adams, 1974). The current status of research on radiosensitization by this compound Ro-07-0582** is summarised below.

SENSITIZATION BY NITROIMIDAZOLES IN VITRO

An investigation of the sensitization of X-irradiated Chinese hamster cells V79-GL$_1$ by both metronidazole and Ro-07-0582, showed that:

(a) sensitization was achieved with hypoxic cells but not in cells which were well oxygenated;

---

* 'Flagyl', May and Baker Ltd., Dagenham, Essex, England.

** Roche Products Ltd., Welwyn Garden City, Herts., England.

(b) full radiosensitization occurred within seconds of mixing the cells with medium containing the drug;

(c) sensitization occurred at much lower concentrations than were cytotoxic after two hours' contact;

(d) for 0582 the maximum X-ray dose enhancement ratio was 2.5, i.e. nearly equivalent to the full oxygen enhancement ratio of 2.7 for this cell line (see Figure 2). Enhancement ratio is obtained from the ratio of X-ray doses without and with the sensitizer which are required to produce the same effect;

(e) for both drugs the sensitization efficiency was independent of the serum concentration in the medium (Figure 2);

(f) The sensitizing efficiency was equally effective on cells at all stages of the mitotic cycle (Asquith et al., 1974a & b).

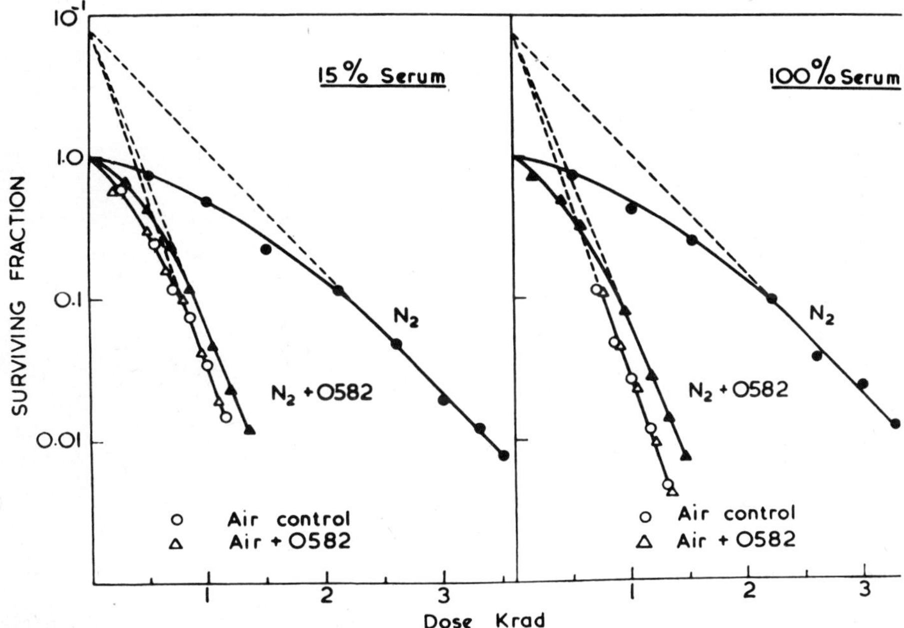

Figure 2. In vitro survival curves for hypoxic and oxic Chinese Hamster cells V79 GL_1 irradiated in the presence of 4mM Ro-07-0582. Sensitization is not diminished by the presence of serum in the culture medium (Asquith et al., 1974). The enhancement ratios achieved (2.5) are almost as high as that of oxygen (i.e. "air control" curves, ER = 2.7).

Other investigations have shown a specific cytotoxicity for hypoxic cells only, if they are exposed to the drugs for periods of many hours (Hall and Roizin-Towle, 1975). This specific killing of hypoxic cells should be a useful contribution to therapy but in animal tumour experiments it has been shown to be a small effect relative to the true radiosensitization.

SENSITIZATION BY NITROIMIDAZOLES IN VIVO

A variety of different test systems has been used to test electron-affinic sensitizers in vivo. Results for the two drugs of present clinical interest will be summarised here.

The first in vivo test system used was the Withers (1967) skin clone method of assessing epidermal cell survival, in the

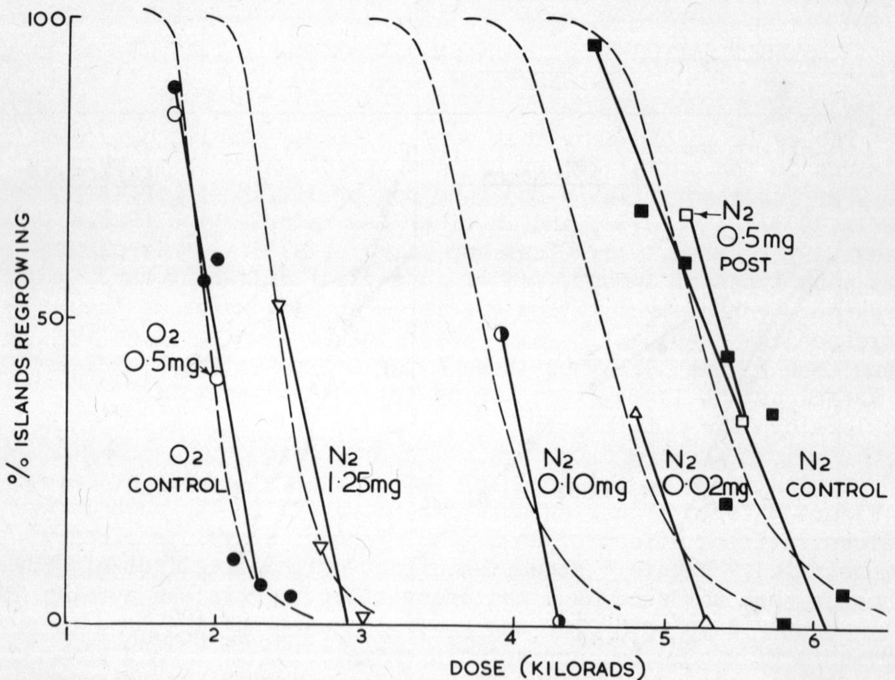

Figure 3. Proportion of epidermal clones (i.e. basal cells) surviving as a function of X-ray dose for various doses of drug in mg per gram bodyweight of Ro-07-0582. The animals were irradiated breathing nitrogen for 35 seconds except for the left-hand curve when they breathed oxygen. Sensitization is shown by the progressive shift to left of the N_2 curves from "control", through increasing drug dosages in mg per gram bodyweight, towards the O_2 curve. The solid lines are 'by-eye' fits. The dashed lines are computer fits (Denekamp, Michael and Harris, 1974).

skin of mice made briefly hypoxic for the tests (Denekamp, Michael and Harris,1974). Figure 3 shows that no enhancement of cell killing in oxygenated cells was caused (left-hand curve), and no sensitizing effect was observed in skin when the drug was given after irradiation (right-hand curve). Enhancement ratios of 2.1 and 1.5 respectively for 0582 and metronidazole (1 mg/g bodyweight) were obtained, as compared with the oxygen enhancement ratio of 2.7 in this system.

Although no significant sensitization has been observed in normal skin, either using skin clones or gross skin reactions (Foster,1975), nevertheless we may expect small but significant enhancement of radiosensitivity in any normal tissues which are hypoxic, such as cartilage. This must be considered when planning the clinical use of these drugs, as is also true with hyperbaric oxygen radiotherapy and neutrons.

SENSITIZATION BY NITROIMIDAZOLES OF SOLID TUMOURS IN EXPERIMENTAL MICE

Tables Ia and Ib show that very promising results have been obtained in ten animal tumour systems investigated by workers at the Gray Laboratory (Table Ia) (Sheldon et al.,1974; Denekamp and Harris,1975; Begg,1975), and in other laboratories too (Table Ib) (Rauth,1975; Brown,1975; Stone and Withers,1975). It is clear that many types of tumour, tested in several different ways, give X-ray dose enhancement ratios greater than 1.7, which is the corresponding therapeutic gain factor for neutrons or negative pions (see Figure 1). Thus these drugs are potentially at least as useful as the large expensive cyclotrons and particle accelerators for radiotherapy.

Typical results obtained for tumour regrowth delay are shown in Figure 4 for a transplantable carcinoma 'NT'. The much larger radiosensitizing effect of Ro-07-0582 than of Flagyl is clearly demonstrated. Figure 5 shows the direct cytocidal effect of 0582 on cells when not used as a radiosensitizer. There was a delay of only about 2 days when 0582 was given to unirradiated mice (top curves in Figure 5) but appreciable extra delay of 7 days when the 0582 was given after 2000 rads. This is probably because the cytotoxic effect is limited to hypoxic cells and these predominate in the response of a tumour after a large single dose of X-rays. The drugs have to be in contact with the hypoxic cells for more than a few hours in order to demonstrate such direct cytocidal effects. A comparison of Figures 4 and 5 shows that a far bigger delay(by 30 days) is caused by the radiosensitizing effect of the drug,i.e.when it is administered before irradiation as in Figure 4 instead of afterwards as in Figure 5.

TABLE Ia
SUMMARY OF ENHANCEMENT RATIOS FOR SOLID MURINE TUMOURS IN VIVO

EXPERIMENTER (a - Gray Laboratory)	TUMOUR	ASSAY	X-RAY DOSE ENHANCEMENT WITH Ro-07-0582 0.2-0.3	1 mg/g
Begg (1975)	CBA Fast Sarc F 1 day >10% hyp	Regrowth Loss of 125-IUdR	1.0	1.5
Denekamp & Harris(1975)	CBA Carcinoma NT 3 d 6%	Regrowth delay	>1.4	2.1
Denekamp & Stewart *	WHT bone Sa 2 2.5d -	Regrowth delay	-	1.8
Denekamp & Stewart *	WHT fibrosarc 2 d -	Regrowth delay	-	1.8
McNally *	CBA Fast Sarc F	Cell diln. in vitro	1.3	2.2
Hewitt *	WHT Squamous Carcinoma D 1 d 18%	Cell diln. in vitro	- 1.0 - (intravenous)	
Hill & Fowler *	WHT Squamous Carcinoma D 1 d 18%	Cure	-	2.1
Peters *	WHT Intradermal Squamous Ca G 1 d 0.3%	Cure	1.9	2.1
Foster, Sheldon & Fowler(1974)	C3H 1st gen trans of spont mamm Ca 6 d 10%	Cure	1.3	1.8
Sheldon *	WHT anaplast.MT line transpl. 1 d 50%	Cure	1.7	2.0
McNally *	WHT anaplast.MT 1 d 50%	Cell diln. in vitro	-	1.5

* Unpublished (private communication)

TABLE Ib
SUMMARY OF ENHANCEMENT RATIOS FOR SOLID MURINE TUMOURS IN VIVO

EXPERIMENTERS (b - other laboratories)	TUMOUR	ASSAY	X-RAY DOSE ENHANCEMENT WITH Ro-07-0582 0.2-0.3	1 mg/g
Rauth (1975) (Toronto)	C3H Sarc KHT 2 d 6%	Cell diln. lung colonies	1.2-1.3	1.8
Kedar, Watson & Bleehen * (London)	EMT 6	Cell diln. in vitro	-	2.2
Brown (1975) (Stanford)	EMT 6	Cell diln. in vitro	-	2.4
Brown (1975) (Stanford)	C3H mamm. Ca	Cure	-	2.3
Stone & Withers (1975) (Houston)	C3H 3rd gen transplant of spont.mamm.Ca	Cure	-	2.4

* Private communication

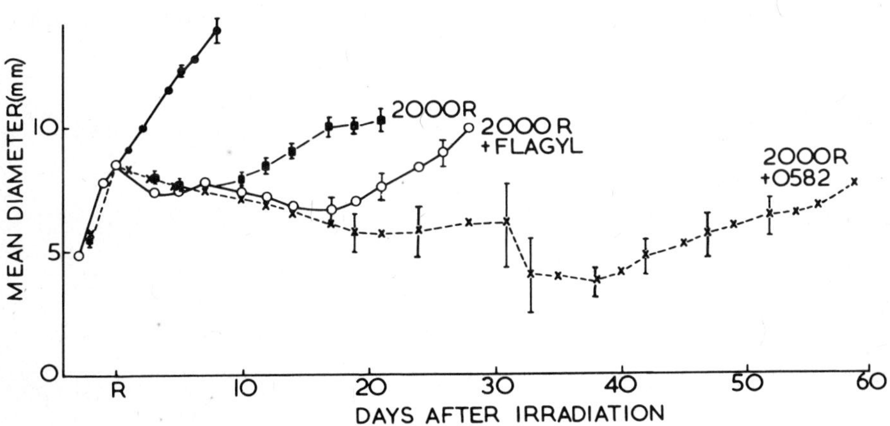

Figure 4. Growth curves for batches of 10-14 mice either untreated (controls), or irradiated with 2000 rads of X-rays alone, 2000 rads 15 min after receiving 0.75 mg/g Flagyl, or 2000 rads 15 min after receiving 1 mg/g Ro-07-0582 i.p. The radiation-induced delay caused by 2000 rads is increased in the presence of the sensitizing drugs (Denekamp and Harris, 1975).

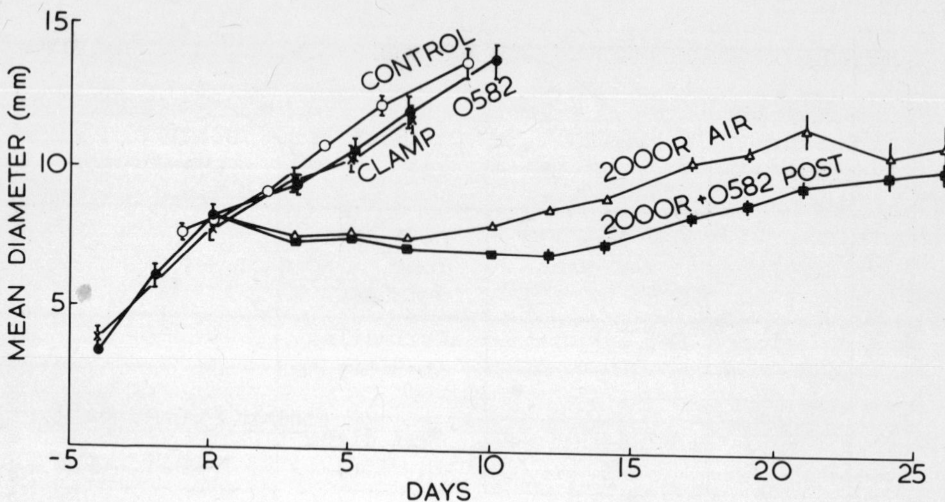

Figure 5. Growth curves for batches of 10-14 mice either untreated with X-rays (controls) or irradiated with 2000 rads, with and without the administration of 1 mg/g 0582 after irradiation or no irradiation. The additional delay of about 7 days in the unirradiated group is due to a direct cytocidal effect of the drug on the hypoxic tumour cells (after Denekamp and Harris, 1975).

Enhancement ratios are somewhat smaller for the lower drug concentrations of 0.2 to 0.3 mg/g bodyweight which correspond in mice to the doses of Ro-07-0582 which can be administered to patients in practice (Tables Ia and Ib).

The results for cure of tumours are more definitive than those for regrowth delay and are also encouraging. Figure 6 shows results for first-generation transplants of spontaneous mammary tumours in C3H/He mice (Sheldon, Foster and Fowler, 1974). The tumours were irradiated at a small size, 6.5 ± 1mm. 1 mg/g bodyweight of Ro-07-0582 was administered intraperitoneally 30 minutes before starting the irradiation. Although the X-ray enhancement ratio of 1.8 is modest compared with other results in the Tables, the use of the drug increases the cure rate from 10% to about 90% at 3200 rads. Further, the dose-response curve was significantly steeper, in the same ratio of 1.8, with the 0582. This finding suggests that the drug was indeed reaching all of the hypoxic cells and sensitizing them efficiently. A similar conclusion was drawn from the results of Denekamp and Harris (1975) on regrowth delay in the carcinoma 'NT' in CBA mice.

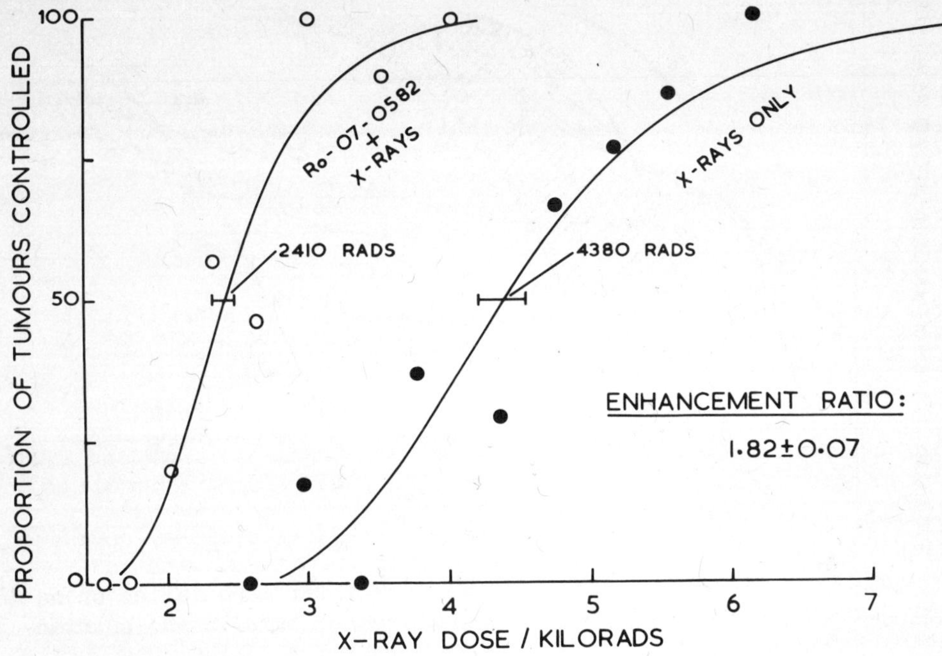

Figure 6. Proportion of C3H mice with transplanted mammary tumours cured versus X-ray dose. "Controlled" means did not recur within 150 days. Right-hand curve, X-rays only. Left-hand curve, X-rays delivered starting 30 minutes after i.p. injection of 1 mg/g bodyweight of Ro-07-0582 (Sheldon, Foster and Fowler, 1974).

Figure 7 shows results for local tumour control of the anaplastic transplanted tumour 'MT' in WHT/Ht mice. For the high drug dose of 1 mg/g, an X-ray dose enhancement ratio of 2.0 was found. This is one of the largest enhancements of local tumour control achieved by any agent in solid experimental tumours.

For the more practical concentrations of 0.1 to 0.3 mg/g the enhancement ratio varied from 1.4 to 1.7. Even at the lowest ER of 1.4, the probability of tumour control was increased from 5% to 95% in this system. The shaded area in Figure 7 shows the range of enhancement ratios in mice for the serum levels that can be achieved in man, for single-dose treatments.

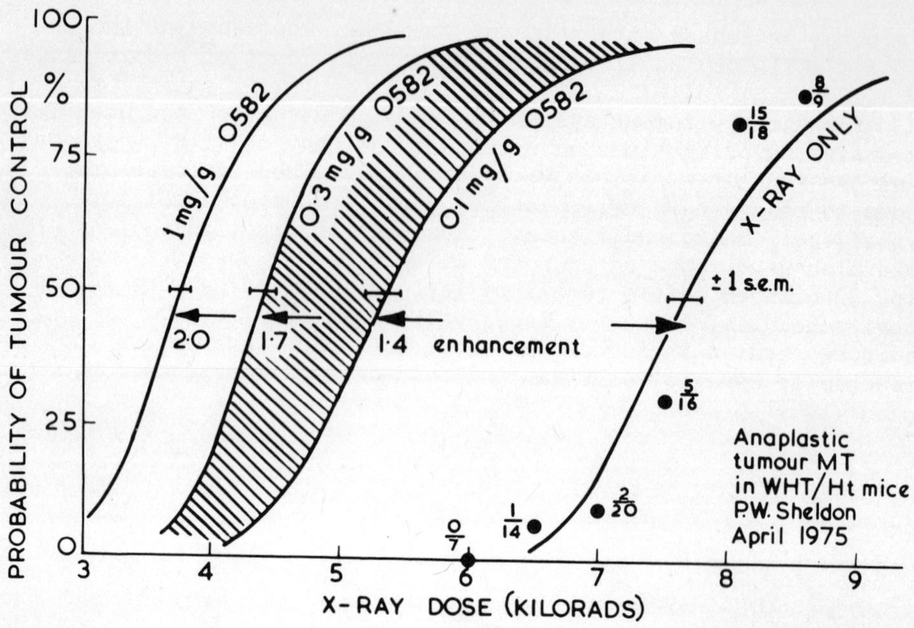

Figure 7. Proportion of WHT mice with transplanted tumours cured at 60 days versus X-ray dose. Right-hand curve, X-rays only. The other three curves are for three different dosages of drug Ro-07-0582 given i.p. 30 minutes before starting X-irradiation. The shaded area represents clinically realistic drug dosages.

Figure 8 shows the way in which enhancement ratios increase with drug dosage for seven of the tumours listed in Tables Ia and Ib. There is more variability of the ER values at the lower, realistic, drug dosages than at the higher dosages of 1 mg/g. This variability may be due to problems of blood flow in some types of tumour. Some of the ER values for tumours are however equally as high as those for skin made artificially hypoxic, so that blood flow is not a problem in all types of tumour. From Figure 8 and Tables Ia and Ib it can be seen that there are no consistent differences in the ER values obtained using the different end points of local control i.e. 'cure', regrowth delay, or cell dilution and assay.

FRACTIONATED X-RAYS PLUS Ro-07-0582

The large enhancement ratios demonstrated above with single doses of X-rays are always reduced in multiple-dose treatments. This is partly because smaller individual X-ray doses yield smaller enhancements, but mainly because reoxygenation occurs to a greater or lesser extent in the tumours. Thus some of the hypoxic cells may be eliminated by multiple doses of X-rays alone.

The mammary tumour system in C3H mice has also been used for extensive investigations on optimum fractionation with X-rays and neutrons (Fowler et al.,1972; 1974; 1975). These tumours are known to reoxygenate well, so they provide a severe test for hypoxic-cell radiosensitizers. Three of the fractionated schedules were repeated with and without Ro-07-0582 (0.67 mg/g i.p. 30 minutes before each irradiation). All three were fairly short schedules, of 4 or 9 days' overall time. The poor or mediocre results in two of the three schedules were due to the presence of hypoxic cells and their inadequate reoxygenation.

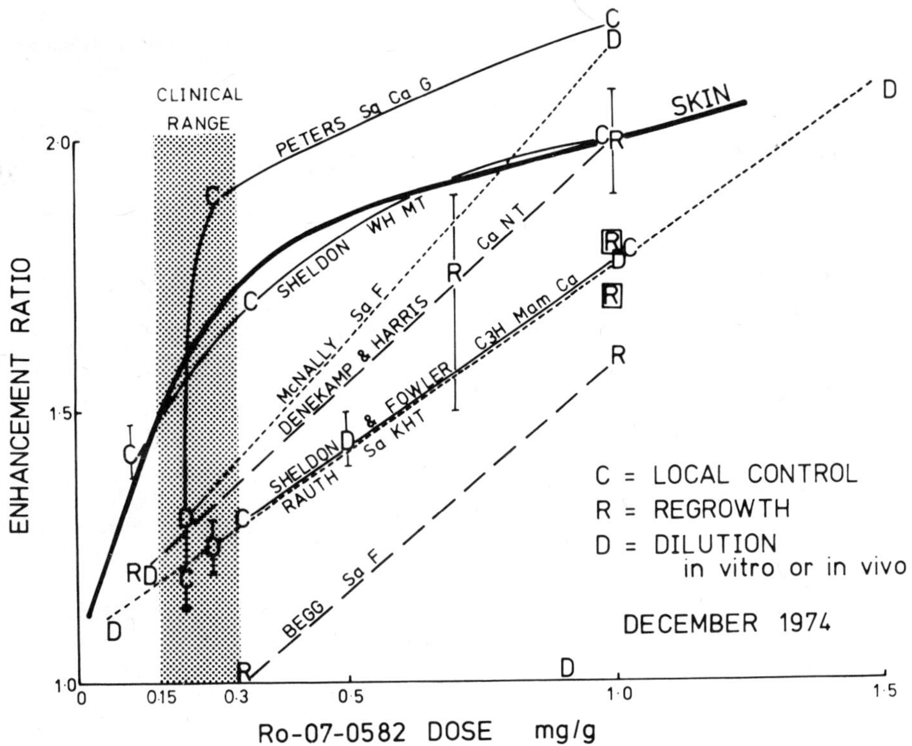

Figure 8. X-ray dose enhancement ratios versus drug dosage in vivo for six types of mouse tumour from Table Ia and one from Table Ib. The heavy line represents the ER for clones in skin made artificially hypoxic (see Figure 3). The shaded area represents the 0582 serum concentrations that can reasonably be achieved in human patients.

For the 5F/4d X-ray schedule in which the response to X-rays alone was poor, a substantial X-ray dose enhancement ratio of 1.3 was obtained. For the other two schedules, smaller enhancement ratios of 1.1 - 1.2 were found (Figure 9). These enhancement ratios were all less than the value of 1.8 found for single doses because reoxygenation had eliminated some of the hypoxic cells in the fractionated schedules and there was less disadvantage to gain back.

Figure 10 shows these results plotted for X-ray doses which give a certain degree of normal tissue damage, viz an average acute skin reaction of 2.0. The vertical arrows show the improvement in local tumour control obtained by the use of Ro-07-0582. It is impressive that all four schedules, including the single dose, bring the tumour control up to the same level of

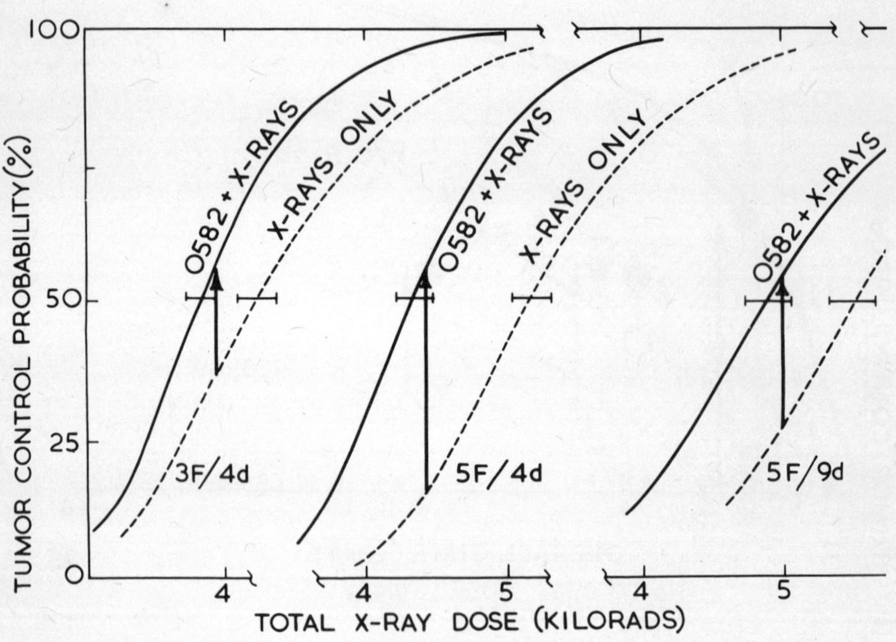

Figure 9. Proportion of C3H mice with transplanted mammary tumours cured for three fractionated X-ray schedules with and without the hypoxic-cell radiosensitizer Ro-07-0582 (0.67 mg/g). The horizontal error bars indicate the standard error of the mean TCD 50's. The vertical arrows show the improvement in tumour control at X-ray doses corresponding to a skin reaction of 2.0 (Fowler et al., 1975).

about 55 - 65%. This suggests that these sensitizers, like neutrons (Fowler et al.,1972), take the variability out of fractionated X-ray schedules. They would be particularly useful for non-standard X-ray schedules which employed fewer and larger fractions, because these appear to give poorer and more variable results than schedules using many small fractions.

A comparison of the effectiveness of fractionated X-rays alone, fractionated X-rays plus 0582 and fractionated neutrons has also been performed on another carcinoma ('NT') using regrowth delay instead of local cure (Denekamp and Harris,1975; Denekamp, Harris and Morris, private communication). As with the C3H carcinoma, this tumour showed a very large enhancement ratio with single doses (2.1) which was reduced with fractionated doses, to 1.6 for 2 fractions in 48 hours and to 1.3 for 5 fractions in 9 days, partly because of reoxygenation and partly because of the reduced drug doses tolerated in repeated treatments (Figure 11).

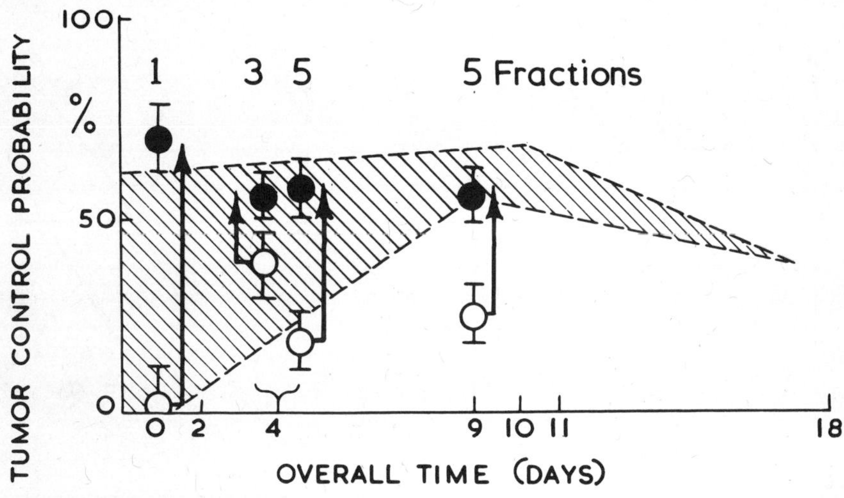

Figure 10. Proportion of C3H mice cured, from Fig. 9,for a skin reaction of 2.0 versus overall treatment time. Open circles: X-rays alone for the same schedules. Solid circles: X-rays with the hypoxic-cell radiosensitizer Ro-07-0582. The vertical arrows indicate the improvements in tumour control with respect to the concurrent X-ray-only experiments. The shaded region represents the envelope of results for other fractionated X-ray-only schedules using 2, 5, 9 or 15 fractions (Fowler et al.,1975).

These enhancement ratios were very close to the gains obtained in the same experiments by using fast neutrons instead of X-rays. In addition, the combination of fast neutrons and 0582 was tested in a single-dose experiment and an added advantage was obtained relative to either fast neutrons alone or to X-rays with 0582.

PROSPECTS FOR CLINICAL APPLICATION

Although basic radiochemical and in vitro research has been in progress for some years, it is only within the last two years that substantial sensitization in vivo has been obtained and

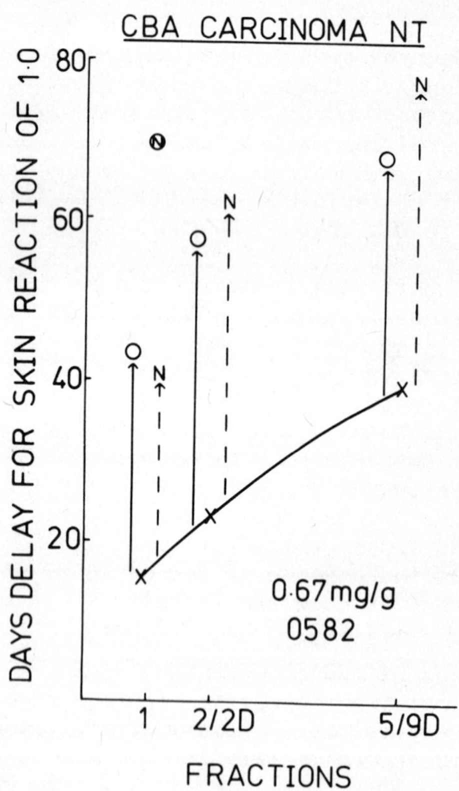

Figure 11. Regrowth delay for a given degree of skin reaction versus fractionation of dose. X: X-rays only. O: X-rays with 0582. N: neutrons only. Ⓝ: neutrons with 0582. (Denekamp, Harris and Morris, unpublished).

progress is now rapid. Preliminary clinical investigations are in progress at Edmonton, Alberta, Canada (Urtasun et al.,1975) and at Mount Vernon Hospital, London, England (Dische et al.,1975). At Edmonton, several dozen patients with brain tumours have been treated using multiple X-ray doses with metronidazole between 3 and about 10 grams orally before each dose. At Mount Vernon, about a dozen patients have been treated using single or repeated doses of metronidazole, and 8 advanced cancer patients have been treated with Ro-07-0582 during single-dose palliative X-ray treatments (Dische et al.,1975). These patients had either multiple skin nodules secondary to breast, cervical or lung cancer, or nodules in the lung observable on X-ray films. The early conclusions are that about 10 - 12 g of metronidazole or about half that quantity of Ro-07-0582 can be administered orally and that the serum concentrations obtained correspond to enhancement ratios which were significant in mouse tumours (e.g. 165 μg/ml after 200 mg/Kg metronidazole and 150-200 μg/ml after 100 - 150 mg/Kg of Ro-07-0582). The tolerance limit of both drugs is set by nausea. Considerably higher concentrations have to be given, at more frequent intervals and continuing for longer periods, to cause the long-term brain damage reported in dogs (Schärer,1972) for some nitroimidazole compounds, including metronidazole. Toxicological and pharmacological studies have been carried out by Johnson and colleages at Roswell Park Memorial Institute, Buffalo, New York, and by Roche Products Ltd. in England.

The serum levels attained in man should be sufficient to produce detectable sensitization of solid tumours, if they contain hypoxic cells for a significant part of the time during fractionated radiotherapy. Results from tumour growth delay measurements are available from four of the eight patients who received Ro-07-0582 at Mount Vernon Hospital (Dische et al.,1975). In three of the four patients some enhancement of delay was observed, in one case the ER being 1.2, which is a significant amount of enhancement. At the same time, research is proceeding to look for radiosensitizers which will give equally good enhancement ratios as those demonstrated by Ro-07-0582 but for smaller drug doses and for no worse toxicity.

ACKNOWLEDGEMENTS

The authors have pleasure in acknowledging the generous help and information given in the preparation of this review by their colleagues, especially Drs. McNally, Watts, Rauth, Bleehen, Urtasun, Dische, Strickland, Alan Gray, Zanelli, Thomlinson, and Messrs. Foster, Sheldon and Begg. We should also like to thank the authors (as acknowledged) and the editors of the following journals for permission to reproduce figures:

Fig. 1, Excerpta Medica (Proc. Int. Congr. of Radiology, Madrid, Oct.1973).

Figs. 2, 3 and 4, Radiation Research.

Figs. 6 and 7, British Journal of Cancer.

Figs 9 and 10, Internat. Journal of Radiation Oncology, Biology & Physics.

Fig. 11, Radiation Research.

REFERENCES

Adams,G.E: 1967. The general application of pulse radiolysis to current problems in radiobiology. In 'Current Topics in Radiation Research'. Vol. 3:35-93. (Ed.Ebert and Howard, North-Holland Pub. Co., Amsterdam).

Adams,G.E: 1973. Chemical radiosensitization of hypoxic cells. Brit. Med. Bull. 29, 48-53.

Adams,G.E., J.C.Asquith, M.E.Watts and C.E.Smithen: 1972. Radiosensitization of hypoxic cells in vitro: a water soluble derivative of paranitroacetophenone. Nature New Biology 239:457-471.

Adams,G.E. and M.S.Cooke: 1969. Electron-affinic sensitization: 1. A structural basis for chemical radiosensitizers in bacteria. Int. J.Radiat.Biol. 15: 457-471.

Adams,G.E. and D.L.Dewey: 1963. Hydrated electrons and radiobiological sensitization. Biochem. Biophysic.Res.Comm. 12: 473-477.

Ashwood-Smith,M.J., D.M.Robinson, J.M.Barnes and B.A.Bridges: 1967. Radiosensitization of bacterial and mammalian cells by substituted glyoxals. Nature (London) 216: 137-139.

Asquith,J.C., J.L.Foster, R.L.Willson, R.Ings & J.A.McFadzean: 1974. Metronidazole ('Flagyl'), a radiosensitizer of hypoxic cells. Brit.J.Radiol. 47: 474.

Asquith,J.C., M.E.Watts, K.Patel, C.E.Smithen and G.E.Adams: 1974. Electron-affinic sensitization: V. Radiosensitization of hypoxic bacteria and mammalian cells in vitro by some nitroimidazoles and nitropyrazoles. Rad. Res. 60: 108-118.

Berry,J.R. and J.C.Asquith: 1974. Cell cycle-dependent and hypoxic radiosensitizers. In 'Advances in chemical radiosensitization'. Proc. of IAEA/WHO meeting on Radiation Sensitization and Protection. IAEA, Vienna: 25-36.

Bridges,B.A: 1969. Sensitization of organisms to ionizing radiation by sulphydyl binding agents. In 'Advances in Radiation Biology' Vol 3:123-176.

Brown,J.M: 1975. Selective radiosensitization of the hypoxic cells of mouse tumours with metronidazole and Ro-07-0582. Rad. Res. (in press).

Catterall, M., I.Sutherland and D.K.Bewley: 1975. A randomised clinical trial of fast neutrons and X or γ-rays in the treatment of advanced tumours of the head and neck. Brit Med.2: 653-659.

Chapman,J.D., A.P.Reuvers, J.Borsa, A.Petkau and D.R.McCalla: 1972. Nitrofurans as radiosensitizers of hypoxic mammalian cells. Cancer Res. 32: 2616-2624.

Chapman,J.D., A.P.Reuvers and J.Borsa: 1973. Effectiveness of nitrofuran derivatives in sensitizing hypoxic mammalian cells to X-rays. Brit.J.Radiol. 46: 623-630.

Denekamp,J. and B.D.Michael: 1972. Preferential sensitization of hypoxic cells to radiation in vivo. Nature New Biology 239:21-23.

Denekamp,J., B.D.Michael and S.R.Harris: 1974. Hypoxic cell radiosensitizers: Comparative tests of some electron affinic compounds using epidermal cell survival in vivo. Rad.Res. 60:119-132.

Denekamp,J. and S.R.Harris: 1975. Tests of two electron-affinic radiosensitizers in vivo using regrowth of an experimental carcinoma. Rad. Res. 61: 191-203.

Dische,S., A.J.Gray, G.D.Zanelli, R.H.Thomlinson, G.E.Adams, I.R.Flockhart and J.L.Foster: 1975. Clinical testing of the radiosensitizer Ro-07-0582. Clinical Radiol.

Emmerson,P.T: 1972. X-ray damage to DNA and loss of biological function: effect of sensitizing agents. In 'Advances in Radiation Chemistry' 3: 209-270.

Foster, J.L. and R.L.Willson: 1973. Radiosensitization of anoxic cells by metronidazole. Brit.J.Radiol. 46: 234-235.

Foster,J.L: 1975. Mouse skin reactions after X-irradiation with the nitroimidazole radiosensitizer Ro-07-0582. Brit.J. Cancer (in press).

Fowler,J.F., J.Denekamp, A.L.Page, A.C.Begg, S.B.Field and K.Butler: 1972. Fractionation with X-rays and neutrons in mice: response of skin and C3H mammary tumours. Brit.J.Radiol.45:237-249.

Fowler,J.F., J.Denekamp, P.W.Sheldon, A.M.Smith, A.C.Begg, S.R.Harris and A.L.Page: 1974. Optimum fractionation in X-ray treatment of C3H mouse mammary tumours. Brit.J.Radiol.47,781-789.

Fowler,J.F., P.W.Sheldon, J.Denekamp and S.B.Field: 1975. Optimum fractionation of the C3H mouse mammary carcinoma using X-rays, the hypoxic-cell radiosensitizer Ro-07-0582, or fast neutrons. Int.J.Radiat.Oncol., Biol. and Physics (in press).

Hall,E.J. and L.Roizin-Towle: 1975. Hypoxic sensitizers: Radiobiological studies at the cellular level. Radiat.Res.(in press).

Henk,J.M: 1975. Does fractionation make hyperbaric oxygen unnecessary? Paper read at 3rd Eur. Sco. Radiol. Congr. at Edinburgh, June 1975.

Rauth,A.M: 1975. In vivo testing of hypoxic cell radiosensitizers in Symposium 'Chemical Radiosensitization of Mammalian Cells'. Proc. 5th Int. Congr. of Radiation Research (Seattle 1974). Academic Press (in press).

Sheldon,P.W., J.L.Foster and J.F.Fowler: 1974. Radiosensitization of C3H mouse mammary tumours by a 2-nitroimidazole drug. Brit.J.Cancer 30: 560-565.

Schärer,K: 1972. Selective injury to Purkinje cells in the dog after oral administration of high doses of nitroimidazole derivatives. Veth.Dtsch.Ges.Path. 56: 407-410.

Sheldon,P.W. and A.M.Smith: 1975. Modest radiosensitization of solid tumours in C3H mice by the hypoxic cell radiosensitizer NDPP. Brit.J.Cancer 31: 81-88.

Stone,H.B. and H.R.Withers: 1975. Enhancement of the radio-response of a murine tumour by a nitroimidazole. Brit.J.Radiol. (in press).

Sutherland,R.M: 1974. Selective chemotherapy of non-cycling cells in an in vitro tumour model. Canc. Res. 34: 3501-3503.

Urtasun,R.C., J.D.Chapman, P.Band, H.Rabin, C.Fryer and J.Sturmwind: 1975. Phase 1 study of high dose metronidazole on in vivo and in vitro specific radiosensitizing of hypoxic cells. Radiology (in press).

Whitmore,G.F., S.Gulyas and A.J.Varghese: 1975. Studies on the radiosensitizing action of NDPP, a sensitizer of hypoxic cells. Rad. Res., 61: 325-341.

Withers,H.R: 1967. Recovery and repopulation in vivo by mouse skin epithelial cells during fractionated irradiation. Rad. Res. 32: 227-239.

BLEOMYCIN AND RADIOTHERAPY

J. Rygard and Hanne S. Hansen
Consultant Radiotherapists
Finsen Institute, Radium Centre
Strandboulevard 49
2100 Copenhagen, Denmark

Bleomycin, BLM, is the generic name for a group of alkaline polypeptides isolated by Umezawa (1965). BLM is a unique cytostatic, concentrating in squamous cell epithelium and its derivatives; it has no bone marrow toxicity and no immunosuppressive effect. Ichikawa's report of curative effect of BLM as the sole modality of treatment has been verified for squamous cell cancers of the head and neck by Rygård and Hansen (1975), who diminished the incidence of lung toxicity without loss of tumor effect by changing from iv to im injections in reduced intensity and total dose. The changes observed clinically in BLM sensitive tumors were similar to those seen during intensive radiotherapy: rather quick resolution of tumor often accompanied by mucositis. There is experimental evidence that BLM acts in much the same way as irradiation. The age of the cell in the reproductive cycle sensitive to BLM has been shown to be M and early S phase (Barranco 1971), whereas cells in G1 are resistant (Barranco 1973). Furthermore, Wharam (1973) showed that the addition of BLM takes the shoulder off the survival curves after irradiation, thus indicating that BLM prevents repair of sublethal irradiation damage. At the Radium Centre, BLM has been used as adjuvants to radiotherapy in 2 groups of previously untreated patients with squamous cell cancer originating in the head and neck regions. Group A: BLM during radiotherapy, DXT. Group B: BLM prior to and during the first part of DXT. The two groups of patients were treated in different periods of time and were not randomized. Group A was treated before Group B and served as a pilot examination of the degree of complications evolving from BLM given during DXT.

Vigorous mucositis, disrupting the treatment, developed in 64% of the 86 patients in Group A, with least incidence when BLM was started within the first week of DXT. The mucositis may have prognostic significance, since it developed in 81% of patients staying free of tumor without further treatment and only in 56% of those with remnant or recurrent tumor; the difference was significant at the 5% level. In Group B the incidence of mucositis was 21: with no difference between patients free of tumor and those with remnant or recurrence.

Table 1. Incidence of Tumor Free Patients at the End of Observation. Previously Untreated Patients

T Class	A. Simultaneous BLM		B. Sequential BLM	
	Tumor/ free/total	Opr. free	Tumor/ free/total	Opr. free
T 1	4/5	1	14/10	1
T 2	7/14	2	31/33	7
T 3	26/41	11	54/68	15
T 4	6/17	3	7/12	3
Other	5/9	1	5/7	-
	48/86 (56%)	18/48 (38%)	111/142 (78%)	26/111 (23%)

The results obtained in the 2 groups are shown in Table 1 for the primary tumors per se, classified according to UICC 1974. The results only concern the primary tumor itself, so that patients in the category "free of tumor" without further treatment may have died with regional or distant metastases. In spite of the series being non-randomized some of the results are outstanding in themselves. In both groups the response among T4 tumors was suprisingly good. By the simultaneous BLM treatment in Group A, 6 patients out of 17 with T4 lesions became tumor free, 3 of them without further treatment, and in Group B, 7 out of 12 became tumor free, 4 without further treatment. Likewise, patients with N3 metastases responded well. In Group A, 6 out of 11 whose primary tumor healed became free of N3 metastases, 3 without further treatment, and in Group B, 6 out of 10 became free of metastases, 5 without further treatment. In spite of no intention of substituting part of the DXT by BLM, 10 patients in the two groups together stayed free of tumor without further treatment after a cumulative radiation dose of from 1600 to 1680 reu and a mean dose of 100 mg of BLM.

A comparison of the results obtained in the two groups is made, in spite of the fact that the proportional number of patients with cancer in the different regions varied. In Group A the tumors originating in larynx and oral cavity constituted 31% and 31% against 42% and 39% in Group B. Tumors originating in pharynx constituted 24% in Group A against 14% in Group B. Also the length of observation was greater in Group A, who thus had a longer time at risk of developed recurrence. However only one patient in Group A did develop recurrence later than one year, which was the minimum length of follow up period for the patients in Group B.

For the largest groups of primary tumors, the T3, a comparison of the results obtained in Group A and B is shown in Table 2 for patients having a full course of DXT. Preoperatively treated patients are left out, as are those who did not carry through the operation and had only palliative treatment.

Table 2. Comparison of Results in T3 Tumors by Simultaneous and by Sequential BLM - DXT (1500 reu) According to Shrinkage of Tumor Prior to Irradiation

Modality of BLM adjuvants		Tumor free no further treatment	Opr. free	Dead with cancer	Tumor free / total	
A Simultaneous BLM adjuvants		15	5	13	20/33	(60%)
B. Pre + Per-irrad BLM						
Degree of Shrinkage	++	19	6	1	25/26	(96%)
	+	9	5	4	14/18	(78%)
	o	8	4	9	12/21	(59%)
Subtotal		36	15	14	51/65	(79%)

The results in Group B are shown for each of 3 subgroups according to the degree of tumor shrinkage obtained by the BLM given before the start of DXT. It is seen that in Group B the relative proportion of patients who were free of tumor at the end of observation did depend upon the shrinkage obtained prior to DXT. Among the 26 patients whose tumors shrank pronouncedly (++), 25 were free of tumor at the end of observation, and only 6 of them were operated free. This subgroup differed significantly at the 1% level from the results obtained by the simultaneous BLM treatment in Group A, whereas the patients whose tumor shrank less by the BLM given prior to DXT in Group B, did not differ significantly from the patients in Group A. In group B, 14 became tumor free of the 18 who had simultaneous BLM and DXT, and 5 had to be operated free of tumor.

The pre-irradiation BLM treatment seemed to preserve larynx in a greater proportion of the tumor-free patients than did simultaneous BLM. Thus of 11 patients with T3 supraglottic tumors in Group B, 9 became tumor free with only 1 laryngectomy against 8 tumor-free patients among 11 T3 supraglottic tumors in Group A, at the cost of 6 laryngectomies.

The lack of bone marrow toxicity and the fact that side effects from skin and hair are transient and lung toxicity rare seem to warrant BLM a place in the treatment of recurrent squamous cell cancers of the head and neck, since long lasting complete regressions are obtained in 25% of patients in this category.

The benefit of using BLM in the primary treatment as adjuvants to DXT has not been established definitely. The present series shows that the best results are obtained in tumors which are diminished pronouncedly by BLM treatment prior to DXT. It remains to be seen if the prognosis could be improved for those patients whose tumor by the present treatment did shrink but less pronouncedly, if the BLM treatment was prolonged or supplemented with vincristin as used by Frei.

EXPERIENCE WITH ICRF 159 AND RADIOTHERAPY IN COMBINATION IN THE TREATMENT OF SOFT TISSUE SARCOMAS

R.D.H. Ryall
Consultant Radiotherapist
Mersey Regional Centre for Radiotherapy & Oncology
Clatterbridge Hospital
Wirral, Merseyside L63 4JY, U.K.

INTRODUCTION

The response of soft tissue sarcomas to radiotherapy treatment is disappointing. Local recurrence of tumour within a year of irradiation occurs in 50% cases or more in most[1] published series. Haematogenous dissemination of tumour is a frequent occurrence and occurs early in the disease. Local recurrence of tumour increases the risk of blood borne metastases which are reported in 65% of such cases. However, radiotherapy has been advocated in the treatment of this group of tumours by a number of authors[2,3,4] either as an adjunct to surgery or on its own. High doses of radiation to large volumes of tissue are required if there is to be any hope of controlling the tumours.

The combination of ICRF-159 with radiotherapy was used in an individual patient with a large neurofibrosarcoma in January 1973. The rapid and impressive response of this tumour to the combination aroused immediate interest and a pilot series was undertaken, the results of which have been published elsewhere[5]. Subsequently, a prospective controlled clinical trial has been undertaken. The effect of radical radiotherapy combined with ICRF-159 being compared with radical radiotherapy alone.

TREATMENT TECHNIQUES

At the Mersey Regional Centre for Radiotherapy and Oncology we have now treated a total of 40 patients with radical radiotherapy combined with ICRF-159. 30 of these patients have soft tissue sarcomas and 10 have tumours of bone or cartilage. The ICRF-159 has been given orally in a fixed dosage of 125 mgms twice daily on the 5 radiotherapy treatment days each week. No drug was given on Saturdays or Sundays. The morning dose was given approximately 4 hours before radiotherapy. All the patients except one have received megavoltage irradiation. The dose of radiation has been the maximum compatible with normal tissue tolerance in each case, adjustments being necessary for volume of tissue irradiated and anatomical site. A dose of 5000 rads in 5 weeks was regarded as the minimum, most patients receiving 6000 rads in 6 weeks.

TOLERANCE

The drug has been well tolerated generally. Gastrointestinal symptoms, mainly anorexia and nausea were experienced by 5/40 patients. In only 2 of them were symptoms so severe that administration of the drug had to be stopped. In both these cases there was a previous history of drug intolerance and nausea, one having a hiatus hernia and the other a peptic ulcer.

Leucopenia and thrombocytopenia were not a problem. The leucocyte count falling to around 2000/cu mm in most cases and stabilising and the platelet count remaining at about 100,000/cu mm. In only one case has there been a sudden and precipitous leucopenia and this reversed at once on ceasing the drug.

Normal tissue responses, especially of the skin, to the combined treatment were reported in the results of the pilot study as being greater than would be expected with radiotherapy alone. In fact this has not been confirmed with more experience in the prospective study, where the patients can be compared with those receiving radical radiotherapy alone. To establish this we have set up a numerical scale to score the severity of the skin reactions, which are plotted against time and have failed to reveal differences between the two groups of patients. This technique is subject to individual variations of skin tolerance, field size and anatomical site. Late normal tissue reactions in patients on the combined treatment are not noticeably more severe than in those treated by radiotherapy alone.

EVIDENCE THAT ICRF-159 BEHAVES AS A SELECTIVE RADIOSENSITISER IN HUMAN TUMOURS

It has been shown that ICRF-159 potentiates the effect of radiation on tumours in experimental animals.[6] If it is proved that the drug improves the response rate of human tumours to radiotherapy without producing more normal tissue damage a selective tumour radiosensitising effect exists. Evidence is accumulating at present to suggest that this may be so in the soft tissue sarcomas. It is, however, too early to come to a definite conclusion. The accrual of these uncommon tumours is inevitably slow.

RESULTS

Only patients with soft tissue sarcomas are included in the prospective controlled trial which is a current study. An analysis of longer term follow up, of patients on study in Liverpool who have been treated for soft tissue and bone and cartilage sarcomas, with the combination of radiotherapy and ICRF-159 is presented. Table I shows that 54% of patients achieved a complete initial response, 32% a partial response with at least 50% reduction of volume and 14% showed no change.

Table II illustrates the numbers of relapses of remissions and their time scales.

In the last table (Table III) the most recent analysis of those patients in the soft tissue sarcoma prospective study is presented.

TABLE I

RTX + 159 IN SARCOMAS - LIVERPOOL

TYPE	No.Pts.	CR	PR	NC	P
BONY	4	1	2	1	-
FIBROS	11	6	3	2	-
OTHER S.T.S.	13	8	4	1	-
TOTAL	28	15	9	4	-
% of TOTAL		54	32	14	-

TABLE II

RTX + 159 IN SARCOMAS - LIVERPOOL

RESPONSE	No.Pts.	RELAPSE within - (MTHS)					NO RELAPSE within - (MTHS)				
		3	6	12	18	24+	3	6	12	18	24+
CR	15/28	-	-	-	1	-	2	2	4	2	4
PR	9/28	3	-	1	-	-	2	2	-	1	-
TOTAL (CR+PR)	24/28	3	-	1	1	-	4	4	4	3	4
RELAPSE OF REMISSIONS		5/24 (21%)					19/24 (79%)				

TABLE III

SOFT TISSUE SARCOMA

31 COMPARABLE PATIENTS

19 RT + 159
12 RT only (some at Westminster)

RESPONSE RATE

RT 3/12 - 25% CR. 4/12 - 33% PR. 3/12- 25%NC. 2-21% P.

RT + 159 9/19- 47%CR. 6/19 - 32% PR. 2/19- 10%NC. 2-10%P.

REC RATE

RT 6/12 - 50% within 1½ yrs. 5/12 within 1 yr.

RT+159 4/19 - 21% within 2 yrs.

NO RELAPSE AT 2 YEARS IN 79%.

PETO TEST. STATISTICS ARE SIGNIFICANT.
P less than 0.05 more than 0.025.

SUMMARY

Initial experience in combining radiotherapy with ICRF-159 in the treatment of sarcomas has been presented. The results are still incomplete but the early data is promising. It is hoped that further clinical study will show that this drug does have a true radiosensitising effect in humans as has been shown in animal studies.

REFERENCES

1. CANTIN.J. et al (1968). Annals of Surgery 168: 47-53.
2. WINDEYER.B.W., DISCHE.S.,MANSFIELD.C.M., (1966) Clin Radiol 17: 32-40
3. CADE.S. (1951). Proc.Roy.Soc.Med. 44:19
4. DEL REGATO.J.A. (1963). J.Amer.Med.Assn. 185:216
5. RYALL.R.D.H.,HANNAM.I.W.F., NEWTON.K.A.,HELLMANN.K., BRINKLEY.D.M. HOERTAAS O.K. (1974) CANCER 34: 1040-1045
6. HELLMANN.K.,MURKIN.G. (1974) CANCER 34: 1033-1039

METRONIDAZOLE (FLAGYL) IN CANCER RADIOTHERAPY

J.L. Foster+ and R.L. Willson*

+Cancer Research Campaign, Gray Laboratory
Mount Vernon Hospital, Northwood, Middlesex, U.K.
*Biochemistry Department, Brunel University
Uxbridge, Middlesex, U.K.

The radiosensitising activity of a wide assortment of oxidising (sometimes termed "electron affinic" or "electrophilic") compounds is now well known. Although they were originally chosen for study for a variety of reasons and have been subsequently somewhat arbitarily divided into particular groups, they have many properties in common. Indeed, all the compounds listed below, and many related compounds, rapidly oxidise organic radicals and many also react rapidly with sulphydryl groups.

<u>Examples of Oxidising ("Electron affinic") Radiosensitisers</u>

Dyes	FLUORESCEIN	Mottram, 1929
	TRYPAN BLUE	Russ and Scott, 1935.
Respiratory Poisons	IODOACETATE	Franks, Shaw & Dickson, 1934
Mitotic Inhibitors	SYNKAVIT (metabolite)	Mitchell, 1948
Paramagnetics	NITRIC OXIDE	Howard-Flanders, 1957
Sulphydryl Reagents	N-ETHYL MALEIMIDE	Bridges, 1960
Conjugated Carbonyls	DIACETYL	Adams & Dewey, 1963
Stable free radicals	DI t.BUTYL NITROXIDE	Emmerson & Howard Flanders, 1964
Complexing metals	COPPER ION	Cramp, 1965
Nitrobenzenes	p-NITROACETOPHENONE	Asquith, Adams & Willson, 1970
Nitrofurans	NITROFURAZONE	Reuvers, Chapman & Borsa, 1972
Nitroimidazoles	METRONIDAZOLE (Flagyl)	Foster & Willson, 1973

Although such studies date back to the 1920's, or earlier, it appears that until recently few compounds of this type have warranted more than a passing interest from the radiotherapist : some are too toxic, others pharmacologically too unstable, others would also sensitise normal tissue.

The recent interest shown by clinicians in metronidazole (Flagyl) has therefore been particularly stimulating and in the time available we would like to elaborate the reasons why Flagyl was originally chosen for study, briefly discuss how it works and present evidence which indicates that in addition to its radiosensitising activity it also has a chemotherapeutic action which could be of considerable clinical value.

WHY FLAGYL ?

In 1972 in the course of a literature search for potential radiosensitisers that were pharmacologically and toxicologically more favourable than those in vogue at the time, our attention was drawn to an article in the May and Baker Bulletin by Dr. J. A. McFadzean entitled "Metronidazole - a review". It was immediately apparent that the drug would probably be of considerable use as a radiosensitiser of hypoxic cells because:-

a) its chemical formula contained a nitro-group
b) it had been widely used clinically, was well tolerated, was rapidly absorbed and a significant percentage was excreted in the urine unchanged

plus c) it was highly toxic to anaerobic but not aerobic microorganisms.

NITRO-GROUP AND RADIOSENSITISATION

The importance of the nitro-group was based on the fact that of all the "electron affinic" radiosensitisers studied, to our knowledge only those containing a nitro-group appreciably sensitised mammalian cells in culture under hypoxic and not under oxygenated conditions. The importance of the nitro-group had also been appreciated by Chapman and colleagues who in consequence had screened various nitrofuran derivatives used for urinary tract infections and had found them to be particularly active *in vitro*. (Raleigh et al 1973, Reuvers et al 1972). It had been proposed that sensitising drugs reacted rapidly with organic free radicals (Willson and Emmerson 1970): pulse radiolysis studies had shown that many nitro compounds such as nitrobenzene and the radiosensitiser p.nitroacetophenone did react rapidly.

Radiosensitisation studies with Flagyl in bean roots, bacteria mammalian cells *in vitro* and *in vivo* progressed rapidly. (Chapman et al 1973, Asquith et al 1973, Asquith et al 1974, Thomson and Rauth 1974, Hall and Chapman 1974, Sutherland 1974, Rauth and Kaufman 1975, Denekamp et al 1974, Denekamp and Harris 1975). Distinct therapeutic advantages gained by administering Flagyl to tumour bearing animals prior to radiation treatment have now been demonstrated: enhancement ratios of 1.2-1.3 have been recorded. (Stone and Withers 1974, Begg et al 1974, Brown 1975). For example in one study following a dose of 4,000 rads only 50% of the mammary tumours of the normal group of animals but over 90% of a group dosed with Flagyl 30 mins before irradiation, were cured (Begg et al 1974).

PHARMACOLOGY AND TOXICOLOGY

Many of the early compounds screened for hypoxic cell activity *in vitro* were unsuitable for extensive study *in vivo* because of their poor pharmacological and toxicological properties. An active drug had to be metabolised slowly relative to its rate of transport to the hypoxic foci of a tumour. Tissue culture studies with Flagyl suggested that for a noticeable therapeutic gain *in vivo*, drug concentrations in the blood of the order of 170 μg per ml would be required. Subsequent pharmacological studies in mice showed that levels of this order could be readily maintained following oral administration (Asquith et al 1974).

It was estimated from published pharmacological data that in man drug levels of the order of 0.2g/kg body weight would need to be administered orally, a dose much higher than the 200 mg t.i.d. normally given for Trichomonad infestations. However, attempted suicides had taken place with doses of this order (Fluker 1961, Lewis and Kenna, 1965) and with the well documented clinical experience of the drug, preliminary clinical studies were begun in Canada and at Mt. Vernon Hospital, Northwood (Urtasun et al 1974, 1975, Deutsch et al 1975).

In summary, results indicate that a dose of 0.2g/kg body weight resulting in serum concentrations of 200 μg/ml could be given 3 x per week for 2 weeks in situations where a clinical gain might be anticipated. As the drug is slowly metabolised with a half-life of approximately 10 hrs. ample time is available for radiation treatment from standard equipment.

Possible contra-indications for the use of Flagyl at high doses which have required consideration are: a) nausea, vomiting, abdominal pain and transient leucopenia reported for man, (b) brain damage observed in dogs but not in other species including primates, (c) mutagenicity observed with bacteria and (d) carcinogenicity reported in rodents. It is considered that of these only nausea and vomiting provide any real drawback to the use of Flagyl at the dose regime suggested for radiotherapy. An increased occurrence of spontaneous tumours in mice given Flagyl has been described, but in this and in a further study in rats where no increased incidence was observed, the number of animals were small and the incidence of tumours in the control group was high (Rustia and Shubik 1972, Cohen et al 1973). The mutagenic effects of Flagyl were observed in experiments in which bacteria were incubated with the drug under conditions where there was a high probability that the oxygen tension was very low (Voogd et al 1974, Legator et al 1974). Since the deleterious effect of Flagyl, as we will discuss later, can be attributed to a toxin which is inactivated by oxygen, mutagenicity is probably unimportant with respect to normally oxygenated cells *in vivo*. In recent studies with rats given 1g/kg Flagyl for 4 days no significant changes in various liver parameters or white cell count were observed relative to control groups although there was a two-fold increase in the weight of the caecum (Eakins et al 1975). Such enlargements are well known in germ-free animals and in animals treated with particular drugs and are probably unimportant in the current context. However, they are associated with marked disturbances in the ecology of the gastrointestinal flora and with changes in the reducing capacity of the intestinal contents. Interestingly, this has led to a possible insight into the mechanisms of the drug's radiosensitising and chemotherapeutic action.

HOW FLAGYL ?

We now believe that at least 3 general types of mechanism may be involved in the hypoxic radiosensitising action of Flagyl :

a) reaction with free radicals.
b) reaction with natural protective agents.
c) formation of an oxygen 'inactivated' toxin under hypoxia (a similar toxin can also be formed biochemically in the absence of radiation which may be useful chemotherapeutically).

a) free radical reactions: like other nitro compounds discussed earlier, Flagyl has been shown to react rapidly with free radicals and may sensitise by increasing the probability of free radical-induced damage (Willson et al 1974a, Willson et al 1974b)

b) reaction with natural protective agents: studies with suspension of rat intestinal contents containing Flagyl showed that the drug's nitro group could be rapidly reduced under hypoxic but not aerated conditions ($t_{\frac{1}{2}} \sim 10$ mins.). Later studies showed that some iron complexing agents and sulphydryl binding agents also lowered the rate of reduction suggesting that an iron-sulphur complex may be involved in its metabolism.

It had been previously found that Flagyl and other nitro-radiosensitisers such as p.nitroacetophenone did not react rapidly, if at all, with sulphydryl compounds suggesting that these compounds did not sensitise by lowering the cells' ability to chemically repair radiation-induced free radical lesions.

In view of the results with the rat intestinal contents it was decided to investigate the possible catalytic effect of iron salts on this reaction. In the presence of ferrous iron the reaction of Flagyl with the sulphur-containing amino acid cysteine was found, in fact, to be very rapid, half-lives for the initial interaction between the drug and an iron-sulphur complex of approximately 1 second being recorded. Other results indicate that faster reactions may occur with other nitro-radiosensitisers. Indeed, for the analogous interaction with oxygen half-lives of $\sim$10 milliseconds have been observed. The rapidity of the reaction can be readily demonstrated by preparing a solution containing 200 mls of water, 1g cysteine hydrochloride, 0.1 g ferrous sulphate and 10 mls of 1M KOH in a 500 ml bottle. A violet colour appears, disappears and rapidly returns on shaking to subsequently decay again (Mathews and Walker 1909, Willson and Searle 1975).

We consider that rapid iron-linked reactions of this type may be of considerable importance in sensitisation generally.

c) formation of an oxygen 'inactivated' toxin: the interaction of iron in haemoglobin with a free radical formed on the reduction of nitrobenzene was suggested as far back as 1948 to explain the compound's toxic action in causing methaemoglobinemia (Huebner 1948). The bactericidal action of some nitrofurans (McCalla et al 1970) and of metronidazole on anaerobic microorganisms has been suggested to be due to a toxic intermediate formed on reduction. Recently it was found that radiation-reduced Flagyl binds to nucleic acid *in vitro* in hypoxic but not in oxygenated conditions. (Willson et al 1974b). We believe these results, together with the recent evidence of a chemotherapeutic action of Flagyl described below, strongly indicate that an important mechanism of the drug's action is through the formation of a reduced toxin, probably RNOH• or a related radical which reacts with a vital molecule in the presence of iron. The toxin is inactivated by oxygen, hence no damage to normal tissue results.

HYPOXIC CHEMOTHERAPEUTIC EFFECT (NO RADIATION)

Flagyl is well known for its ability to kill anaerobic but not aerobic microorganisms at concentrations of ~1 μg per ml. It has also been found to be toxic to *E.coli* B/r when incubated under nitrogen. (Cramp unpublished). Recent results now indicate an analogous selective cytocidal action in mammalian systems which could provide an additional method of overcoming the hypoxic tumour cell problem. An increased rate of cell loss from murine sarcomas has been observed when animals were given Flagyl (Begg et al 1974). The drug has also been shown to selectively kill non-cycling mammalian cells in spheroid culture (Sutherland 1974). Results of a recent experiment in which the days of death were recorded for groups of mice injected i.p. with 4×10^6 Ehrlich ascites cells are shown below. The cells had been previously incubated under hypoxia in the absence of presence of Flagyl (Conroy, Searle and Willson unpublished).

Incubation (hours)	Flagyl (mM)	Day of death	Mean
0	0	18,18,19,21,21	19.4
	10	18,19,20,21,21	19.8
2	0	20,20,22,22,23	21.4
	10	21,22,22,24,24	22.4
4	0	19,23,23,24	22.3
	10	22,48,54,54,56	46.8
6	0	13,21,24,24,24	21.2
	10	> 60	> 60

Clearly incubation under hypoxia in the presence of Flagyl leads to a considerable decrease in the number of viable cells injected: after 6 hours insufficient cells remain to cause death of the animal within 60 days. Below are also shown the percentages of mice originally bearing carcinomas that show no sign of tumour 60 days after radiation treatment. One group was given 0.3 mg per kg of Flagyl for 36 hours at 6-hourly intervals. The tumours were irradiated 6-8 hours after the last drug dose. Whilst this is a preliminary result and further tumours will undoubtedly recur before 130 days when results are usually assessed, it is clear that the cure rate of the Flagyl treated group is likely to be significantly higher than that of the controls. This particular tumour is thought to contain some 10% hypoxic cells as estimated from tumour regrowth data (Denekamp and Harris 1975). Since the Flagyl blood level at the time of irradiation was less than 30 μg per ml we conclude that the increase in cure rate is principally due to a hypoxic chemotherapeutic effect on the drug in the absence of radiation.

X-ray dose (rads)	% controlled at 60 days	
	X-rays only	X-rays + Flagyl
4450	-	57(4/7)
4750	7(1/15)	89(8/9)
5050	11(1/9)	100(7/7)
5350	37(3/8)	91(10/11)

Further experiments of this type are in progress. However, the evidence to date indicating that Flagyl has a chemotherapeutic effect as well as a radiosensitising effect on hypoxic cells is sufficient to warrant serious consideration in the design of any clinical trial in which it is used as an adjunct in radiotherapy. It may well be beneficial to treat the patient with Flagyl for several days before, as well as immediately before, radiation therapy. Modification of established radiation fractionation schemes due to its intolerance of the high drug doses required for radiosensitisation, may be unnecessary if the drug is also used as a chemotherapeutic agent.

Preliminary clinical trials using Flagyl as a radiosensitiser are in progress in Canada (Urtasun et al 1974,1975). Others are under consideration in this country. No increase in normal tissue damage has so far been detected. It is probable that other compounds will subsequently be shown unequivocally to offer greater therapeutic promise in man. However, any anticipated increased sensitising and/or chemotherapeutic activity will have to be balanced against possible unfavourable pharmacological and toxicological properties and the possibility of an effect on normal oxygenated tissue. For nitrocompounds in particular, a marked increase in oxidising properties may lead to a more active drug *in vitro* but in total it may be clinically less favourable.

At the present time we believe that Flagyl provides an acceptable compromise between these effects. Since stationary cells are relatively resistant to cytotoxic drugs, the possibility that Flagyl may also be a useful adjunct in chemotherapy is particularly exciting.

References

Adams, G.E. and Dewey, D.L.(1963) Biochem.Biophys.Res.Comm.12,473.

Asquith,J.C., Willson,R.L.and Adams,G.E. (1970) 4th Int.Cong. Radiation Research,Evian, France.

Asquith,J.C.,Foster,J.L.and Willson,R.L.(1973) Brit.J.Radiol.46,648.

Asquith,J.C.,Foster,J.L.,Willson,R.L.,Ings,R.M.J. and McFadzean, J.A. (1974) Brit.J.Radiol., 47,474.

Begg,A.C.,Sheldon,P.W.,and Foster,J.L.(1974) Brit.J.Radiol.47,399.

Bridges,B.A. (1960) Nature 188, 415.

Brown,J.M. (1975) Radiat.Res., in the press.

Cohen,S.M.,Erturk,F.,Von Esch,A.M.,Crovetti,A.J. and Bryan, G.T. (1973) J.Nat.Cancer Inst.,51,403.

Cramp, W.A. (1965) Nature 206, 636.

Denekamp,J.D. and Harris, S.R. (1975) Radiat.Res.,61, 191.

Denekamp,J.D.,Michael,B.D.and Harris,S.R.(1974) Radiat.Res.60,119.

Deutsch,G., Foster, J.L., McFadzean,J A. and Parnell,M.(1975) Brit.J.Cancer 31,75.

Eakins,M.,Conroy,P.,Searle,A.F.J.,S ater,T.F. and Willson, R.L. (1975) to be published.

Emmerson,P.T. and Howard-Flanders,P. (1964) Nature 204, 1005.

Fluker,J.L. (1961) Brit.J.Vener.Dis.36, 280.

Foster,J.L. and Willson,R.L. (1973) Brit.J.Radiol. 46,234.

Franks,W.R.,Shaw,M.M.and Dickson,W.H.(1934) Am.J.Cancer 22, 601.

Hall,G.J. and Chapman,J.D. (1974) Brit.J.Radiol. 47, 513.

Howard-Flanders, P. (1957) Nature 180, 1191.

Huebner (1948) Arch.Exp.Path.Pharmac.,205,310.

Legator,M., Connor,T., and Stoeckel,M. (1974) Proc.XI Int.Cancer Cong.Florence. Excerpta Medica, Elsevier Americal, p.77.

Lewis,B.V. and Kenna,A.P.(1965) J.Obst.and Gynaec.Brit.Comm.72,806.

Mathews,A.P. and Walker,S. (1909) J.Biol.Chem.,6,299.

McCalla,D.R.,Reuvers,A.and Kaiser,C.(1970)J.Bact., 104, 1126.

Mitchell,J.S. (1948) Brit.J.Cancer 2, 351.

Mottram, J.C. (1929) Brit.Med.Journ. p.149.

Raleigh,J.A., Chapman,J.D., Borse, J., Kremers, W. and Reuvers, A.P. (1973) Int.J.Radiat.Biol., 23, 377.

Rauth, A.M. and Kaufman, K. (1975) Brit.J.Radiol. 48, 209.

Reuvers, A.P., Chapman, J.D. and Borsa, J. (1972) Nature 237, 402.

Russ, S. and Scott, G.M. (1935) Proc.Roy.Soc. 118, 316.

Rustia,M. and Shubik, P.J. (1972) J.Nat.Cancer Inst. 48, 721.

Scharer, K. (1972) Verh.Dtsch.Ges.Path. 56, 407.

Stone, H.B. and Withers, H.R. (1974) Radiology 113, 441.

Sutherland, R.M. (1974) Cancer Research 34, 3501.

Thomson, J.E. and Rauth, A.M. (1974) Radiat.Res. 60, 489.

Urtasun, R.C., Chapman, J.D., Band, P., Rabin, H., Fryer, C. and Sturmwind, J. (1975) Radiology, in the press.

Urtasun, R.C., Sturmwind, J., Rabin, H., Band, P.R. and Chapman, J.D. (1974) Brit.J.Radiol. 47, 297.

Voogd, C.E., Van der Stel, J.J. and Jacobs, J.J.J.A.A. (1974) Mutation Res. 26, 483.

Willson, R.L. and Emmerson, P.T. (1970) in Radiation Protection and Sensitisation (Moroson and Quintiliana eds.) Taylor and Francis, London p.73.

Willson, R.L., Gilbert, B.C., Marshall, P.D.R. and Norman, R.O.C. (1974a) Int.J.Radiat.Biol. 26, 427.

Willson, R.L., Cramp, W.A. and Ings, R.M.J. (1974b) Int.J.Radiat. Biol. 26, 557.

Willson, R.L. and Searle, A.J.F. (1975) Nature 255, 498.

POSSIBILITIES OF THE HUMAN TUMOUR/NUDE MOUSE SYSTEM IN CANCER CHEMOTHERAPY RESEARCH

Carl O. Povlsen

University Institute of Pathological Anatomy

Juliane Mariesvej 16, Copenhagen
DK-2100 Denmark

Nude mice suffering from congenital thymus aplasia will regularly accept transplants of human malignant tumours. Tumours grow locally and metastases have not been observed. Serial growth has been obtained for up to 53 generations during a 5 year period. The human nature of these tumours is preserved as judged by microscopic appearance, chromosome analyses, isozyme patterns and demonstration of antihuman antibodies in sera of tumour bearing mice.
Cancer chemotherapeutic assays in the human tumour/nude mouse system have shown a pattern of drug susceptibility of the mouse grown tumours which is in accordance with experiences from clinical practice. The possibilities for practical application of this model in testing the sensitivity of individual human tumours for various cancer chemotherapeutic agents will be discussed.

CHEMOTHERAPY OF TRANSPLANTABLE COLON TUMOURS IN MICE

John A. Double

Department of Experimental Pathology and Cancer Research

University of Leeds, School of Medicine, Leeds. LS2 9NL

A series of transplantable mouse adenocarcinomas of the colon (MAC) have been developed from primary tumours induced by dimethylhydrazine. The tumours are all moderately to well differentiated and retain their histological appearance and growth characteristics through successive generations. The tumour lines were originally obtained by transplanting whole tumour nodules from the colons of donor mice subcutaneously, in syngeneic mice, and in this way we obtained several lines from a succession of transplant attempts. It is interesting to note the longer the donor animals were left following cessation of the dimethylhydrazine treatment the more successful were the attempts at obtaining transplantable lines. This is illustrated in Table 1 and probably reflects the progression toward greater malignancy with time observed by Haase et al., (1). A protocol for determining the chemosensitivity of the tumours has been developed, and to date eleven standard drugs have been tested, and from the results it would appear that the model has considerable disease specificity.

The histopathology of the tumour lines has already been described (2), but one line, MAC 13, is characterised by large cysts occupying up to 40% of the tumour volume, and it was thought that this might present a complication in evaluation of chemotherapy effects, in that false positive antitumour action might be seen if the drug simply decreased the production of cystic fluid, however, preliminary morphometric analysis of the cystic space in treated and control groups from chemotherapy experiments showed no such drug induced alteration with agents studied so far.

Table 1

Transplantation of DMH induced colon tumours

Group	No. injections*	Age of donors	Take rate	Tumour line	Present transplant generation (1. 7. 75)
A	17	27	0/6	-	-
B	17	33-36	1/33	MAC 7	6
C	17	45-49	6/37	MAC 10	10
				MAC 13	20
				MAC 14	12
				MAC 15	21
				MAC 41	4
				MAC 59	14

TOTAL TAKE RATE 7/76

* 15mg/kg dimethylhydrazine sub-cutaneously at weekly intervals

Table 2

Characteristics of tumour lines

Line	'Growth rate' (weeks)	Approx. volume doubling time (days)	'Mucin'	Labelling index
MAC 7	16	n. d.*	-	n. d.
MAC 10	6	7	+	21
MAC 13	3	4	+++	12
MAC 14	8	10	+	19
MAC 15	3	5	++	24

*not determined

Some characteristics of five of the lines are shown in Table 2. "Growth rate" is the time in weeks for a fragment implant to grow to a 5 x 5 mm nodule. Volume doubling times have been estimated from growth curves established using caliper measurements. Pulse tritiated thymidine labelling indices for four tumours are shown and have a similar range to those observed in colo-rectal tumours in man (3). These preliminary measurements of course give little insight into the cell kinetics of this type of tumour. More detailed analyses are complicated by the complex morphological structure of each tumour. For example preliminary morphometric analysis of MAC 15 shows 34% of its volume is occupied by tumour cells, 29% by connective tissue cells and 26% is acinar fluid containing space. The mitotic index of the tumour cell population was 1.1%. Semicontinuous tritiated thymidine label (11 injections at 4-hourly intervals) has shown the growth fraction of this tumour to be around 90%. Clearly, since the labelling index is 24%, and the volume doubling time 5 days, there must be considerable cell death in the tumour populations.

It is seen from Table 2 that the lines MAC 13 and MAC 15 are the two fastest growing and the majority of the chemotherapy studies have been carried out on these two lines.

In early experiments size changes in both control and treated groups of tumours were followed by caliper measurements at 3 or 4 day intervals. Volumes were calculated in the standard manner and related to the volume of the individual tumours at the start of the experiments to give a 'relative tumour volume'. The results of a typical experiment, with single dose treatment with 5-fluorouracil, are shown in Figure 1. It was seen that over a limited range, control curves were exponential (Figure 1a) and from this plot volume doubling times were obtained. Although it was possible to evaluate therapeutic effects by the drug induced delay in tumours reaching a certain size (Figure 1b) this procedure requires frequent caliper measurements and is difficult to quantitate. However, the growth characteristics observed in these experiments enabled us to develop a simpler protocol based on tumour weight measurements. Survival time experiments were not practical as large tumours tended to ulcerate through the skin.

The primary problem in establishing statistically sound protocols for this type of tumour system is that using fragment implants for transplantation, tumour load in the fragment is variable and as a result the size range of tumours growing in large groups transplanted at the same time is quite wide. Using tumour homogenates for transplantation did not appear to overcome this problem and had the added disadvantage that continual passage in this way might induce dedifferentiation. From growth curves it was clear that growth rates in a group of tumours were closely similar even when their absolute sizes has a significant range. Also it was observed that

Table 3

Chemotherapy results

Drug	Schedule	Maximum tolerated dose (mg/kg)	Tumour inhibition*	
			MAC 13	MAC 15
5-fluorouracil	q.d. x 5	40	+	-
Cyclophosphamide	single	450	+	++
Methotrexate	q.d. x 5	4.5	-	-
Mitomycin C	single	6.7	+	-
BCNU	single	56	++	-
CCNU	single	40	++	+
Me-CCNU	single	30	+	+
Vincristine	single	2.6	-	-
Adriamycin	single	8	-	-
Melphalan	single	12	-	-
Chlorambucil	single	30	-	-

* Tumour inhibition at Maximum tolerated dose

-; <65% tumour inhibition

+; >65% but less than 90% inhibition

++; >90% tumour inhibition

in a group of transplanted animal tumours sizes were approximately a normal distribution. A method was established to select tumours (by caliper measurements) from a transplanted group such that the median volume was about 150 mm^3 and the volume range less than five-fold. Eighty-five to ninety per cent were selected by this means, randomised and treated the same day in the chemotherapy test. The control groups had fifteen mice and treated groups eight. The 95% confidence limits of the control tumour group, selected in this way with a five-fold size range, indicated that the % T/C of a treated group has to be <35% (i.e. >65% inhibition) before it is statistically significant.

So that the results for different tumour lines would be assessed by similar criterion, it was decided that all experiments would

Table 4

Chemotherapy Results

Tumour line	MAC 10	MAC 13	MAC 14	MAC 15	MAC 59
FU	-	+	+	-	+
MeCCNU	+	+	-	+	+
Cyclophosphamide	-	+	-	+	n. d.

n. d. - not determined

\- - no significant effect

\+ - significant inhibition at MTD or less

be terminated, and the tumours excised and weighed, when the control had increased ten times in volume from the start of the experiment. All tests consisted of three drug dose groups with 1.5 fold dose spacing (eg. 40, 60, 90 mg/kg) such that the top dose had some toxicity. The maximum tolerated dose (MTD) was defined as the maximum dose at which no animals died and in which weight loss at day 5 post-treatment did not exceed 15%. Although dose response curves were carried out in this way, in most cases significant anti-tumour action was only seen at maximum tolerated dose. Lower doses were ineffective, reflecting the general insensitivity of both tumour lines to chemotherapy. Tumour inhibition results are therefore, for clarity, presented for the maximum tolerated dose only (Table 3). In only three drug-tumour combinations out of 22, was there significant therapeutic effect at a dose lower than MTD - for cyclophosphamide against both lines, and for CCNU against MAC 13.

If we are considering the possible value of tumour lines of this type as secondary screening systems to select drugs for colo-rectal disease, it is possible to view cur results in at least two ways. In Table 3, the most clinically effective drugs are in the upper half of the table, the dividing line from inactivity being around the level of CCNU. It is important to note that no positive results were obtained amongst the four clinically inactive drugs tested. Clearly we must test more negative drugs to confirm that the tumours have a real pedictive value. It is also seen that some agents, (eg. FU) do not inhibit both tumours. This point is illus-treated in Table 4 on preliminary tests of five tumour lines for

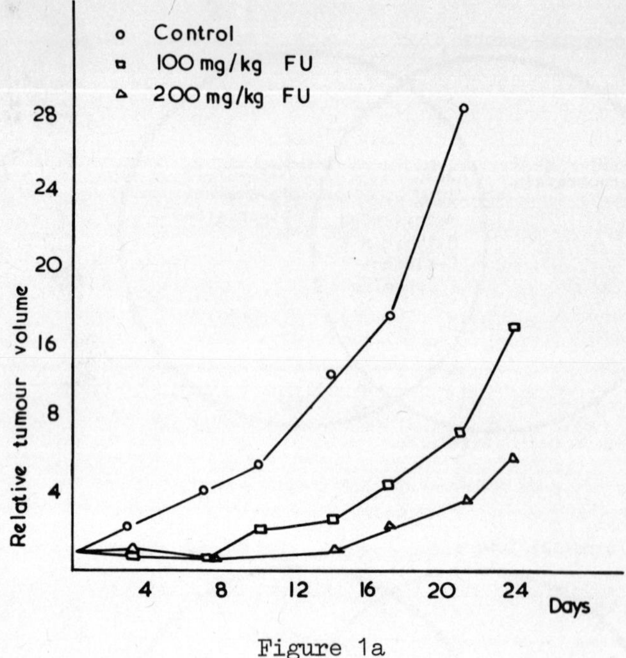

Figure 1a

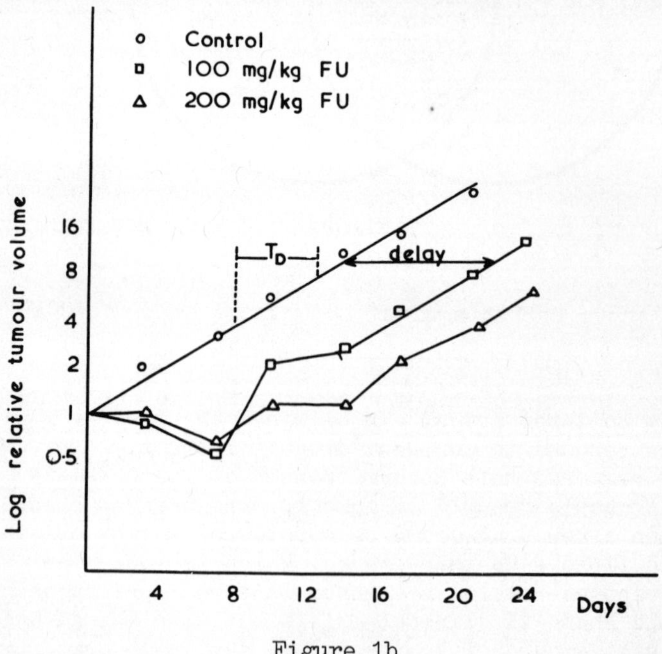

Figure 1b

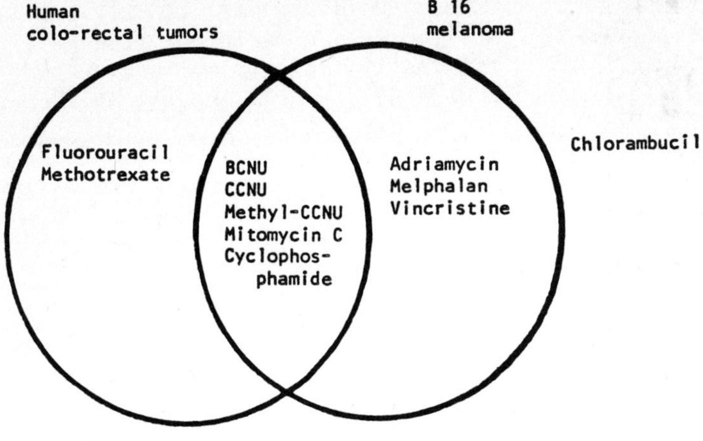

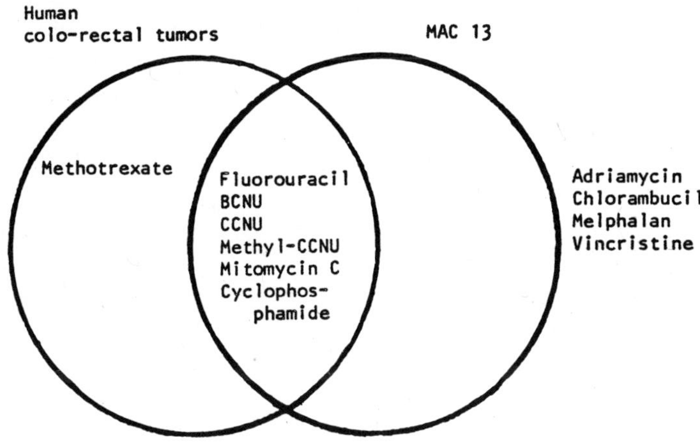

Figure 2

sensitivity to three drugs. In clinical practice no more than 25% of patients respond to our best drugs. There similarly will be a percentage response rate in our "panel" of mouse tumours (eg. 3/5 for FU), if such a "panel" of tumours were used as a screening system, then a new drug could be considered worthy of examination if it could improve on this figure, which is equivalent to the clinical response rate. In essence this would be an animal equivalent of the Phase II clinical trials but with the advantage of using the same groups of "patients" to test each new drug.

Although this way of looking at the data clearly raises the question of whether it is valid to use on tumour line as a screening syste, if we examine the data on our most sensitive line, MAC 13, and compare the results from the B16 Melanoma, which has been introduced as a secondary screen in an attempt to isolate better drugs for solid tumour therapy it can be seen in Figure 2, that as far as colo-rectal tumours are concerned, the MAC system is a far more efficient screen on the current results. Each tumour is represented by a circle and the drugs with activity against that tumour placed within the circle. The B16 would make five false predictions our of eleven had it been used for large bowel cancer, the line MAC 13, only one - a flase negative - Methotrexate.

Only 11 out 29 standard drugs have been tested so far, and by single dose schedules, but results indicate that these tumour lines may have some value as secondary screening systems in the search for drugs active against large bowel cancer. An extension of this type of analysis for the remaining drugs and comparisons with the effects of new drugs in Phase II clinical trials would establish whether a screening system of this type would be superior to those currently used.

UTILIZATION OF NITROSAMINE-INDUCED TUMORS AS MODELS FOR CANCER CHEMOTHERAPY*

D. Schmähl

Institut für Toxikologie und Chemotherapy am

Deutschen Krebsforschungszentrum, Heidelberg

Chemotherapeutic studies on transplanted tumors have only little relevance for the cancer in man. The reason for this is first the biological differences between transplanted tumors and autochthonous tumours, and second, that the malignant tumors in man are of autochthonous character. It is not surprising, therefore, that positive chemotherapy findings in rats on transplanted tumors (2) first carried out in the 1950's, were later proved to be unsuccessful when used as therapy for human cancer. It is well known that in rats and mice a great number of transplanted tumors can be cured today by various chemotherapeutic agents, whereas malignant tumors in man are mostly resistant to chemotherapy or are only partially responding. Therefore, for the last few years we have tried to use chemically-induced autochthonous tumors (predominantly in rats) in chemotherapeutic studies (1, 4, 7-12). These tumors appear to be ideal test models because most of the human tumors are also considered to be induced by chemical carcinogens (12). The following essentials are required for the use of autochthonous animal tumors in chemotherapeutic studies:

a) the tumor must be reproducible in high yield and if possible should be developed in only one organ (unilocular occurrence);
b) the tumors must occur at almost the same time in all animals (use of inbred strains);
c) the tumors must be diagnosable in time;
d) a chemotherapeutically untreated control, as large as possible, is particularly important.

*Dedicated to Professor Huggins (Chicago) on the occasion of his 75th birthday.

Since at the present stage of experimental chemotherapy we cannot expect complete cure, the prolongation of life-span of treated animals as compared to the untreated controls serves as the decisive parameter for the chemotherapeutic efficiency.

In principle, all substances with marked organotropy of the carcinogenic effect are suitable to induce autochthonous tumors by chemical carcinogens. N-nitroso compounds appear to be a particular interesting group in this connection because they have relatively organospecific effects and are able to induce high yields of tumours (3). In table 1 I have listed the most essential data, which is based on my personal experience, for the induction of such tumors in rats of the BD- and Sprague-Dawley-strain. Besides N-nitroso compounds, there are some other substances regarded to be able to induce malignomas well-suited for chemotherapeutic studies, which cannot be easily produced by nitroso compounds.

Now I will report our practical experiences in tumor diagnosis and the design of experiments. Since all tumors do not occur simultaneously the animals have to be examined twice weekly during the critical induction period, and those animals bearing tumors at random are to be integrated into the experimental groups and control.

Local fibrosarcomas induced by 3,4-benzpyrene can be detected easily by palpation of the site of injection. We start the chemotherapy at a tumor weight of $\simeq$2g and kill the rats when the tumors are $\simeq 3\frac{1}{4}$g in weight. If left untreated the tumors develop to this weight after $\simeq$5 weeks. The determination of tumor growth and plotting of growth curves can be done initially by means of respective plastic reproductions (having the same specific weight as the tumors) and later on by personal experience during the palpation process.

Carcinomas of the ear duct induced by 4-dimethyl-aminostilbene can be detected most readily by palpation of the angles of mandible, where the tumour growth can be seen initially by small, solid bulgings. In most cases the animals show a decrease in weight. This is the point of time to start the therapy. When left untreated some of the carcinomas show monstrous forms after 4-6 weeks. The histological examination predominantly shows keratinised squamous cell carcinomas.

Adenocarcinomas of the breast, which frequently occur multilocularly, can be induced in female Sprague-Dawley rats by 9,10-dimethyl-1,2-benzanthracene. Besides carcinomas there frequently occur fibroadenomas which in most cases can be distinguished easily from carcinomas (solid, grown together with the substratum) by palpation. We start the treatment at a tumor weight of $\simeq$2g and take into account only the growth of the module diagnosed first, that means, we do not consider the growth of mammary carcinomas developing during or after the therapy.

Table 1: Chemically-induced autochthonous malignomas in rats suitable for chemotherapy studies

substance	mode of application	daily dose mg/kg body wt.	induction time days	type of tumors	incidence %	diagnosis
3,4-benz-pyrene	s.c.	6 (one time)	90-140	local fibrosarcoma	> 90	palpation
4-dimethyl-amino-stilbene	orally	1,5	350-400	carcinoma of the ear duct	>90	palpation
9,10-dimethyl-1,2-benz-anthracene	i.v.	8^{+}	60-120	mamma carcinoma	>90	palpation
diethyl-nitrosamine	orally	3	150-210	hepatoma	>90	palpation
phenyl-ethyl-nitrosamine	orally	1	180-250	carcinoma of the oesophagus	>80	X-rays, control of body weight
acetoxy-methyl-methyl-nitrosamine	orally	2	160-200	carcinoma of the forestomach	>90	operation and inspection X-rays
methyl-acetyl-nitroso-urea	orally	2	400-500	carcinoma of the glandular stomach	>90	operation and inspection X-rays
butyl-butanol-nitrosamine	orally	10	350-450	carcinoma of the urinary bladder	>90	operation and inspection haematuria
ethyl-nitroso-urea	dia-placentally i.v.	30^{++} (one time)	170-230	brain glioma peripheral neurilemmoma	>90	neurological symptoms
methyl-vinyl-nitrosamine	inhalation	2^{+++}	250-300	carcinoma of the para-nasal sinus	>80	inspection

+ = injected in female Sprague-Dawley-rats on day 48, 50 and 52 of life

++ = injected in pregnant rats on day 19 of pregnancy; tumors arising in the offsprings

+++ = inhalation twice weekly

Diethylnitrosamine-induced hepatomas are detected by palpation of the epigastrium, after the animals have been starved for 24 hours. If a resistance is palpated and scybala or the right kidney can be excluded, it must be a tumor of the liver. In the diagnosis of such tumors the personal experience plays a decisive role. Here, as well as in the following cases the treatment is started immediately after diagnosis.

Early diagnosis of oesophagus carcinomas is most difficult. These tumors can be detected only by x-ray examination (5). The tumor growth frequently is indicated by a decrease in weight. These tumors can be used as test models, if one has the necessary radiodiagnostic facilities and experience (6).

Carcinomas of the stomach can be similarly detected by x-ray examination, but we also detect those with laparotomy during the critical induction period and exact inspection of the stomach walls from outside. For that purpose the animals have to be starved sufficiently long (12 hours). In the thin gastric walls small tumorous changes can be mostly detected without difficulty. The same applies to external inspection of the urinary bladder after laparotomy. In this case the beginning of the tumor growth can also be indicated by hematuria.

Tumors of the central or peripheral nervous system can be frequently detected relatively early by the respective neurological symptoms, the type and appearance of which depends on the tumor localization. This type of diagnosis requires considerable practical experience.

The diagnosis of tumors of the paranasal sinus, however, is relatively easy. These tumors can be indicated by bulgings of the nasal region as well as by secretion and sometimes bleeding from the nose.

The 10 autochthonous tumor types of the rat presented in this lecture are suitable, in principle, for all chemotherapeutic studies. The amount of work involved is of course much higher than in working with transplanted tumors, and it is unavoidable that in some cases relatively advanced tumors have to be treated. This disadvantage however, applies to the experimental groups as well as to the control in the same way. Similarly, the treatment of advanced tumors in animal experiments is also comparable with the realities in human cancer treatment, where frequently the tumors are treated only in advanced stages.

In my lecture I did not mention the nitrosamine-induced autochthonous rat leukemia. We are at present investigating this model, but have still some methodical difficulties. Therefore we cannot recommend this leukemia for routine investigations. I think that in about one year we will be able to report on this.

As I have pointed out in my present lecture the success of chemotherapeutic studies in autochthonous tumours depends on the practical experience of the investigator in the field of chemical carcinogenesis. A close connection between these two working fields is therefore necessary. Chemically-induced, autochthonous animal tumours should be used more than before in chemotherapeutic studies since these finding are of great significance for the treatment of human cancer.

REFERENCES

1. Brune, H., Henning, S., Schmähl, D. Der Einfluß von Glukokortikoiden auf das Wachstum und die chemotherapeutische Beeinflußbarkeit autochthoner Benzpyren-Sarkome bei Mäusen Z. Krebsforschung 72, 213-218 (1969).

2. Druckrey, H., Schmähl, D., Dischler, W. Endgültige Heilung großer Yoshida-Sarkome durch N-oxyd-Lost. Dtsch. med. Wschr. 83, 489-492 (1958).

3. Druckrey, H., Preussmann, R., Ivankovic, S., Schmähl, D. Organotrope carcinogene Wirkungen bei 65 verschiedenen N-Nitroso-Verbindungen an BD-Ratten. Z. Krebsforschung 69, 103-137 (1967).

4. Fretz, J., Rohde, D., Schmähl, D., Thomas, C. Therapieversuche am autochthonen Mamma-Carcinom der Ratte Arzneimittelforschung 19, 1291-1293 (1969).

6. Bürkle, G. Fortschr. Röntgenstrahlen (in press).

5. Burkle, G. Möglichkeiten röntgendiagnostischer Untersuchungen und therapeutische Perspektiven bei chemisch induzierten Tumoren Fortschr. Röntgenstrahlen 122, 352-364 (1975).

7. Schmähl, D., Schrick, G., König, K. Chemotherapie-Versuche an Hepatomen. Arzneimittelforschung 13, 370-371 (1963).

8. Schmähl, D. Wert und Gefahr der Krebs-Chemotherapie. Dtsch. med. Wschr. 88, 1463-1468 (1963).

9. Schmähl, D., Osswald, H., Brune, H. Chemotherapieversuche mit Endoxan an autochthonen Benzpyren-Sarkomen bei Ratten und Mäusen. Z. Krebsforschung 68, 293-302 (1966).

10. Schmähl, D., Osswald, H., Brune, H. Einfluß von Dosis und Tumorgröße für das Ansprechen autochthoner Benzpyren-Sarkome bei Ratten und Mäusen auf chemotherapeutische Behandlung mit Endoxan. Z. Krebsforschung 70, 246-251 (1968).

11. Schmähl, D. Autochthone Tiertumoren als Testmodelle für Krebs-Chemotherapeutika. Mitteilungen der Deutschen Pharmazeutischen Gesellschaft 40, 173-175 (1970).

12. Schmähl, D. Entstehung, Wachstum und Chemotherapie maligner Tumoren, 2nd Edition 1970, Editio Cantor Aulendorf.

THE PRODUCTION OF OSTEOLYTIC SUBSTANCES BY HUMAN BREAST TUMOURS

G.C. EASTY, T.J. POWLES, M. DOWSETT, D.M. EASTY AND A.M. NEVILLE
Unit of Human Cancer Biology, London Branch, Ludwig Institute for Cancer Research and Royal Marsden Hospital Fulham Road, London, England.

Patients with cancer of the breast frequently develop abnormalities of calcium metabolism which sometimes result in death. These abnormalities are usually associated with osteolytic bone metastases and are mainly caused by excessive mobilisation of skeletal calcium. This raises the possibility that the mobilisation of skeletal calcium and erosion of bone to provide space for tumour growth may depend on the production of osteolytically active substances either by tumour cells or as a result of interactions between tumour and host cells.

In order to investigate this phenomenon in human breast cancer we have used a bioassay system for osteolytic activity based on that developed by Reynolds (1968) in which neonatal mouse bones labelled with radioactive calcium *in vivo* are maintained in organ culture, and the effects of agents which can stimulate calcium release from bones are detected by measuring the quantities of radioactive calcium left in bones and released into the culture medium. Such a system will reproducibly detect nanogram amounts of osteolytically active substances such as parathyroid hormone or prostaglandins.

Using this bioassay, we have examined over 60 samples of breast cancer removed from patients at operation and found that about 60% of them had significant osteolytical activity, while all benign tumours of the breast and uninvolved regions were quite inactive. We were impressed with a number of similarities between rheumatoid arthritis and osteolysis associated with bone metastases, and as aspirin and indomethacin are widely used for treatment of rheumatoid arthritis, we decided to investigate its effectiveness on our *in vitro* tumour-associated osteolysis. Both agents were found to be quite ineffective in inhibiting calcium release, indomethacin being about 100 to 1,000 times more active than aspirin. It was also observed that these agents were only effective if they were added to the medium in which the breast tumours were maintained at the beginning of the culture. If they were added to the medium after culturing, they were almost completely ineffective, implying that they were inhibiting the synthesis or release of osteolytically active substances by the tumour tissue.

It was obviously desirable to have an in vivo system in order to ascertain whether or not the in vitro observations were relevant to an animal or human situation. We had previously established that the osteolytic activity of the Walker rat tumour cells in vitro could be inhibited by non-toxic concentrations of aspirin and indomethacin, and this tumour in the form of a cell suspension was therefore injected intra-aortically into 300g rats, resulting in the growth of extensive tumour in both hind limbs, significant hypercalcaemia, and considerable erosion and loss of calcium from the distal ends of both femurs and the proximal ends of the tibias, giving four sites of bone erosion which could be detected by X-ray analysis or xeroradiography. Daily force feeding with aspirin or indomethacin from the day of tumour cell injection, or beginning one week after tumour cell injection resulted in complete abolition of bone erosion and hypercalcaemia, but was without significant effect on the quantity of soft tissue tumour. The in vivo effects of the drugs were therefore comparable with the in vitro effects in that they appeared to affect the metabolism of the tumour and inhibit its osteolytic capacity but did not significantly influence tumour proliferation.

As aspirin and indomethacin are anti-inflammatory drugs which are considered to act mainly by their ability to inhibit the synthesis of prostaglandins by cells, investigations of the identity of the osteolytic substances produced by human tumours were directed towards the search for prostaglandins. Extraction of the medium in which tumours have been cultured by ether at neutral pH has never yielded an active factor, but if the pH of the medium is adjusted to pH 3.5 and then extracted with ether, variable amounts of activity have been extracted and subsequently identified as prostaglandins PGE and PGF. In very few cases has all the osteolytic activity of the tumours been identified as prostaglandins, and we have recently isolated a high molecular weight, non-dialysable factor(s), which is almost certainly a protein. It should, perhaps, be emphasised that inhibition of osteolytic activity by indomethacin does not necessarily identify the factor as a prostaglandin as we have recently observed that the highly osteolytically active enzyme, collagenase, is almost completely inhibited by indomethacin and we have obtained some evidence that it acts by stimulating prostaglandin synthesis within the bone cells.

The extension of these observations to human tumours other than those of the breast has recently been made by Robertson and Baylink (1975) who found that patients with renal and lung carcinomas had elevated levels of prostaglandin E in their plasma, and that treatment of some patients who had hypercalcaemia and elevated plasma prostaglandin levels with aspirin or indomethacin decreased the levels of calcium and prostaglandins in the blood.

Similarly, Seyberth *et al* (1975) have measured the quantities of prostaglandin metabolites in the urine of patients with cancer and hypercalcaemia, and have successfully reduced the levels of urinary prostaglandin metabolites and plasma calcium by treating the patients with aspirin or indomethacin.

A much wider role for tumour-derived prostaglandins than bone erosion and hypercalcaemia has recently been suggested by the work of Plescia *et al* (1975) and Strausser and Humes (1975) who observed some inhibition of the growth rates of mouse tumours by treating the animals with aspirin or indomethacin, and Plescia *et al* obtained some evidence that prostaglandins may act as immunosuppressants, thus facilitating tumour growth.

References

Reynolds, J.J. (1968). *Proc. Roy. Soc. B*. *170*, 61

Robertson, R.P. and Baylink, R. (1975). *Clin. Res*. *23*, 329A

Seyberth, H.W., Morgan, J.L., Sweetman, B.J. and Oates, J.A. (1975). *Clin. Res*. *23*, 423A

Plescia, O.J., Smith, A.H. and Grinwich, K. (1975). *Proc. Nat. Acad. Sci. U.S.A*. *72*, 1848

Strausser, H.R. and Humes, J.L. (1975). *Int. J. Cancer*, *15*, 724

THE BIOLOGICAL BASIS OF COMBINATION CHEMOTHERAPY

Abraham Goldin

National Cancer Institute

Bethesda, Maryland 20014, U.S.A.

The biological rationales employed to increase antitumor specificity with combination chemotherapy are reviewed here.

I. Increased antitumor effectiveness relative to host toxicity: Combinations of drugs have been selected for investigation on the basis that: a) they are effective individually; b) they exert differing qualitative toxicities or pharmacologic activities; c) they act via differing biochemical mechanisms. For a series of chemotherapeutically synergistic drug combinations the host toxicity of the drugs was usually less than additive, thereby permitting the use of higher total dosage (Schabel 1975). An example in which a combination of drugs exerted therapeutic synergism involves methotrexate (MTX) plus 1,3-Bis-(2-chloroethyl)-1-nitrosourea (BCNU) (Venditti et al. 1965) in the treatment of systemic leukemia L1210. Over a series of dosage ratios the increase in survival time with the drug combination was considerably greater than that for the drugs individually. Here too the host toxicity of the drugs was less than additive, permitting a higher total dosage. Cyclophosphamide plus melphalan or thioTEPA are highly synergistic combinations in the treatment of leukemia L1210 (Johnson et al. 1975; Schabel et al. 1975), arguing for the further investigation of congeners.

Rationales for obtaining classical synergism in which the summation of activity with respect to a single parameter such as host toxicity or antitumor effect exceeds that observed for the drugs individually, usually have a biochemical basis. Types of multiple biochemical blockade may be listed (a) sequential blockade in which two drugs act at separate loci in a series of biochemical transformations (Potter 1951). Sequential blockade resulting in therapeutic synergism for leukemia L1210 was observed with hydroxyurea, 5-hydroxypicolinaldehyde thiosemicarbazone or guanazole as inhibitors of ribonucleotide reductase (Krakoff et al. 1968; Sartorelli et al. 1969; Brockman et al. 1970a; Brockman et al. 1970b) plus cytosine arabinoside as an inhibitor of DNA polymerase (Furth and Cohen, 1968). (b) Concurrent blockade (Elion et al. 1954) in which two alternate metabolic pathways must both be blocked to prevent product formation. (c) Complementary inhibition (Sartorelli and Booth 1967; Sartorelli and Creasey 1973; Sartorelli 1974) involves the combination of one agent which inhibits the biosynthetic pathway to a macromolecular structure (DNA, RNA, protein) with an agent that directly damages the macromolecular polymeric target. An example would be a combination of an antimetabolite to inhibit purine or pyrimidine nucleotide biosynthesis plus an alkylating agent that damages DNA directly (Sartorelli 1974). (d) The combination of mutagens with drugs that cause a deficiency of thymine deoxyribonucleotides may lead to error amplification (Sartorelli and Creasey 1973; Sartorelli 1974).

Consideration of multiple biochemical blockade mechanisms must take into account the inhibitory action for the host as well as the tumor. Synergistic action against tumor must not be accompanied by proportionate limiting damage to the host.

II. Decreased host toxicity with retention of antitumor effect: Examples of this include MTX plus delayed administration of citrovorum factor (Goldin et al. 1955), cytosine arabinoside plus 6-thioguanine (Schmidt et al. 1970), ICRF-159 plus daunomycin (Woodman et al. 1972), N-acetylcysteine plus iphosphamide (Kline et al. 1972; Goldin et al. 1973; Venditti and Goldin 1974). In all of these instances because of reduced host toxicity it was possible to employ higher dosages of the active drugs.

III. Identification of optimal dosages and dosage ratios: The dosages employed with drug combinations may influence therapeutic effectiveness. Also, the utilization of optimal ratios may improve the therapeutic outcome. With BCNU plus MTX (Venditti et al. 1965) maximum therapeutic synergism against leukemia L1210 was observed with no reduction in optimal dose for MTX but a 50 percent decrease in optimal dose for BCNU. With MTX plus 5-fluorouracil optimal therapy resulted with optimal dosage of MTX and markedly reduced levels of 5-fluorouracil (Kline et al. 1966a).

IV. Determination of optimal scheduling: Scheduling may influence the results with combination chemotherapy. Schedule dependency with combinations of drugs was observed with the combination of 6-mercaptopurine plus azaserine in the treatment of leukemia L1210. For this combination, treatment every two days was optimal for obtaining therapeutic synergism (Goldin et al. 1958). MTX daily plus cyclophosphamide weekly was more effective than MTX daily plus cyclophosphamide daily in increasing the survival time of leukemic animals (Venditti and Goldin 1964). The sequence of drug administration may alter the therapeutic response. Therapeutic synergism for leukemia L5178Y was observed with MTX treatment on days 3-7 followed by L-asparaginase on days 10-14. The reverse sequence provided no therapeutic advantage (Vadlamudi et al. 1972).

V. Delay in origin and treatment of tumor cell resistance: Combination chemotherapy may delay the origin of spontaneous or drug-induced resistant mutants and permit improved therapeutic response once resistance has occurred. For example, treatment with cytosine arabinoside plus cyclophosphamide delayed the appearance of resistance to cytosine arabinoside by at least two transplant generations (Goldin and Johnson 1975).

VI. Treatment of metastatic disease including sequestered tumor: Combinations of drugs may provide a basis for the treatment of metastatic and sequestered tumor cells. BCNU and cytosine arabinoside are therapeutically synergistic against leukemia L1210 and this has been attributed at least in part to their ability to cross the blood-brain barrier (Kline et al. 1966b). BCNU plus cytosine arabinoside was therapeutically synergistic against intracranial leukemia (Tyrer et al. 1967). Cyclophosphamide plus methyl-CCNU elicited therapeutic synergism against advanced Lewis lung carcinoma in which there was bronchial metastasis (Mayo et al. 1972).

VII. Kinetic considerations: Tumor cell synchronization may be employed to therapeutic advantage. Vinblastine and also colcemid have been employed to synchronize leukemia L1210 cells and therapeutic synergism was observed when cytosine arabinoside was administered at the time the cells were traversing S-phase (Vadlamudi and Goldin 1971). Therapeutic synergism may occur with drugs that stimulate G_0 cells to divide to increase tumor cell susceptibility to a second drug active during the cell cycle.

VIII. Loading dose chemotherapy of advanced disseminated tumor: A loading dose regimen of one drug may reduce the body burden of tumor cells sufficiently so that the second drug may become highly effective. By reducing the tumor cell population it may increase the proportion of actively dividing cells, thereby making them more sensitive to a cell cycle specific agent. Examples of therapeutically synergistic loading dose protocols against leukemia L1210 may be cited (Straus and Goldin 1972; Goldin 1973).

IX. Combined modalities: (a) Surgery may be employed to reduce the body burden of tumor cells and this reduction plus an increase in the pool of actively dividing cells may markedly improve drug effectiveness. Surgery plus cyclophosphamide (Karrer et al. 1967) and surgery plus cyclophosphamide plus methyl-CCNU (Mayo et al. 1972) have proven to be more effective than surgery alone or chemotherapy alone in the treatment of Lewis lung carcinoma. (b) There has not been extensive investigation at the preclinical level with the combined modality of radiation plus chemotherapy. In one study (Johnson 1964) it was observed that whole body radiation plus chemotherapy with cyclophosphamide was more effective than either modality alone for leukemia L1210. (c) There is considerable interest in immunochemotherapy. Non-specific immunostimulants such as BCG or Corynebacterium parvum have been employed alone and in conjunction with chemotherapy (Fisher et al. 1970; Pearson et al. 1972; Bast et al. 1974). Adoptive immunochemotherapeutic approaches are receiving current attention such as with the transplantable Moloney leukemia (LSTRA) in BALB/c mice. In one study (Glynn et al. 1969) treatment with cyclophosphamide followed by inoculation of specifically sensitized allogeneic spleen cells yielded marked increases in survival time. The immunogenicity of tumor cells may be altered by treatment _in vitro_ with substances such as neuraminidase (Simmons and Rios 1971) or _in vivo_ by administration of antitumor agents such as DIC (Bonmassar et al. 1970). Such alteration of tumor cell immunogenicity may result in collateral sensitivity to chemotherapy (Law et al. 1954; Hutchison 1963; Venditti and Goldin 1964; Mihich 1967). A variety of sublines of leukemia L1210 resistant to various antitumor agents showed immunocollateral sensitivity to BCNU (Nicolin et al. 1972). Active and passive immunization procedures have also been attempted.

X. _Drugs that assist active compounds_: Drugs may be investigated to prevent detoxification, maintain blood and tissue levels, improve penetration to target tumor sites, or otherwise increase concentration and time of tumor cell exposure to active drugs. Drugs may be sought that will prevent immunosuppressant action of antitumor agents.

XI. _Antiviral plus antitumor agents_: Where there is a viral etiology of tumor, drugs may be sought that act against tumorigenic virus, viral induction of tumor or reinduction, to be employed in conjunction with antitumor agents.

XII. _Polychemotherapy_: Methodology has been developed for the investigation of three-drug combinations (Goldin et al. 1968) but has not been used extensively. Very few studies have been conducted at the preclinical level with combinations of four or more drugs.

In summary it may be stated that there is extensive animal data, as well as clinical data, showing that combination chemotherapy may provide a considerable advantage in the therapeutic outcome in the cancerous patient.

REFERENCES

1. Bast, R.C., Jr., Zbar, B., Borsos, T. and Rapp, H.J. (1974), New England J. Med., 290, 1413.
2. Bonmassar, E., Bonmassar, A., Vadlamudi, S. and Goldin, A. (1970), Proc. Natl. Acad. Sciences, 66, 1089.
3. Brockman, R.W., Shaddix, S., Laster, W.R., Jr. and Schabel, F.M., Jr., (1970a), Cancer Res., 30, 2358.
4. Brockman, R.W., Sidwell, R.W., Arnett, G. and Shaddix, S. (1970b), Proc. Soc. Exp. Biology, New York, 133, 609.
5. Elion, G.B., Singer, S. and Hitchings, G.H. (1954), J. Biol. Chem., 208, 477.
6. Fisher, J.C., Grace, W.R. and Mannick, J.A. (1970), Cancer, 26, 1379.
7. Furth, J.J. and Cohen, S.S. (1968), Cancer Res., 28, 2061.
8. Glynn, J.B., Halpern, B.L. and Fefer, A. (1969), Cancer Res., 29, 515.
9. Goldin, A. (1973), Cancer Chem. Rep., 4, 189.
10. Goldin, A., Humphreys, S.R., Venditti, J.M. and Mantel, N. (1958), Ann. N.Y. Acad. Sci., 76, 932.
11. Goldin, A. and Johnson, R.K. (1975), Excerpta Medica International Congress, Series No. 353, 5, Proc. XIth Int. Cancer Cong., Florence, Italy, 1974, 308.
12. Goldin, A., Venditti, J.M., Humphreys, S.R., Dennis, D. and Mantel, N. (1955), Cancer Res., 15, 742.
13. Goldin, A., Venditti, J.M., Mantel, N., Kline, I. and Gang, M. (1968), Cancer Res., 28, 950.
14. Goldin, A., Venditti, J.M. and Mantel, N. (1973), Handbook of Experimental Pharmacology, Antineoplastic and Immunosuppressive Agents, Berlin, Springer-Verlag, 411.
15. Hutchison, D.J. (1963), Advances in Cancer Research (edited by A. Haddow and S. Weinhouse), 7, 235.
16. Johnson, R.E. (1964), J. Natl. Cancer Inst., 32, 1333.
17. Johnson, R.K., Kline, I., Venditti, J.M. and Goldin, A. (1975), Proc. Amer. Assoc. Cancer Res., 16, 75.
18. Karrer, K., Humphreys, S.R. and Goldin, A. (1967), Internatl. J. of Cancer, 2, 213.
19. Kline, I., Gang, M. and Venditti, J.M. (1972), Proc. Amer. Assoc. Cancer Res., 13, 29.
20. Kline, I., Venditti, J.M., Mead, J.A.R., Tyrer, D.D. and Goldin, A. (1966a), Cancer Res., 26, 848.
21. Kline, I., Venditti, J.M., Tyrer, D.D., Mantel, N. and Goldin, A. (1966b), Cancer Res., 26, 1930.
22. Krakoff, I.H., Brown, N.C. and Reichard, P. (1968), Cancer Res., 28, 1559.
23. Law, L.W., Taormina, V. and Boyle, B.J. (1954), Ann. N.Y. Acad. Sci., 60, 224.
24. Mayo, J.G., Laster, W.R., Jr., Andrews, C.M. and Schabel, F.M., Jr. (1972), Cancer Chem. Rep., 56, 183.

25. Mihich, E. (1967), Proc. of the 5th International Congress of Chemotherapy, (edited by K.H. Spitzy and H. Haschek), Wiener Medizinischen Akademie, Vienna, 3, 327.
26. Nicolin, A., Vadlamudi, S. and Goldin, A. (1972), Cancer Res., 32, 653.
27. Pearson, J.W., Pearson, G.R., Gibson, W.T., Chermann, J.C. and Chirigos, M.A. (1972), Cancer Res., 32, 904.
28. Potter, V.R. (1951), Proc. Soc. Exp. Biol. Med., 76, 44.
29. Sartorelli, A.C. (1974), Biochemical Pharmacology, 23, Supplement 2, 129.
30. Sartorelli, A.C. and Booth, B.A. (1967), Cancer Res., 27, 1614.
31. Sartorelli, A.C., Booth, B.A. and Moore, E.C. (1969), Proc. Amer. Assoc. Cancer Res., 10, 76.
32. Sartorelli, A.C. and Creasey, W.A. (1973), Cancer Medicine, (edited by J.F. Holland and E. Frei, III), Philadelphia, Lea and Febiger, 707.
33. Schabel, F.M., Jr. (1975), Pharmacological Basis of Cancer Chemotherapy, The Williams and Wilkins Co., Baltimore, Md.,595.
34. Schabel, F.M., Jr., Laster, W.R., Jr., Trader, M.W. and Witt, M.H. (1975), Proc. Amer. Assoc, Cancer Res., 16, 24.
35. Schmidt, L.H., Montgomery, J.A., Laster, W.R., Jr. and Schabel, F.M., Jr. (1970), Proc. Amer. Assoc. Cancer Res., 11, 70.
36. Simmons, R.L. and Rios, A. (1971), Science, 174, 591.
37. Straus, M.J. and Goldin, A. (1972), Cancer Chem. Rep., 56, 19.
38. Tyrer, D.D., Kline, I., Venditti, J.M. and Goldin, A. (1967), Cancer Res., 27, 873.
39. Vadlamudi, S. and Goldin, A. (1971), Cancer Chem. Rep., 55,547.
40. Vadlamudi, S., Subba Reddy, V.V. and Goldin, A. (1972), Proc. Amer. Assoc. Cancer Res., 13, 31.
41. Venditti, J.M. and Goldin, A. (1964), Advances in Chemotherapy, Volume 1, Academic Press Inc., New York, 397.
42. Venditti, J.M. and Goldin, A. (1974), Biochemical Pharmacology, 23, Supplement 2, 141.
43. Venditti, J.M., Kline, I., Tyrer, D.D. and Goldin, A. (1965), Cancer Chem. Rep., 48, 35.
44. Woodman, R.J., Kline, I. and Venditti, J.M. (1972), Proc. Amer. Assoc. Cancer Res., 13, 31.

COMBINATION CHEMOTHERAPY OF ADVANCED GASTROINTESTINAL CARCINOMA

Allan J. Schutt and Charles G. Moertel

Mayo Clinic and Mayo Foundation

Rochester, Minnesota USA

In most areas of the world the annual incidence of gastrointestinal cancer is greater than that of any other organ system. It is estimated that 102,000 Americans will die of gastrointestinal cancer in 1975 (1).

FLUORINATED PYRIMIDINE THERAPY

Since its introduction 17 years ago, 5-Fluorouracil (5-FU) has been the only widely accepted chemotherapeutic agent for advanced gastrointestinal cancer. Early reports in the English literature claimed objective regression rates in gastrointestinal cancer with 5-FU therapy which varied from 85 to 8%.

We define objective tumor response as a 50% or more decrease in the product of the two longest diameters of the most clearly measurable area of tumor, no increase in size of known areas of malignant disease, no new areas appearing, and a response lasting two months or more. Our controlled studies have been stratified so primary indicator lesions, patient performance status, and presence or absence of previous chemotherapy are equally represented in each treatment group.

Despite trials of numerous dosage schedules and routes of administration we have found that 5-FU produces only partial tumor regression, usually for 15-20% of the patients without increasing patient survival at any stage of the disease. The Central Oncology Group has reported that 5-FU given by loading course produces a regression rate superior to weekly injections (2). Several randomized, controlled comparisons of oral and intravenous routes have demonstrated that the IV route produces a significantly higher incidence of tumor regression and a longer duration of regression. (Table 1)

In the search for other agents of value in the treatment of advanced gastrointestinal cancer we have observed many interesting toxicological patterns. Unfortunately no single drug has been found which exceeds or even equals the limited activity of 5-FU.

COMBINATION CHEMOTHERAPY

In view of the success of combination chemotherapy in other malignant disease increased attention has been more recently given to trials of this approach in advanced gastrointestinal cancer.

Colorectal Carcinoma

Single agents which we have found to have therapeutic activity in large bowel cancer are listed in Table 2. Our initial attempts at combination chemotherapy of advanced large bowel cancer were quite disappointing (Table 3). Only 5-FU and Mitomycin C equaled the activity of 5-FU alone, while the other combinations were less active.

The nitrosoureas (BCNU, CCNU, and Methyl CCNU) combine well with 5-FU at about 75% of the full dose of each agent. At this dose of 5-FU less mucocutaneous toxicity is observed. The bone marrow suppression of the nitrosoureas is delayed until after that of 5-FU.

In 1974 Professor Geoffrey Falkson and his co-workers in Pretoria (3) reported a 43% response rate of colorectal cancer treated with a four drug combination utilizing 5-FU, BCNU, Dimethyl imidazole carboxamide, and Vincristine compared to 25% with 5-FU alone. This is the only report of significant activity in colorectal cancer with a combination including 5-FU and BCNU.

Table 1
5-FU Therapy
Randomized, Controlled Comparisons of Oral and IV Routes

Schedule	Group	Pts.	Objective Response Rate IV	Objective Response Rate Oral
Weekly	Western	190	24%	13%
Loading → weekly	Central	136	39%	18%
Intense Course	Mayo	100	26%	13%
		426	29%	14%
				($p<0.001$)

Table 2
Chemotherapy of Colorectal Carcinoma
Single Agents with Therapeutic Activity

Agent	No. of Patients	Objective Response Rate at 2 Months (%)
5-Fluorouracil	359	17
FUDR, rapid IV	147	22
Mitomycin C	69	12
ICRF-159	25	12
CCNU	75	9
BCNU	69	10
Methyl CCNU	38	18

Methyl CCNU seems to be more active and has the advantage of oral administration. Table 4 summarizes our controlled trial and that of the Southwest Oncology Group with 5-FU plus Methyl CCNU combinations compared to 5-FU alone in advanced colorectal carcinoma. In our study despite a statistically significant difference in regression rate with combination therapy, patient survival was not significantly enhanced. Our current controlled study is evaluating the role of Vincristine in this combination.

Gastric Carcinoma

Table 5 lists the single agents we have found to demonstrate significant activity against advanced gastric carcinoma. In our initial studies with 5-FU and a nitrosourea combination we found 5-FU plus BCNU to yield high regression rates in a small number of advanced stomach cancers. In a larger controlled study (comparing the combination to each drug used alone) objective regressions

Table 3
Chemotherapy of Colorectal Carcinoma
Combination Chemotherapy

Regimen	No. Pts.	Objective Response Rate at 2 months (%)
Actinomycin D + Cyclophosphamide	11	0
5-FU + BCNU	25	4
5-FU + BCNU + Mitomycin C	22	5
Sequential CCNU + 5-FU	28	7
BCNU + Mitomycin C	25	8
5-FU + Mitomycin C	23	17

Table 4
Controlled Trials of 5-FU - Methyl CCNU Combinations in Advanced Colorectal Cancer

Investigating Group	Regimen	Pts.	Objective Response Rate %	
Mayo Clinic	5-FU* + Methyl CCNU + VCR	39	43	
	5-FU* alone	41	19	$p<0.05$
Southwest Oncology Group	5-FU** + Methyl CCNU	128	30	
	5-FU** alone	36	14	$p<0.05$

* 5-FU given by intensive course
** 5-FU given by weekly schedule

occurred in 41% (14 of 34) of advanced gastric cancers with a median duration of 7 months. A substantial increase in long-term survivors was observed. At 18 months 26% of patients treated with 5-FU plus BCNU were alive compared to 9% with BCNU alone, 7% with 5-FU alone and 7% in untreated patients. More recent studies have utilized Methyl CCNU in combination with 5-FU. In a preliminary report (6) using 5-FU by intensive course the Eastern Cooperative Oncology Group reported a 52% response rate to 5-FU plus Methyl CCNU combination in advanced gastric carcinoma compared to 13% with Methyl CCNU alone. Median survival times were 27 weeks (combination) and 14 weeks (Methyl CCNU alone). Both response rate and survival duration reached statistical significance at the $p<0.05$ level.

Table 5
Chemotherapy of Advanced Gastric Carcinoma
Single Agents

Regimen	No. of Pts.	Objective Response at 2 months	Duration (median, months)
5-FU	72	19 (26%)	4.5
BCNU	33	6 (18%)	4.0
Adriamycin	14	5 (36%)	5.0
Mitomycin C	11	3 (27%)	2.7

Pancreatic and Hepatocellular Carcinomas

In our controlled study 5-FU alone produced only very brief (median duration 2.5 months) objective regressions in 16% (5 of 31) of patients with advanced pancreatic carcinoma. No regressions were seen in the 21 patients who received BCNU alone. Combination of 5-FU plus BCNU yielded a 33% (10 of 30) objective regression rate but no significant increase in survival.

We have noted objective responses in 37% of (7 of 19) patients with primary hepatocellular carcinoma treated with 5-FU plus BCNU. Three of these patients have had extraordinarily long lasting total regression (3, 4, and 6 years).

Gastrointestinal Endocrine Carcinomas

Islet cell carcinoma of the pancreas has proved to be among the most responsive to chemotherapy of all gastrointestinal cancers. In cumulative experience Streptozotocin has produced objective regression in 37% of patients and functional improvement in 64%. (7) Streptozotocin can be combined with 5-FU in full dose of both drugs. This combination produced objective regressions in 6 of the first 8 patients we treated compared to 3 of 6 treated with Streptozotocin alone.

Objective responses of metastatic carcinoid tumors to 5-FU were observed in 40% (6 of 15) of patients treated. Regression rates in carcinoid tumors to Streptozotocin alone (3 of 6) and in combination with 5-FU (7 of 9) are similar to rates observed in islet cell carcinoma. Clinically the responses in islet cell carcinoma are more dramatic (particularly relief of hormone hypersecretion syndromes).

Discussion

The more active combination chemotherapy regimes for gastrointestinal cancer have now produced objective regression rates of 30 to 52% in several hundred patients. For colorectal carcinoma the combination of 5-FU with Methyl CCNU seems most favorable. For upper gastrointestinal cancer (stomach, pancreas, and liver) combinations utilizing 5-FU plus either BCNU or Methyl CCNU have produced similar activity, and three consecutive studies of the combinations have shown objective response rates superior to the single component drugs. Two of these studies have demonstrated substantially prolonged survival of gastric carcinoma patients. This is the first well-documented improvement in the chemotherapy of advanced gastrointestinal cancer in nearly 20 years. Still it must be recognized that while combination 5-FU and nitrosourea therapy appears hopeful, only about half these patients benefit and these only transiently. Our current recommended dose is Methyl CCNU 130 mgm/m^2 in a single oral dose on day 1, 5-FU 325 mgm/m^2 by rapid IV injection days 1 through 5 and 5-FU alone, 375 mgm/m^2 on days 36 through 40. The entire cycle is commenced again on day 71 with dose modifications if excessive toxicity is experienced.

Controlled surgical adjuvant studies of these combinations are currently underway in several large cooperative groups. Until any positive benefit has been proven in these experimental settings, patients resected for cure should not be routinely exposed to the expense, morbidity and possible carcinogenic risks of combination nitrosourea and 5-FU therapy.

REFERENCES

1. Third National Cancer Survey, National Cancer Institute: Cancer Statistics, 1975. CA 25:8-21, 1975.

2. Ansfield, F. J.: A Randomized Phase III Study of Four Dosage Regimens of 5-Fluorouracil. Proc. Am. Ass. Cancer Res. 16:224, 1975.

3. Falkson, G., Van Eden, E. G., and Falkson, H. C.: Fluorouracil, Imidazole Carboxamide Dimethyl Triazeno, Vincristine, and Bis - Chlorethyl Nitrosourea in Colon Cancer. Cancer 33:1207-1209, 1974.

4. Moertel, C. G., Schutt, A. J., Hahn, R. G., and Reitemeier, R. J.: Therapy of Advanced Colorectal Cancer with a Combination of 5-Fluorouracil, Methyl - 1, 3 - Cis (2-Chlorethyl) -1- Nitrosourea, and Vincristine. J. Natl. Cancer Inst. 54:69-71, 1975.

5. Baker, L. H., Matter, R., Talley, R., Vaitkevicius, V.: 5-FU vs. 5-FU and MeCCNU in Gastrointestinal Cancers. Proc. Am. Ass. Cancer Res. 16:229, 1975.

6. Moertel, C. G., and Hanley, J. A.: Phase II-III Studies in Chemotherapy of Advanced Gastric Cancer. Proc. Am. Ass. Cancer Res. 16:260, 1975.

7. Broder, L. E., and Carter, S. K.: Pancreatic Islet Cell Carcinoma: Results of Therapy with Streptozotocin in 52 Patients. Ann. Int. Med. 79:108-118, 1973.

COMBINATION CHEMOTHERAPY IN BREAST AND LUNG CANCER

C.G. Schmidt

Department of Medical Oncology

University of Essen, Essen, West Germany

It is now well established that chemotherapy can exert a significant degree of palliation in women with advanced breast cancer lesions. Secondary drug therapy is ultimately required in most women with disseminated breast cancer. Alkylating agents, antimetabolites, vinca alkaloids, cytostatic antibiotics and miscellaneous agents have been used either as single drugs or in more modern combination regimes.

TABLE 1: Results of single drug chemo. in advanced br. ca.

	No. of patients	CR +PR
Alkylating agents		
Cyclophosphamide (Endoxan)	165	31.5%
Nitrogen Mustard	92	35%
Melphalan	86	23%
Thio-TEPA	162	30%
Chlorambucil	54	20%
Antimetabolites		
5-Fluorouracil	1052	29%
Methotrexate	259	33%
Vinca-Alkaloids		
Vincristine	164	20%
Vinblastine	95 (Carter '72)	20%
Tumor-Antibiotics		
Adriamycin	345	37%

Table 1 summarizes the results of single drug treatment in advanced breast cancer. Adding complete and partial remissions, it is quite obvious that the results obtained with alkylating agents and the antimetabolities are reaching remission rates of about 30% while the vinca alkaloids are less active. Adriamycin is the most important tumour antibiotic with a remission rate of 37%.

The alkylating agentswere the first group of non-hormonal chemotherapeutic agents shown to be effective in the treatment of metastatic carcinoma of the breast. Cyclophosphamide (Cytoxan, Endoxan) has been most extensively investigated and is generally regarded to be the alkylating agent of choice. This compound is available in both parenteral and oral formulations and has been used in a wide variety of dosage schedules. Other alkylating agents such as nitrogen mustard, thio-TEPA and chlorambucil are of less importance and not so widely used. Daily administration has resulted in an overall response rate of 35%, although this varies widely between investigators from a low rate of 10% to a high rate of 62%. This large variation in response rates among various investigators occurs for all the agents discussed and is due to several factors such as patient selection, intensity of treatment, definition of response and definition of the study population.

Other alkylating agents, for instance phenylalanine-mustard (Melphalan, Alkeran) and Chlorambucil (Leukeran) have been used with response rates no better and perhaps a bit less than cyclophosphamide. However, the total number of patients are far less than the group treated with cyclophosphamide.

Antimetabolites: 5-Fluorouracil has been most extensively studied, and was introduced in the treatment of breast cancer by Ansfield and co-workers. Its testing has been on a five-day loading course schedule. On this schedule the drug is administered intravenously at a dosage of 15 mg/kg/day x 5, and then half the dosage was given every other day until toxicity was seen. Severe toxicity has frequently been observed, and many clinicians now use the lowered dose of 12-13.5 mg/kg/day x 5. From 1,000 treated patients the overall response rate was 27% with a great variation in response rates reported.

Recently, weekly administration of 5-FU without a loading course has been used more frequently. The dosage schedule takes 15 mg/kg/week x 4, then if tolerated 20 mg/kg/week x 4 or using 20 mg/kg/week x 4 from the very beginning of the course. The overall response rate is 30% which is comparable to that reported for the loading course. The weekly course is probably less toxic and should be preferred. Additional schedules of 5-FU have been used with no imporvement or clear cut advantage and need not be discussed in detail. When the total 5-FU experience is evaluated, a response rate of 25.7% has been observed.

Methotrexate has also been extensively studied in breast cancer. Following experimental data in mouse L1210 leukaemia, an intermittent dosage schedule has been shown to be optimal. In early studies, MTX was used as a dose schedule of a single daily dose chronically administered in most cases orally. The response rate was strikingly high, reaching 41.5%. Fractionation of the daily dose or infusion therapy gives also high response rates. It is quite remarkable that loading dose-therapy with 0.2-0.4 mg/kg/day x 4 and repetition of the course at 3 or 4 weeks later resulted in rather low response rates. Only one study group has reported on MTX administered twice weekly (0.4 - 0.6 mg/mg/2 x weekly) and found an impressive response rate of 40%. In summary it does appear that on an optimal schedule MTX could be the single agent with the greatest potential for achieving tumour regression.

6-Mercaptopurine, arabinosyl-cytosine and hydroxyurea are less important in the treatment of breast cancer since their response rates are very low.

Vinca Alkaloids: An overall response rate for vincristine of 20% has been obtained. There is a dose response effect for regression. At a dose level of 12.5 μg/kg, no responses were observed in these series and the response rate increases as the dose is increased until at 75 μg/kg a response rate of 33% is observed. Hormone treatment and endocrine ablation have had no apparent effect on the rate of partial remission from vincristine. The response rate for vinblastine is exactly that observed for vincristine (20%).

The goals of most combination drug programmes have been to increase the percentage of complete remission rates to therapy and to inhibit or to retard drug induced resistance. In case of a successful combination, the length of time the patient remains free of his disease after all therapy is discontinued can be used as an indication of the magnitude of the volume of tumour reduction. Finally, if these indications of successful treatment are valid, survival should be improved.

The prerequisites for a successful combination for a given tumour are: 1) the drugs used should be active as single agents; 2) the drugs used should have independent mechanisms of action and 3) the drugs used should not have overlapping toxicity.

As has been shown, most of these conditions can be met for the chemotherapy of breast cancer. Drugs with different mechanism of action include cyclophosphamide, 5-FU, MTX, vincristine and adriamycin, and all have demonstrable activity as single agents in breast cancer. There is some degree of overlapping toxicity.

	No. of patients	CR+PR
MTX, End, Pred.		
Brunner et al, 1969	76	62%
C.G. Schmidt et al 1974	49	57%
End, Vi, Pred, 5-FU, MTX		
Cooper et al, 1969	60	90%
Ansfield et al, 1971	18	61%
Carter et al, 1972	91	56%
Brunner et al, 1973	91	75%
Kaufman et al, 1973	42	54%
Spigel et al 1973	23	43%
Davis et al, 1974	74	42%
C.G. Schmidt et al 1974	66	65%

TABLE 2: Results of combination chemotherapy in advanced Breast cancer.

Table 2 summarizes the results of several oncology groups with either a three or five drug combination regime. By comparing theseresults with the single drug treatment it is obvious that the remission rates are much higher reaching in most study groups a level of doubling the CR and PR.

RESULTS	PATIENTS	95% CONFIDENCE
CR	5	57
PR	23	(42-71)
No Change	5	43
Failure	16	(29-58)

TABLE 3: Triple drug chemotherapy (CYT, MTX, PRED) in 49 patients with breast cancer.

The results of the triple drug therapy are demonstrated in Table 3 compared with the remission rates to be obtained by the five drug combination regime demonstrated in Table 4.

RESULT	PATIENTS	95% CONFIDENCE
CR PR	12 31	65 (52-76)
No change Failure	8 15	35 (24-48)

TABLE 4: Five drug combination chemotherapy (CYT,MTX,VI, FU,PRED) in 66 patients with breast cancer.

From our own group 115 women with far advanced breast cancer were treated. The triple drug regime was only slightly less active than the five drug combination, the remission rates being 57% and 65% respectively. Although there was a good response rate, quite a few patients belong to the no-change category. As will be seen, this category is of a prognostic significance. Several series have correlated response to chemotherapy with site of dominant lesions. This procedure is rather important since response rate may vary greatly depending on the type of lesion. The range in response rates reported is probably due to different criteria in patient selection. Our results are taken from unselected cases including every patient regardless of former treatment, site of dominant lesions, hormonal status or age.

METASTASES	RESULTS	PATIENTS
loco-regional	CR	2
	PR	8
	No change	1
	failure	3
bone	CR	0
	PR	0
	No change	7
	failure	3
visceral	CR	11
	PR	10
	No change	7
	failure	9

TABLE 5: Triple drug chemotherapy (CYT,MTX,PRED) in 49 patients with breast cancer-response of different tumors

Soft tissue and osseous lesions appear to be equally responsive, while visceral lesions are the least responsive and patients with hepatic manifestations rarely respond. Ansfield's large series of mono-chemotherapy shows the lowest response rate (18%) in the visceral category and the highest rate (29%) in the osseous category. The break down of our results with triple drug combination therapy - seen in Table 5 - and the five drug combination regime - demonstrated in Table 6 - show quite a remarkable response of visceral metastases. This is mainly due to the high response rate of pulmonary metastases. Patients with major hepatic involvement respond less frequently and sometimes poorly to systemic therapy.

METASTASES	RESULTS	PATIENTS
loco-regional	CR	7
	PR	13
	No change	3
	failure	3
bone	CR	0
	PR	0
	No change	9
	failure	7
visceral	CR	13
	PR	13
	No change	3
	failure	11

TABLE 6: Five drug combination chemotherapy (CYT,MTX,VI,FU, PRED) in 66 patients with breast cancer—response of different tumor sites.

Our results as far as bone metastases are concerned are rather disappointing and probably underestimated, because of the difficulty in measuring objective response. The only quick and convincing method would be the follow-up of bone scintigram for instance with 85 Sr and the normalisation of the former abnormal high uptakes of radioactivity.

Hypercalcaemia, which is usually associated with extensive skeletal metastases and sometimes induced by the acceleration of tumour growth following hormone treatment should be regarded as an absolute indication for combination chemotherapy. The results are remarkably good, reaching response rates of more than 90%.

Marrow reserve may be limited in such patients and

systemic chemotherapy should be initially reduced. But I wish to emphasise that these cases respond remarkably well to chemotherapy. These patients should not be left without systemic chemotherapy under the assumption of reduced bone marrow reserves. On the contrary, it is well-established that despite a rather low level of white blood cells in the peripheral blood and the presence of immature precursors, there is a tendency for a rather quick normalisation under combination chemotherapy.

Although in our series of 115 unselected cases there has been no significant difference between the response to the two forms of treatment, we should like to point out that we do prefer the five drug combination regime due to the fact that in quite a few cases in which secondary resistance to chemotherapy has occured with the triple drug combination, these respond well to the five drug combination regime.

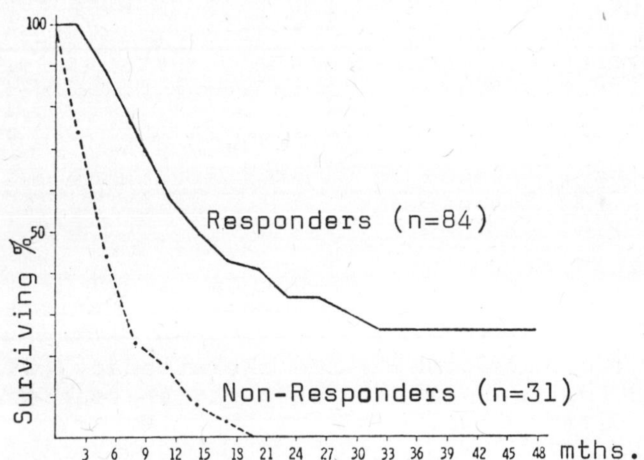

FIG 1 : SURVIVAL OF RESPONDERS AND NON-RESPONDERS AFTER CHEMOTHERAPY OF BREAST CANCER.

There is ample evidence that the responders have a significant advantage in median survival as is demonstrated in Fig 1 . Mean survival time was 13 months in the remission group and 6 months in the failure group. Furthermore, no patient of the non-responders survived more than 18 months, but about 30% of the responders are still living more than 48 months later.

One of the interesting results regarding the median survival of breast cancer are to be seen in Table 7, which gives the clear evidence for the fact that the no change

RESULT	SURVIVAL (MONTHS)
CR	17
PR	11
No Change	14
Failure	6

TABLE 7 : Medium survival of mammary carcinoma patients.

group has a far better prognosis than the non-responders even reaching the survival levels of the partial responders It is for this reason, that the category of no change in cases of widely disseminated breast cancer under systemic treatment, can be regarded as a worthwile attainment.

Adriamycin is one of the most important recently developed single agents with remarkably high response rates in breast cancer reached. It is therefore worthwhile to exploit the activity of this compound by combination with other drugs. To obtain an additive or even synergistic effect we should consider that Adriamycin belongs to the inducer-compounds with rather quick but not very long-lasting effect. It is for this reason that we now combine cyclophosphamide, vincristine and adriamycin for the induction of complete or partial remission and try to continue the treatment as consolidation and maintenance by using 5-FU and methotrexate.

1)	Induction	:Cyclophosphamide Vincristine Adriamycin
2)	Consolidation and maintenance	:5-Fluorouracil Methotrexate

TABLE 8 : BREAST CANCER - CHEMOTHERAPY
Rationale of a new combination chemotherapy program in advanced breast cancer.

Quite similar approaches have been performed by the M.D. Anderson group using adriamycin, cyclophosphamide and 5-FU (FAC) as triple drug treatment reaching high overall response rates of 84% (CR + PR) as is demonstrated in Table 9 . It is our experience that the duration of response to FAC treatment is rather short. In a recent attempt to improve quality and duration of response as well as survival, a sequential combination chemotherapy with systemic immunotherapy was used by Cardenas and co-workers to treat 32 patients with advanced breast cancer. Three courses of vincristine, adriamycin and cyclophosphamide administered sequentially on day one and two and

Adriamycin	50 mg/qm	day 1
Cyclophosphamide	500 mg/qm	day 1
Fluorouracil	500 mg/qm	days 1 and 8
CR	3/25	(3/13)+
PR	15/25	(8/13)
CR + PR	72%	84%

TABLE 9: FAC Chemotherapy for Breast Cancer

+ Patients completing 3 courses
G.R. Blumenschein, J.O. Cardenas, E.J. Freireich, J.A. Gottlieb.
Proc. Amer. Ass. Cancer Res. + Amer. Soc. Clin. Oncol. 15, Abstr. 839, 1974.

repeated every 28 days. BCG (6×10^8 organisms) was given by scarification between the courses. The overall response rate being 69% includes three complete and 19 partial remissions. Response according to site of metastatic involvement were: nodal - 91%, skin and breast - 81%, lung and pleura - 71% and liver - 43% response rate. It is too early to evaluate final response but the sequential program was introduced to prevent early development of drug resistance.

Chemotherapy of Bronchogenic Cancer

The pathology of bronchogenic cancer and especially the microscopic pattern of these tumours are important for the chemotherapist because they might reflect tumours with small or large growth fraction, slow or fast proliferation kinetics and a different response to cytostatic drug.

For practical reasons it is worthwhile to concentrate on the main classifications of the W.H.O. histological typing.

1. Epidermoid carcinomas (squamous cell carcinoma)
2. Small anaplastic carcinomas (including the oat-cell type)
3. Adenocarcinomas (either bronchogenic or bronchiolo-alveolar)
4. Large cell carcinomas (with or without mucin like content including also the giant and the "clear" cell carcinoma)
5. Combined epidermoid and adenocarcinoma

Single drug or combination chemotherapy is, at present, the

major option for systematic treatment of bronchogenic cancer. It has been pointed out that combination chemotherapy should include such drugs which have shown to be active against the tumour when given as a single drug. A short review about the data on chemotherapy with single agents is therefore in order.

Alkylating agents are among the most effective against lung cancer, including cyclophosphamide and mechlorethamine, reaching response rates of 23% and 36% respectively. But melphalan, chlorambucil, Thio-TEPA and busulfan are much less active.

From the class of tumour inhibitory antibiotics, mitomycin and adriamycin are active against bronchogenic carcinoma. Differentiation by cell type is rather important, because both compounds are active against small cell carcinomas, but virtually without any influence on the squamous cell carcinoma. Bleomycin is remarkably disappointing, even against epidermoid carcinoma and despite its well known pulmonary toxicity. Agents such as vinblastine and vincristine are also mainly active against small cell carcinoma and only to a rather limited extent against squamous cell carcinoma.

Methotrexate shows a good overall activity against all four major cell types of bronchogenic cancer with the expected preference for small cell carcinoma. The other antimetabolites, such as mercaptopurine and the fluorinated pyrimidines are disappointing, while cytarabine needs further study. Procarbazine is remarkably effective against small cell carcinoma and the nitrosoureas have been studied recently including a randomized study comparing CCNU and methyl-CCNU in unresectable, advanced bronchogenic carcinoma. The response rate for CCNU as far as tumour regression is concerned was 3.5% and for methyl-CCNU 7.8%. Combining the regressions with the group of stable disease, there was no difference, the results being 36.5% and 36.1%.

It is quite obvious that tumour measurement at its present stage in clinical medicine is a rather unsophisticated method for evaluating effectiveness. From this the obvious question arises of the correlation between survival and objective response rate. A statistically significant correlation has been reported by several groups. No objective regressions were noted in patients who had prior chemotherapy including cyclophosphamide, 5-FU, mechlorethemine and methotrexate. The response rates for both drugs by cell types were as follows: epidermoid - 5.6% for

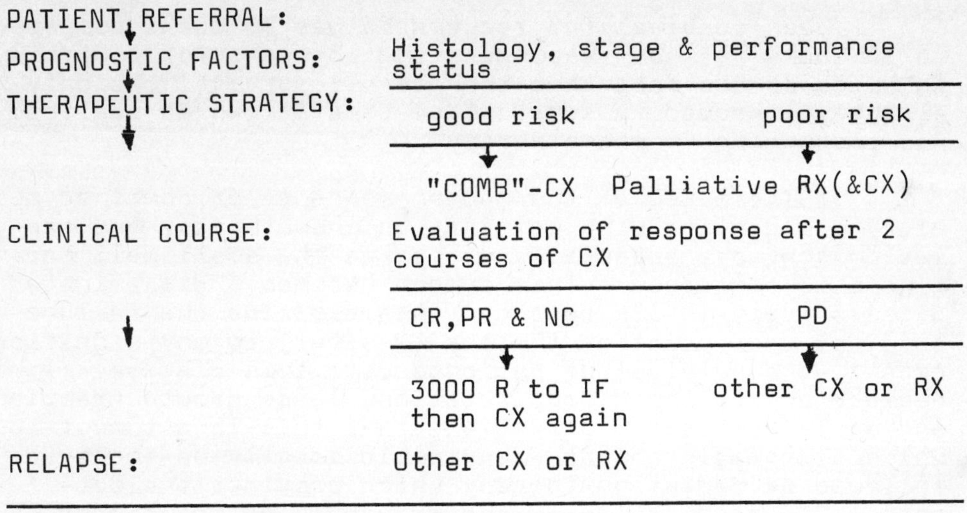

PATIENT REFERRAL:		
↓		
PROGNOSTIC FACTORS:	Histology, stage & performance status	
↓		
THERAPEUTIC STRATEGY:	good risk	poor risk
↓	↓	↓
	"COMB"-CX	Palliative RX(&CX)
CLINICAL COURSE:	Evaluation of response after 2 courses of CX	
↓	CR,PR & NC	PD
	↓	↓
	3000 R to IF then CX again	other CX or RX
RELAPSE:	Other CX or RX	

FIGURE 2

By and large, the effect of the treatment on survival is rather disappointing in contrast to the promising results in the induction of objective remissions. The responders and non-responders have mean survivals which are not very different considering the different combination regimes. But it is important to realize that more responders are alive while only a very small number of non-responders survive.

It is quite obvious that the induced remission may dramatically improve symptoms of the disease and the performance status of the patients. Since a definite cure is not available at the time, this is perhaps the most important advantage of combination chemotherapy over single drug chemotherapy for bronchogenic cancer.

CHEMOTHERAPY OF CNS TUMORS

Michael D. Walker

Baltimore Cancer Research Center, National Cancer Institute
22 S. Greene Street, Baltimore, Maryland, USA

The use of chemotherapy in the treatment of malignant glioma is not new. Since the earliest days of using nitrogen mustard, a few score of patients have been treated with whatever was the agent of interest at the time. The problem has always been to assess the value of these compounds which obviously have modest efficacy and an extremely low therapeutic index. These evaluations were usually carried out in patients who were seen at anytime during the course of their disease, but frequently upon recurrence and at a time when they were deteriorating. Thus, we have multiple reports within the literature which are, at best, discouraging and, at worst, inconclusive.

Over the course of the last several years, the treatment of brain tumor has gradually shifted from a purely clinical art, to becoming a more vigorous scientific discipline. In order to approach the treatment of brain cancers on a more rational basis, one must assess where we have been in the past, where we are at this point in time, and whither we should take our therapeutic endeavors.

Little attention has been paid to the treatment of malignant brain tumor as they were frequently thought of as hopeless. They have not been recorded in epidemiologic surveys until lately, and the best data available indicates a crude incidence rate of approximately 4.5/100,000 patients. In the United States, one could then expect approximately 8,000 new brain tumors per year. Compared to other cancers (lung, gastrointestinal, breast, etc.) cancer of the brain is not frequently seen. However, placing it in perspective with other cancers with which we have had therapeutic success, brain tumor is seen more frequently than Hodgkin's Disease, and about half as frequently as leukemia. It, therefore, is realistic to devote considerable energy to the treatment of this disease. Recent trends tend to indicate that as the control of cancer elsewhere becomes a greater reality and life is prolonged, we will begin to see an increasing number of cases of intracranial metastatic disease. At this time, we are poorly prepared to cope with this event.

One major problem thus far identified is that "brain tumor" is an organ location rather than a specific biologic and histologic disease, such as Hodgkin's Disease or leukemia. We, therefore, should not refer to CNS tumors, but rather should use terms of specific biologic and histologic relevance. For the purposes of further discussion, this paper will utilize the term malignant glioma, indicating that continuum of glial neoplasms, including glioblastoma multiforme, astrocytoma III and IV, etc. Primary malignant glioma is a completely lethal disease. Survival has been variably reported, but the median survival is approximately six months from time of operation. At the end of one year, less than 20% of patients so afflicted are alive, and at the end of two years, approximately 10% are alive (Walker 1974). From the survival point of view, malignant glioma is not dissimilar from bronchogenic carcinoma.

The therapeutic approaches used in the past had specific limits, assets, and liabilities. Surgery, since the initial intracranial operation of Bennett and Godley in 1884, has been utilized to decrease the tumor burden and, thereby, to reduce the pressure within the closed cranial vault. In addition, surgery provides tissue for histopathologic examination. Resection of a malignant glioma is never complete, as unseen nidi of tumor remain, and within a brief period of time regrow. The virtually complete lethality and survival statistics mentioned above attest to our inability to surgically extricate these tumors. Nevertheless, a subtotal resection is of paramount importance, as it provides a decompression of the already troubled brain, as well as the time needed to apply additional therapy.

Radiation therapy has been utilized for over forty years in the treatment of intracranial malignancy (Bouchard 1966). There are a multitude of clinical observations indicating its efficacy. However, it has not been subjected to carefully controlled studies which define precisely its value, as well as the most efficacious time-dose relationship. In addition, the effects of radiotherapy are cumulative, and, therefore, its use is limited by the total dose delivered.

Chemotherapy has similarly been used for many years (Goldsmith 1974). The list of agents employed is essentially the Oncologist's Pharmacopeia, as virtually every drug has been employed utilizing multiple routes of administration. Such studies have been frequently carried out in critically ill patients, which do not allow for comparative evaluation of the efficacy of these various modes of therapy and, hence, the frustration of our current day situation. Drug treatment of malignant glioma is further compromised by the lack of specificity of the agents employed, the low therapeutic index of available drugs, and problems of the blood-brain barrier and pharmacodynamics of agents which are known to be effective in the treatment of other tumors.

Combined modalities therapy attempts to put together in a rational approach all of the above modalities of therapy both to maximize the efficacy of each and minimize the amount of overlapping toxicity. Little experimental work has been carried out in this field, and it is just recently being applied to the treatment of man.

Several recent preliminary reports have shed light on new therapeutic trials. Bond et al (1974) reported a study in which CCNU (130 mg/m2/day every 6 weeks) was compared to radiotherapy (4500 rads over 25 days) and the combination of the two. In the interim report of this controlled, randomized study, utilizing patients harboring astrocytoma Grade III and IV, there was no significant difference demonstrated either in the response rate or the median survival of the patients so treated. However, the trend tends to favor combination therapy. BCNU and vincristine, with and without radiotherapy, has been evaluated by Shapiro and Young (1974). In this controlled study, BCNU (80 mg/m2 on 3 successive days every 6-8 weeks), and vincristine (1.4 mg/m2 on day 1 and 8) were utilized alone and with radiotherapy (6000 rads). The majority of the 34 patients entered were considered as evaluable. Although at the median survival time there is an apparent difference, this is not statistically significant, and is artifactual as the surivival curves tend to overlap both before and after the median point. The authors, however, favor this combination.

Procarbazine, CCNU and vincristine have been evaluated in a Phase II study carried out by Gutin et al (1975). The doses of drugs were those which were conventionally utilized, and the hope of this study was to capitalize on the combined modalities therapy approach. The response rate was considered to be about 60% of the patients so treated, with the duration of response greater than 30 weeks. The conclusions of the authors, however, were that the combination is not significantly better than procarbazine or CCNU alone.

Hydroxyurea, with and without radiotherapy, was studied by Irwin et al (1975). It was anticipated that hydroxyurea (800 mg/m2 in divided doses every other day might potentiate radiotherapy (5000 rads whole brain with a 1000 rad tumor boost). The median survival of patients receiving radiotherapy alone was 35 weeks, while those who received both drug and radiotherapy was 52 weeks. The difference was considered statistically significant and the study needs to be validated.

Radiation therapy, with or without BCNU or CCNU, was evaluated in a preliminary report by Crivelli et al (1974). The doses of drug and radiotherapy are similar to those mentioned above, and a significant number of patients have been entered into the study for preliminary evaluation.The median survival between the various groups is not yet significantly different; however, the trend is in favor of CCNU and radiotherapy.

These recent studies clearly show progress toward a systematic evaluation of the treatment of malignant glioma. A few years ago, the first multi-institutional controlled, prospective, and randomized study for the treatment of malignant glioma was reported by Leventhal et al (1969). This study evaluated patients with known glioblastoma multiforme who were treated with mithramycin (25 mcg/kg/day x 21 days I.V.) as compared with those who had best conventional therapy, and indicated no difference between these two groups. The results of this study are not so significant in that they demonstrate the failure of mithramycin in the treatment of this disease, but rather that one can carry out large multi-institutional studies of this nature and generate significant factual information.

During the course of this study, several Phase II evaluations of the nitrosureas were being carried out, which indicated their potential value. This led to a carefully controlled study evaluating BCNU (80 mg/m2/day I.V. x 3 days every 6-8 weeks with and without radiotherapy 5000-6000 rads whole brain) as compared to best conventional care in patients harboring malignant glioma who had undergone definitive surgical resection. Some 303 patients were entered into this study, and an analysis of population characteristics indicated no difference between the various therapeutic arms. Patients who received at least two full doses of BCNU and 5000 or more rads of radiotherapy had a median survival of 40.5 weeks, while those who received radiotherapy alone had a median survival of 37.5 weeks. Patients who had at least two doses of BCNU only showed a median survival of 25 weeks, as compared to those who received neither radiotherapy nor BCNU who had a median survival of 17 weeks. This study has been the first to specifically indicate the efficacy of adjuvant therapy, and that radiotherapy increased median survival by approximately 120%. However, an analysis of the survival curves tends to indicate that the efficacy of radiotherapy diminishes with time.

A series of current ongoing studies are evaluating the newest of the nitrosoureas Methyl CCNU with and without radiotherapy, as compared to radiotherapy with and without BCNU as in the previous study. Trends are becoming apparent, although the data remains coded at this time. In addition, carefully controlled Phase II studies are being carried out in order to identify new chemotherapeutic agents which might be of value for more prolonged definitive studies. Procarbazine, streptozotocin, dibromodulcitol and adriamycin are all being evaluated in comparative randomized studies, and pilot studies are investigating the use of epipodophyllotoxin, dianhydrogalactitol, imidazole carboxamide, and corticosteroids.

The chemotherapeutic treatment of malignant glioma is advancing by virtue of the use of controlled studies. Specific problem areas which remain are: (1) To identify effective therapeutic agents which have reasonable therapeutic indices. (2) To define more clearly the biology of the tumor and, hence, how best to treat it. (3) To select the optimum dose-time combination schedules of chemotherapeutic agents and their relationship with radiotherapy. (4) To determine better methods of measuring tumor biologic activity and, hence, response, so that studies are not dependent upon survival. (5) The development of experimental model systems which may provide better predictive information for the treatment of man.

References

Bennett, A.H. and Godlee, R.J. (1884) Lancet, 2, 1090.

Bouchard, J. (1966) Radiation Therapy of Tumors and Diseases of the Nervous System, Phila. Lea & Febiger, 244.

Crivelli, G., Monfardini, S., Morello, G., and Bonadonna, G. (1974), Presented at the XIth International Cancer Congress, Florence.

Goldsmith, M.A. (1974) Cancer Treatment Reviews, 1, 153.

Gutin, P.H., Wilson, C.B., Kumar, A.R.V., et al (1975) Cancer, 35, 1398.

Irwin, L., George, F., Pitts, F., and Davis, R. (1975) Amer. Assoc. Cancer Res. 16, 1088, p. 243.

Shapiro, W.R. and Young, D.F. (1974) Neurology, Minn., 24, 380.

Walker, M.D. (1973) in Cancer Medicine, edited by Holland & Frei, Philadelphia, Lea & Febiger, 1385.

NITROSOUREAS: CLINICAL AND EXPERIMENTAL CONSIDERATIONS IN THE TREATMENT OF BRAIN TUMORS

Victor A. Levin and Charles B. Wilson

Department of Neurosurgery, University of California

San Francisco, California, USA 94143

CLINICAL EXPERIENCE

The nitrosoureas have been in clinical usage in the treatment of primary and secondary brain tumors since 1969. Either as a tribute to the activity of these drugs or as an example of our ineptness in discovering other active drugs, the nitrosoureas, particularly BCNU, remain our most active agents.

$$R_1-N(NO)-C(=O)-N(H)-R_2$$

$$\downarrow$$

$$\left[\ R_1-N \quad C(=O) \quad N-R_2;\ N{=}O \quad H\ \right]$$

$$R_1-N=N-OH \rightarrow \text{Alkylation} \qquad O=C=N-R_2 \rightarrow \text{Carbamoylation}$$

Figure 1. Nitrosourea Structure and Chemical Transformation

The general structure of the nitrosoureas is shown in Figure 1. In the case of BCNU both R_1 and R_2 are chloroethyl groups while for CCNU and MeCCNU the R_2 group is replaced by a cyclohexyl and methyl cyclohexyl moiety, respectively. The mode of action of these compounds is not entirely understood although clearly monofunctional alkylation or carbamoylation are likely to be important factors in any consideration of their mode of action (1,2,3,4).

Before expanding on laboratory studies with the nitrosoureas and brain tumor models, I would like to review our clinical experience with the nitrosoureas in the treatment of recurrent and unbiopsied brain tumors. For the sake of discussion, I will confine myself to primary malignant gliomas of the brain as these constitute the most frequent and homogeneous group of tumors we encounter.

In general, entry into our Phase II studies over the years required all of the following criteria. Patients must have evidence of tumor (re)growth resulting in clinical neurological deterioration and supported by neuroradiologic studies such as isotope brain scan, arteriography, pneumonencephalography, and recently, computerized axial tomography. To avoid later confusion in evaluating response to chemotherapy, the patients must have been more than 2 months post-operative (unless biopsy only was performed) and 3 months post-radiotherapy. In addition, complicating medical illness and infections must be absent.

"Response" to chemotherapy was rigidly defined as <u>unequivocal</u> improvement in clinical neurological status <u>and</u> isotope brain scan while the patient was on non-escalating doses of glucocorticoids. Although these have been the criteria for determining response used in all of our studies to date, it is likely that we may change the neurodiagnostic criterion after we have completed a study currently in progress comparing the clinical neurological exam, isotope brain scan, CAT scan, and EEG to response and to deterioration following response.

"Probable responders" were defined as those patients who demonstrated improvement in either clinical neurological status <u>or</u> isotope brain scan without deterioration in the other parameter while on non-escalating doses of glucocorticoids; or patients harboring anaplastic tumors who maintained a status quo for at least 3 months. Most patients in this category had short-term responses.

Table 1 summarizes our results with six protocols which utilize BCNU or CCNU alone and in combination with other drugs. It has been our impression that BCNU, 80 mg/m^2 q.d. x3 every 6-8 wks., is more effective than CCNU, 120 mg/m^2 q.d. x1 every 6-8 wks. (5). Since we previously found procarbazine to be an effective agent in brain tumor therapy (6), we combined it with CCNU and later with BCNU (7, 8). The combination of procarbazine, CCNU, and vincristine resulted in a 60% response rate with a median duration of clinical response of 9 months. This was similar to BCNU alone and better than CCNU alone. The combination of BCNU with procarbazine had a lower response rate and an inferior median duration of response. In both cases, it appeared as though myelotoxicity was the response rate limiting factor as all our patients who demonstrated a response recurred after dose reduction.

TABLE 1. Nitrosoureas: Phase II Chemotherapy Study Results in Malignant Gliomas

Treatment	Responders* Evaluable	Mdn Duration of Response(Mos.)
1) BCNU	22/43(51%)	9
2) CCNU	10/23(43%)	6
3) BCNU & Vincristine	7/17(41%)	4
4) Procarbazine, CCNU, & Vincristine	18/30(60%)	9
5) Cyclophosphamide, CCNU, & Vincristine	2/8 (25%)	2
6) BCNU - Procarbazine	21/45(47%)	7

*Includes "Responders" and "Probable Responders"

Against recurrent medulloblastoma, there have been anecdotal reports of activity with CCNU but not BCNU (5). We have found the combination of procarbazine, CCNU, and vincristine to be quite effective (9). Recent analysis of 13 patients with recurrent medulloblastoma indicate an unequivocal response rate of 58%, a probable response rate of 33%, and median duration of response ≃10 months. As with the patients harboring malignant gliomas, myelotoxicity was dose-limiting and tumor regrowth frequently occurred after prolonged dose-reduction.

EXPERIMENTAL STUDIES

It is because of the activity of the nitrosoureas and our limited understanding of these agents, that our laboratory has been studying these drugs in depth. The studies that I will mention briefly are the result of investigations by Kenneth Wheeler, Mark Rosenblum, Marvin Barker, Takao Hoshino, Charles Wilson, Pokar Kabra, and myself. We have relied primarily upon the 9L gliosarcoma brain tumor model and secondarily on the murine glioma 26 model.

In cell culture 9L cells exposed to differing concentrations of BCNU for varying time periods demonstrate a predictable first-order cell-kill effect. When BCNU pharmacokinetics are utilized to determine the integrated exposure dose to BCNU, a shoulder region exists before cell kill becomes manifest (10). In terms of a time-dose relationship the shoulder region occupies approximately

5-8 minutes of exposure. This corresponds to approximately .2nMoles of BCNU bound to 10^6 (1 mg) cells. Thus accumulation of sublethal cell damage precedes cell death following exposure to BCNU.

If rats bearing intracerebral (i.c.) 9L tumors are treated with varying doses of BCNU followed by a colony-forming efficiency assay for tumor cell kill, a first-order cell-kill relationship is also found (11). However, at doses of BCNU ranging from 1 to 2 times the LD_{10} there is a plateau in cell-kill indicating a resistant cell population. Based on reculture experiments, this does not appear to represent a biochemically resistant cell population. We have hypothesised that a small number of cells (*i.e.* 0.01%) may not receive enough drug by virtue of their location.

Following treatment with BCNU, the tumor does not appear to begin repopulation for several days. This is presently being exploited in an effort to introduce cell cycle specific drugs during exponential tumor cell repopulation.

Of the many questions which arise concerning the antitumor activity of the nitrosoureas, two have been of particular interest to us. First, what mode of drug action is the most important for activity? And second, what are the characteristics of the most active agents *vis a vis* brain tumor therapy: particularly lipophilicity; and must active nitrosoureas cross the normal blood-brain barrier?

TABLE 2. Nitrosourea Treatment of I.C. Gliosarcoma 9L

Drug	Log P	T/C
Urea,1-2(2-chloroethyl)-1-nitroso-3(tetrahydrothiopyran-4-yl)-,S,S-dioxide(NSC-105763)	-0.41	117
Urea,1-(2-fluoroethyl)-1-nitroso-3-(tetrahydrothiopyran-4-yl)-,S,S-dioxide(NSC-106767)	0.19	136
PCNU: Urea,1-(2-chloroethyl)-3-(2,6-dioxo-3-piperidyl)-1-nitroso- (NSC-95466)	0.37	189
BCNU: Urea,1,3-bis(2-chloroethyl)-1-nitroso-(NSC-409962)	1.53	160
CCNU: Urea, 1-(2-chloroethyl)-3-cyclohexyl-1-nitroso- (NSC-79037)	2.83	152
Methyl-CCNU: Urea, 1-(2-chloroethyl)-3-(4-methylcyclohexyl)-1-nitroso- (NSC-95441)	3.3	139

To answer these questions we undertook structure-activity studies with 6 nitrosoureas of varying lipophilicity (12). Table

2 shows the six compounds studied, their lipophilicity (log P), and antitumor activity against i.c. 9L tumors. We have plotted the log P against the log 1/C where C is the drug dose giving T/C values of 130-160%. A parabola could not be fitted to the data for a Hansch analysis since the two most polar drugs showed no activity. The drug with log P =.37 was clearly the most active. It was a glutaramide nitrosourea which we called PCNU.

In Table 3 we have compared the six drugs in terms of lipophilicity, antitumor activity, spontaneous chemical transformation, alkylation, and carbamoylation. The first three are directly related and the last one indirectly related to antitumor activity. Against i.c. glioma 26, the relationship, in general is similar; however, CCNU is more active than BCNU but PCNU remains the most active.

TABLE 3. Relationship of Antitumor Activity, Log P, Drug Half-life, Alkylating Activity, and Carbamoylating Activity (All comparisons are relative to PCNU which has been taken as 100%)

Drug	Log P	Antitumor Activity	$T_{1/2}$*	Alkylating Activity*	Carbamoylating Activity*
NSC-106767	-0.41	--	72	162	108
NSC-105763	0.19	--	85†	128†	--
PCNU	0.37	100	100†	100†	100
BCNU	1.53	48	163	75	285
CCNU	2.83	21	201	28	417
Methyl-CCNU	3.30	15	201	28	379

Half-life $T_{1/2}$ (ethanol/phosphate buffer), relative alkylating activity, and relative carbamoylating activity from Wheeler *et al.* (3)

†Kindly determined by Dr. G.P. Wheeler, Southern Research Institute, Birmingham, Alabama, USA.

In an effort to further understand structure-activity relationships, we compared the amount of ^{14}C-labeled BCNU and CCNU bound to rat brain and 9L tumor 30 minutes after i.v. administration of varying doses of the two drugs (13). On an equimolar dose, BCNU attains a higher soluble concentration and binds to nucleic acid to a greater extent than does CCNU. At doses of 10-120 μM/kg the differences are greater than 10-fold. To explain this we studied the plasma pharmacokinetics of free BCNU and CCNU. We found that CCNU was cleared from the plasma faster than BCNU. Calculating the area on the plasma curve, BCNU was over 3-fold that of CCNU. The volume of distribution at steady-state for CCNU was >5 times that for BCNU and the plasma elimination constant for CCNU was almost 7 times that for BCNU.

Thus, to explain the greater amount of BCNU in brain and tumor compared to CCNU we concluded that it is, to a great extent, a function of the greater amount of BCNU in the plasma available to diffuse into the brain and tumor. As a result of these studies, it becomes less clear that alkylation is the major antitumor action of the nitrosourea; a lesser action such as carbamyolation or some unknown process may well be of importance since tissue levels of the less lipophilic drugs are significantly higher than those of more lipophilic drugs.

These laboratory studies indicate some of the progress made in elucidating the action of the nitrosoureas in brain tumor chemotherapy. We have indicated certain pitfalls to our increased understanding and elaborated upon the current status of clinical chemotherapy of primary malignant brain tumors.

This work was supported by NIH Center Grant CA-13525, NIH Grant CA-15435, The Association for Brain Tumor Research, the Joe Gheen Medical Foundation, and the Phi Beta Psi Sorority.

REFERENCES

1. Wheeler GP: Recent advances in the biochemical pharmacology of selected alkylating agents. *Transplant Proc.* 5:1167-1170, 1973.
2. Montgomery JA and Struck RF: The relationship of the metabolism of anticancer agents to their activity. *Prog Drug Res* 17:320-409, 1973.
3. Wheeler GP, Bowdon BJ, Grimsley JA, *et al.*: Interrelationships of some chemical, physicochemical, and biological activities of several 1-(2-haloethyl)-1-nitrosoureas. *Cancer Res* 34:194-200, 1974.
4. Levin VA and Wilson CB: Pharmacological considerations in brain tumor chemotherapy. IN: *Brain Tumor Chemotherapy*, D Fewer, CB Wilson, VA Levin (eds) Charles C Thomas, Springfield, Chapter 3 (in press).
5. Levin VA and Wilson CB: Chemotherapy: The agents in current use. *Seminars in Oncology* 2:63-67, 1975.
6. Kumar AVR, Renaudin J, Wilson CB, Boldrey EB, Enot KJ and Levin VA: Phase II study of N-isopropyl-OC-2(methyl-hydrazine)-toluamide hydrochloride (Matulane, Procarbazine HCl; NSC-77213) in the treatment of brain tumors. *J Neurosurg* 40:365-371, 1974.
7. Gutin PH, Wilson CB, Kumar AVR, Boldrey EB, Levin VA, Powell M, and Enot KJ: Phase II study of procarbazine, CCNU and vincristine combination therapy in the treatment of malignant brain tumors. *Cancer* 35:1398-1404, 1975.
8. Levin VA, Crafts D, Wilson CB, Boldrey EB, Enot KJ, Pischer T, and Seager M: A phase II study of BCNU-Procarbazine in recurrent malignant gliomas (in preparation).
9. Crafts D, Wilson CB, Levin VA, Boldrey EB, Pischer T, and Enot KJ: Chemotherapy of recurrent medulloblastoma with combined procarbazine, CCNU and vincristine (submitted).
10. Wheeler, KT, Tel N, Williams M, Sheppard S, Levin VA, and Kabra

PM: Factors influencing the survival of rat brain tumor cells following *in vitro* treatment with 1,3 bis(2-chloroethyl)-1-nitrosourea (BCNU). *Cancer Res* 35:1464-1469, 1975.
11. Rosenblum ML, Wheeler KT, Wilson CB, Barker M, and Knebel KD: *In vitro* evaluation of *in vivo* brain tumor chemotherapy with 1,3 bis(2-chloroethyl)-1-nitrosourea (BCNU). *Cancer Res* 35: 1387-1391, 1975.
12. Levin VA and Kabra PM: Effectiveness of the nitrosoureas as a function of their lipid solubility in the chemotherapy of experimental rat brain tumors. *Cancer Chemother Rep* 58:787-792, 1974.
13. Levin VA and Kabra PM: Brain and tumor pharmacokinetics of BCNU and CCNU following i.v. and intracarotid artery (i.c.a.) administration. *Proc Amer Assoc Cancer Res* 16:19, 1975.

EFFECT OF CCNU ON SURVIVAL, OBJECTIVE REMISSIONS AND FREE INTERVAL IN PATIENTS WITH MALIGNANT GLIOMAS

EORTC Brain Tumor Group, presented by L.Calliauw

Department of Neurosurgery

Saint Jans Hospital, Brugge, Belgium

Three nitrosourea derivatives have been shown to be active against malignant brain glioma. The EORTC Brain Tumor Group is concerned with the therapeutic effects of one of them - CCNU (1-2-chloroethyl-3-cyclohexyl-1-nitrosourea) - on three clinical parameters; total survival time, objective remission rates and free interval between surgery and relapse. To meet the difficulties encountered in measuring these different criteria two parallel trials were performed. The aim of trial 26741 was to study the rate of objective remissions and free interval, the purpose of trial 26742 was to measure the effect of CCNU on survival time.

Patients had to satisfy the following criteria to be admitted to either trial. Operation had to be performed 3 weeks before start of chemotherapy. The diagnosis had to be based on histology. Patients were expected to have a survival of 8 weeks or more and normal hematopoietic, liver and renal function and no major medical disease. Two additional criteria had to be fulfilled for admission to trial 26741 (a) steroid therapy must have been stopped on the 10th day after surgery, and (b) the neurological findings had to be either normal or show only a minimal deficit. The schedules of both trials are shown on figure 1. CCNU was given p.o. 130 mg/m2 every 6 weeks. Of 100 patients admitted to trial 26741, 81 are evaluable. The purpose of this trial was to answer 4 questions:
(a) Can we measure the free interval? The answer is yes, at least in a selected group of patients and if they are seen regularly. (b) Does CCNU prolong the free interval?The

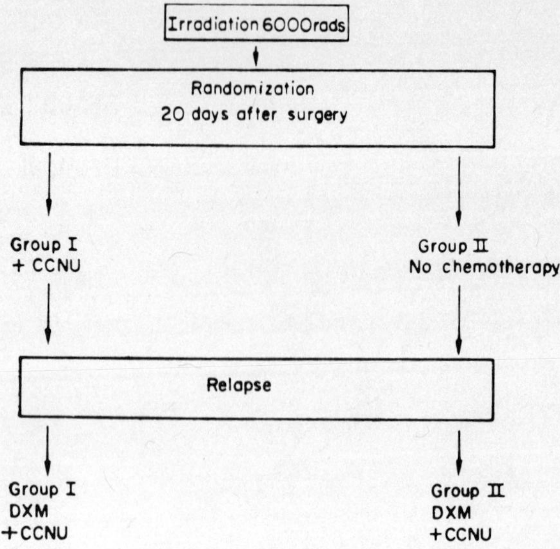

TRIAL 26741

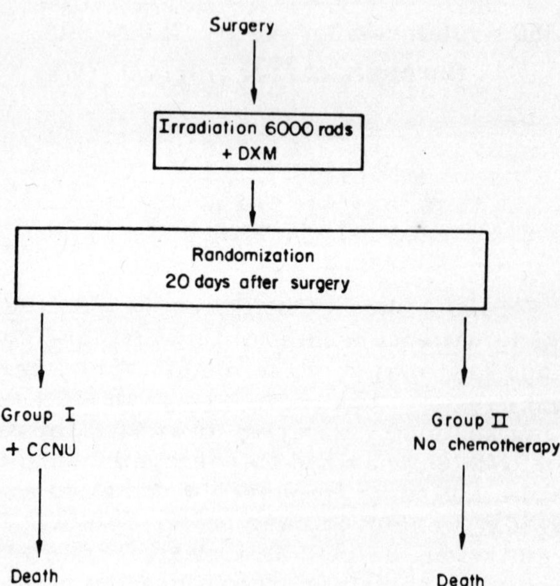

TRIAL 26742

Figure 1

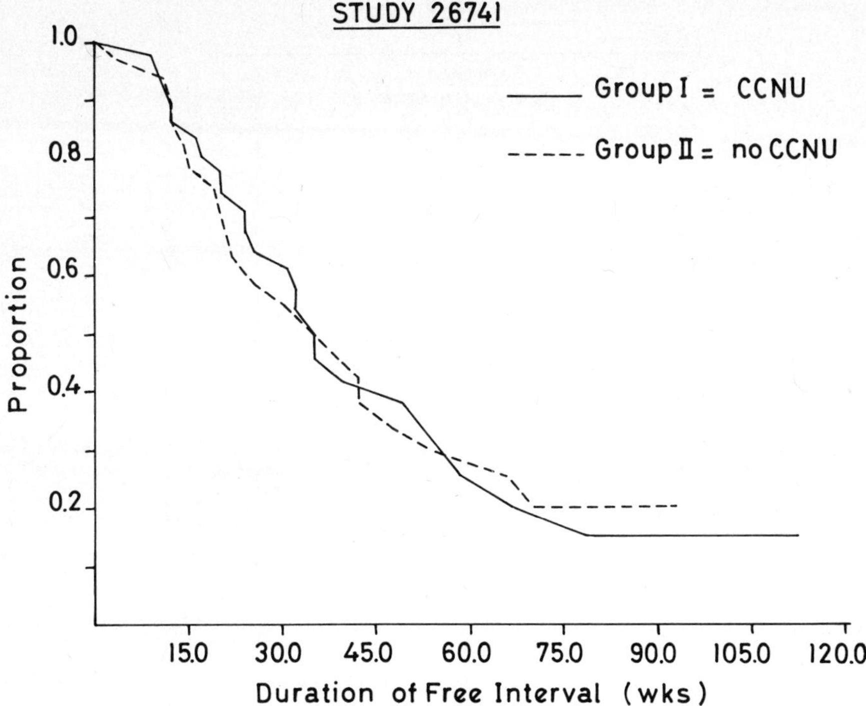

Figure 2

answer is no. Figure 2 shows that the curves of free interval are almost identical in patients treated with CCNU and controls. The maximal likelihood estimated of the median free interval is about 34 weeks in both groups. The mean dosage of CCNU actually given was about 106 mg/m2 every 6 weeks, over 80 % of the scheduled dosage. It should be emphasized that the patients of the two groups were followed with the same frequency and that no supportive therapy, especially steroids, were ever used before relapse.

(c) Objective remission, defined as a clinical improvement persisting 6 weeks or more after complete discontinuation of steroids could be observed in 4 patients out of 16 evaluable for that parameter. The duration of this remission ranged from 4+ to 53 weeks (mean 34+ weeks)

(d) Finally, the total survival time was 50 weeks in patients who received CCNU after operation (early CCNU) and 77 in this group treated only after relapse. This difference is significative at a 5 % level, and is due to a longer survival of late CCNU-treated patients after relapse.

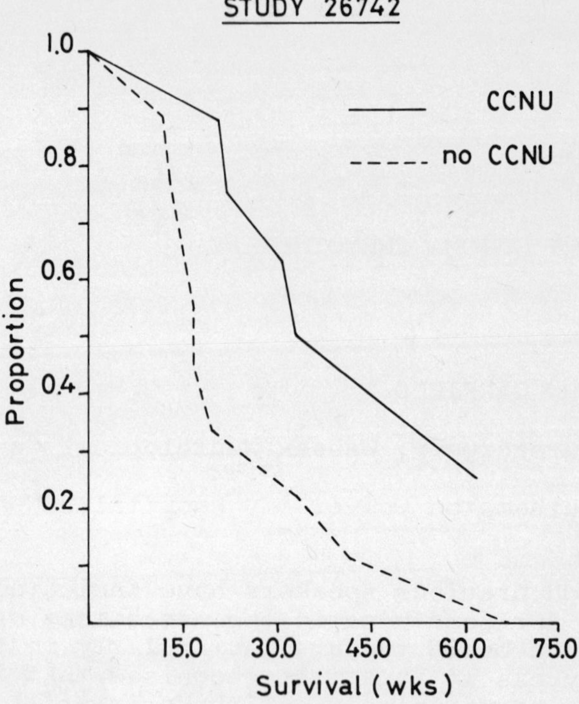

Figure 3

The aim of the trial 26742 was to compare the total survival time of patients receiving CCNU to controls. As shown in figure 3 the estimated median survival of those receiving CCNU was 33 weeks, compared to 17 weeks in controls. Even though only 17 patients were analyzed in this trial, the observed difference is significant at the 5 % level.

To conclude, the combined results of the two trials suggest that CCNU adds something to the treatment of human malignant gliomas : (a) it prolongs the survival time, (b) it is able to produce objective remissions in about 25 % of treated patients. In patients with free interval it seems that CCNU should be given only after relapse.

INTRACAVITARY GLIOMA CHEMOTHERAPY

JOHN GARFIELD

Neurosurgery, Wessex Neurological Centre

Southampton University Hospital, ENGLAND

Although previous speakers have indicated that there are grounds for some hope in the management of patients with malignant brain tumours particularly in the trials of the nitrosoureas it is still recognised that in the management of the individual patient there is still much work to be done before any significant prolongation of survival and improved quality of survival can be achieved. Neurosurgeons must still rely upon the conventional methods of management which include surgical decompression with or without radiotherapy and chemotherapy. This paper reports a small preliminary study using the intracavitary method of chemotherapy. It is open to several points of criticism which will be discussed but the workers were led to introduce this method of therapy by the poor results they obtained by conventional methods of therapy in previous years. The administration of chemotherapeutic agents directly to a brain tumour cavity is attractive for several reasons. First the malignant supratentorial gliomas rarely metastasise either widely or elsewhere in the nervous system, recurrence is usually at the same site as the first growth, the method would allow administration of very high dosage of the agent at its required site of action and the route might surmount some of the problems of the blood brain barrier. Obvious criticisms of the method are the lack of knowledge of diffusion in the brain of the substance administered, the inactivation of the substance within the cavity before entering the brain and the timing of administration in relation to cell kinetics of the malignant tissue. It is accepted that these questions are largely unanswered. More immediate problems concern the technique of repeated administration, the immediate neurological and septic complications which might be severe and systemic toxicity. Therefore, the objects of the study were restricted to determining the feasibility of the method of administration with particular reference to the duration that the catheter system could remain in situ, immediate and delayed neurological complications, systemic toxicity and the determination of maximum tolerable dosage. By obtaining all surgical and autopsy material assessment was made of pathological changes produced by the agents. Because it was a preliminary study of an entirely new method of administration the work was not designed as a clinical trial and no attempt was made to compare one substance with another or with previously used methods of treatment. Table 1 summarises the clinical material employing first methotrexate and later BCNU.

The usual indications for craniotomy for supratentorial malignant gliomas were employed, and the use of chemotherapy did not influence the prime decision. Standard craniotomy under general anaesthesia with controlled respiration and without the use of Mannitol was performed and a macroscopically complete removal of tumour attempted, with a generous internal decompression. A spigotted red rubber catheter was then positioned so

Table 1

Series I - Methotrexate

Supratentorial Astrocytoma grade 3/4		7 patients
Oligodendroglioma grade 3		1
Metastatic adenocarcinoma		1
Survival:	Max.	56 weeks
	Minimum	12 days
	Average (gliomas)	20 weeks

Series II - BCNU

Supratentorial Astrocytoma grade 3/4		10 patients
Survival:	1 alive at 4½ years	
	9 dead: Max. survival	141 weeks
	Minimum	1 week
	Average	32 weeks

that its tip lay in the resultant cavity the spigotted end being brought out through one burr hole of the craniotomy and covered by the craniotomy dressings. Through this catheter the chemotherapeutic agents were administered post operatively, precautions for sterility being within the compass of a ward dressing room. Full post operative observations of neurological studies and systemic toxicity were continued throughout the period of hospitalization. Catheters were left in place in the methotrexate series for up to 44 days the average being 14 days, 2 patients developing meningitis one of which was treated successfully. In the BCNU series the maximum was 27 days with an average of 16 days without any case of infection. The dosages of methotrexate are shown in table 2. Despite the administration of folinic acid (Leucovorin) in doses varying between 18 and 36 mg. per day systemic toxicity characterized by fever, rash and leucopaenia occurred with a delay of up to 14 days following the administration of methotrexate in an average dose of 580 mg. maximum of 1150 mg. and minimum of 150 mg. Toxicity cleared within a few days of stopping therapy.

The dosages of BCNU used are shown in table 3, these dosages being of a high order given in a short space of time compared with its use by other routes. Systemic toxicity did not occur in terms of haematologic or liver function disturbance, these parameters being monitored for up to 3 weeks after cessation of chemotherapy. The absence of any systemic toxicity is a valid criticism of the method of administration in that the agent may have

Table 2

Methotrexate:

Total dosage in mg.	Number of doses	Days of therapy
300	7	9
325	7	12
350	7	9
1000	10	16
500	10	13
1250	9	15
750	5	6
1250	13	44
700	7	7
1150	9	9

Table 3

BCNU

Total dosage in mg.	Number of doses	Days of therapy
400	4	12
650	7	24
1000	5	16
200	2	4
500	5	18
1000	5	12
540	3	6
600	2	3
1050	11	40
1000	6	17

become inactive shortly after its administration. Local adverse neurological change immediately following or during injection of both methotrexate and BCNU occurred. In the methotrexate series the position of the catheter tip and its pressure on or entry into the brain substance appeared to be more important than the volume or concentration of the fluid administered. On several occasions patients became deeply unconscious, but all recovered consciousness within 2 hours but in some patients residual hemiparesis took several more hours to clear. The immediate neurological complications could be prevented at the next injection by withdrawing the catheter so that its tip lay free within the tumour cavity. Methotrexate in dosages of up to 1150 mg. in 15 days in volumes of 10 or 15 ml. did not produce neurological toxicity either immediate or delayed beyond that produced by an unsatisfactory position of the catheter tip. With BCNU adverse neurological reaction appeared to occur at concentrations greater than 100 mg. in 10 ml. or at single doses of 300mg. As well as surgical biopsy specimens the brains of all patients in both series who died were obtained at autopsy. It proved difficult to draw conclusions about the pathological changes following administration of these substances due to the passage of time between operation, chemotherapy and death, the effects of surgery itself and the change in tumour characteristics such as neurosis. Neither methotrexate nor BCNU appeared to produce pathological changes remote from the site of administration. With methotrexate the surrounding zone of necrosis was greater than that usually seen following craniotomy but it was impossible to quantify. With BCNU with patients dying early after its administration there was an acute necrosis of the surrounding brain and residual tumour tissue to a depth of 0.8 to 1.5 cms. about twice the depth of the zone following methotrexate administration. In cases examined at autopsy after a relatively long survival varying from 6 months to nearly 3 years there was a noticeable increase in pleomorphism with abnormal mitoses and many multinucleate giant cells. The pleomorphic cells were found mainly in the centre of the main tumour mass whereas neoplastic cells diffusely infiltrating the cortex and distant white matter usually showed less pleomorphism and a greater number of normal mitoses.

One of the criteria for admission to the studies was the exclusion of other forms of therapy. It was felt that any accurate assessment of a new chemotherapeutic method would be vitiated by other methods of therapy which in themselves were still undergoing trial. This was considered especially relevant in the use of Dexamethasone which is known to have a beneficial effect in patients with malignant gliomas. Furthermore the remarkable variation in effect even with constant dose schedules makes it impossible to discount their influence in any chemotherapeutic trial. The exclusion of patients on dexamethasone is a controversial but very significant point in this work.

The studies have not shown any significant improvement in survival although one survivor alive 4½ years after treatment for a verified Kernohan grade 3/4 glioma is encouraging. However the method of administration is feasible and without the anticipated immediate adverse neurological effects and sepsis. The use of methotrexate and BCNU in this way can be criticised on many grounds and the substance may well have been inappropriate to the tumours. However the method does offer a means of achieving high drug levels at the tumour site and should be considered in combination with other methods of drug administration.

SCREENING OF ENZYME INHIBITORS WITH POTENTIAL ANTITUMOR ACTIVITY

Hamao Umezawa

Institute of Microbial chemistry
Kamiosaki 3-chome, Shinagawa-ku, Tokyo, Japan and
Department of Antibiotics, National Institute of
Health, Tokyo

Antitumor antibiotics have been discovered by screening of microbial culture filtrates for activity to inhibit experimental animal tumors which can be conveniently utilized. However, there is no direct relationship between a particular type of human tumor and such experimental animal tumors, and all antitumor antibiotics thus found exhibit cytotoxic action. Methods of testing activity against animal tumors, methods of testing cytotoxic action against cancer cells in culture or in disc plate agar (1), methods of testing mutagenic action, for instance, testing activity to cause induction of lyzogenic phage (2) or to cause mutation of T_2 phage from h^+ to h (3), have been devised. Biochemical methods (4) to test activity of culture filtrates to inhibit synthesis of protein, RNA and DNA in cancer cell homogenates were also presented.

About 15 years ago, I tried an in vivo screening of antibacterial antibiotics, testing activity of culture filtrates against bacterial infection in mice. However, this study did not lead to finding of any interesting compounds. It suggests that screening of activity against experimental animal tumors would not be the best method for screening of antitumor agents. As previously reported (5), I initiated the study of enzyme inhibitors produced by microorganisms in 1965, and confirmed that microorganisms produce not only inhibitors of proteases but also inhibitors of enzymes involved in animal physiology. Although cancer biochemistry has not yet progressed enough, if we assume that a specific enzyme plays a role in cell division of cancer cells, it is possible to screen microbial culture filtrates for inhibition against such an enzyme. Along these lines, I and one of my colleagues, T. Takeuchi, attempted to find glyoxalase inhibitors and found two types of compounds.

Glyoxalase consists of the enzymes I and II and reduced glutathione as the cofactor and catalyzes the reduction of α-ketoacids to hydroxy acids. This enzyme reaction can be shown as follows:

$$CH_3COCHO + GSH \rightleftarrows CH_3COCH(OH)SG \xrightarrow{\text{Glyoxalase I}} CH_3CH(OH)COSG$$

$$\xrightarrow{\text{Glyoxalase II}} CH_3\text{-}\overset{OH}{\underset{H}{C}}\text{-}COOH\ (D) + GSH$$

Szent-Györgi postulated a hypothesis that cancer cells might have lost the ability to maintain a proper balance of methylglyoxal and continue to grow at an uncontrolled rate (6,7). Although it is hypothesis, we attempted to search for inhibitors of this enzyme in microbial culture filtrates. Glyoxalase activities were measured by a method based on the principle described by Alexander and Boyer (8). An active agent (I) was isolated from culture filtrate of a mushroom. Type of inhibition by this compound was competitive with the hemiacetal adduct ($CH_3COCH(OH)SG$) produced from methylglyoxal and glutathione and Ki was 4.6×10^{-6}M. It inhibited Yoshida rat sarcoma cells with a 50% inhibition concentration 85 μg/ml. However, the ester bond in this compound is easily hydrolyzed, and (I) showed no inhibition against Ehrlich carcinoma.

The other inhibitor (II) was obtained from S. griseosporeus. It was clarified that the inhibition is due to the following chemical reaction:

I

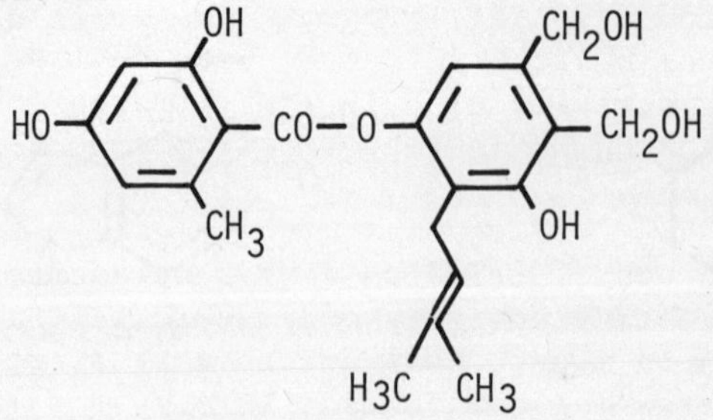

HO–(ring: OH, CH_3)–CO–O–(ring: CH_2OH, CH_2OH, OH, $CH_2CH=C(CH_3)_2$) [H_3C CH_3]

II

(cyclohexenone with HO, OH, OH, =O and CH_2–O–C(=O)–CH=CH–CH_3) + RSH ⟶ (cyclohexenone with HO, OH, OH, =O and CH_2–SR) + CH_3CH=CH–COOH

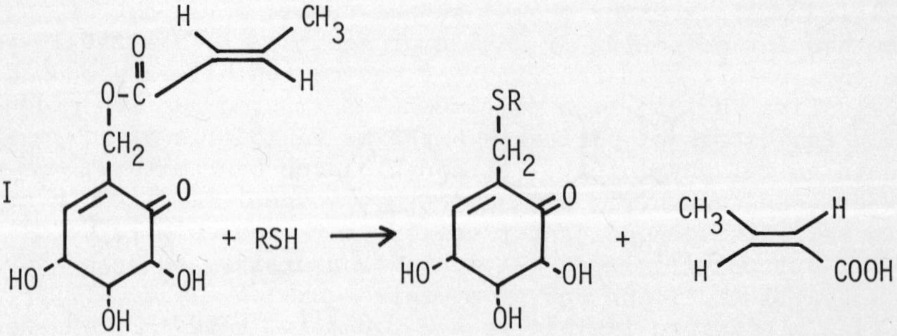

This inhibitor exhibited inhibition against animal cells. Fifty percent inhibition of growth of HeLa cells in cell culture was shown by 18.0 μg/ml (7.25×10^{-5}M) of the inhibitor. It exhibits inhibition against ascites and solid types of Ehrlich carcinoma. Daily intraperitoneal injection of 10 mg/kg prolonged the survival period. However, the ascites started to increase 7 days after the last injection of this compound. It prolonged also the survival period of L-1210 leukemia: 77% by 35 mg/kg/day, 40% by 25 mg/kg/day, 27% by 15 mg/kg/day, 24% by 10 mg/kg/day. These results suggest a possibility to find antitumor agents in screening of glyoxalase inhibitors.

Lack of contact inhibition is a characteristic of cancer cells and in general, when contact inhibition occurs, cAMP increases. In the screening of inhibitors of cAMP phosphodiesterase prepared from rabbit brain, three compounds (III, IV, V) were isolated from streptomyces. III (IC_{50} 4.1×10^{-5}M) was identified to be reticulol previously reported by Mitscher et al. (9) as a metabolite of streptomyces. The others (IC_{50}: IV, 2.0×10^{-5}M; V, 1.0×10^{-6}M) are new compounds containing indole skelton. The other two compounds found in aspergillus and streptomyces were isoflavones which were identified to be genistein (VI)(IC_{50} 2.4×10^{-5}M) and orobol (VII) (IC_{50} 1.8×10^{-5}M). However, these inhibitors showed no inhibition against Yoshida rat sarcoma cells in vitro and Ehrlich ascites carcinoma. Their effect on plaque formation is now under study.

We also confirmed that microorganisms produce inhibitors of reverse transcriptase, though the inhibitor would not have activity to suppress growth of already transformed cells.

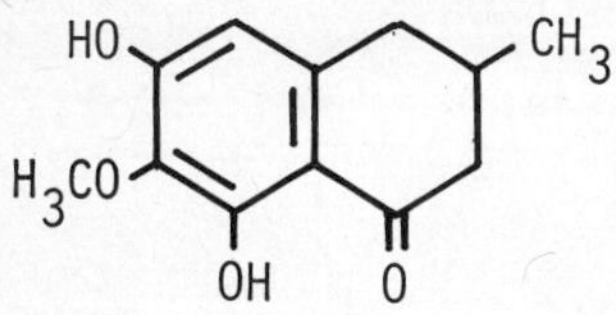

HO, H_3CO, OH, O, CH_3

III

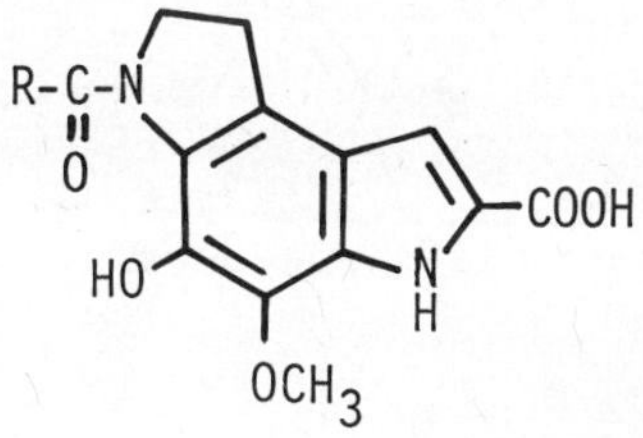

R-C(=O)-N, HO, OCH_3, N-H, COOH

IV: $R=NH_2$

V: $R=CH_3$

HO, O, R, OH, HO, O

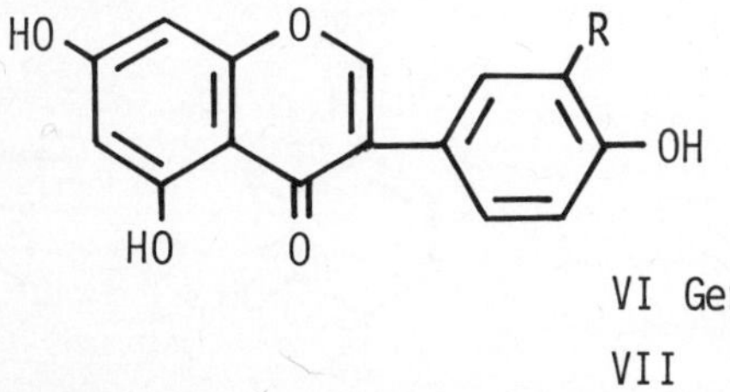

VI Genistein: R=H

VII Orobol: R=OH

As described above, if we assume roles of some enzymes in cancer growth, we can establish a screening method on enzyme level, and we are able to find their inhibitors in microbial culture filtrates. I think, along the progress in biochemistry of each types of human tumor, the study of inhibitors of enzymes involved in cancer cells will become more and more useful to approach cancer chemotherapy. The compound I will be reported in Agricultural Biol. Chem., 1975 and compounds II, III, IV, V, VI, VII will be reported in J. Antibiot. in 1975.

References

1. Yamazaki, S., Nitta, K., Hikiji, T., Nogi, M., Takeuchi, T., Yamamoto, T. and Umezawa, H.: Cylinder plate method testing the anti-cell effect. J. Antibiot., 9, 135-140, 1956
2. Lein, J., Heinemann, B. and Gourevitch, A.: Induction of lysogenic bacteria as a method of detecting potential antitumor agents. Nature, 196, 783-784, 1962
3. Nakamura, S., Omura, S., Hamada, M., Nishimura, T., Yamaki, H., Tanaka, N., Okami, Y. and Umezawa, H.: Application of mutation of T_2 phage from h^+ to h to screening of antitumor antibiotics produced by actinomycetes. J. Antibiot., 20, 217-222, 1967
4. Nitta, K., Mizuno, S. and Umezawa, H.: Biochemical method of screening of microbial products exhibiting antitumor activity. J. Antibiot., 19, 282-284, 1966
5. Umezawa, H.: Enzyme Inhibitors of Microbial Origin. Published by the University of Tokyo Press, 1972
6. Együd, L. G. and Szent-Györgi, A.: Cell division, SH, keto-aldehydes and cancer. Proc. N.A.S., 55, 388-393, 1966
7. Együd, L. G. and Szent-Györgi, A.: On the regulation of cell division. Proc. N.A.S., 56, 203-207, 1966
8. Alexander, N. M. and Boyer, J. L.: A rapid assay for the glyoxalase enzyme system. Analyt. Biochem., 41, 29-38, 1971
9. Mitscher, L. A., Andres, W. W. and McCrae, W.: Reticulol, a new metabolic isocoumarin. Experientia, 20, 258-259, 1964

RECENT EXPERIENCE WITH MICROBIAL SYSTEMS AND CANCER CELLS IN VITRO IN THE SCREENING FOR ANTITUMOR ANTIBIOTICS

G.F. Gause
Institute of New Antibiotics
Academy of Medical Sciences
Moscow, USSR

Summary

New mutants of *E. coli* with altered cytoplasmic membrane and increased permeability have been profitably employed for the detection of new antimetabolites synthesized by microorganisms. Mitochondrial mutants of yeast also represent considerable interest in the screening for new antimetabolites synthesized by actinomycetes, since they can detect products which remain unnoticed with the aid of many other tests. Ascites tumor cells, after numerous alternating passages through the primary culture in the test tube and through the abdominal cavity of mice, are also useful in the screening of antitumor antibiotics.

Microbial systems are rather widely used at present for early detection of new products of microbial biosynthesis possessing cytostatic action. Many cytostatic compounds have demonstrated antimicrobial activities as well. Therefore, to detect a "correlative" antimicrobial activity, cytostatic compounds are tested against a broad spectrum of microorganisms. Correlative microbiological assays have been recently discussed by Hanka (1972). The principal advantages of a microbiological assay are its extreme sensitivity and a high degree of specificity It is not unusual to find microorganisms that can detect accurately concentrations of 0.1 mcg/ml or less of a drug in biological material. Microbiological assays offer several additional advantages. As a rule, the amount of sample required is very small. Such assays are rather fast and easy to perform. Another advantage is that they help to recognize early any known drugs that might be present in fermentation liquors. This identification of drugs is done by paper chromatography of such samples in several solvent systems, followed by bioautography against a sensitive microorganism.

In our laboratories microbial systems have been used widely in the screening for antitumor antibiotics. More recently, new mutants of *E. coli* with altered cytoplasmic membrane and increased permeability have been profitably employed (Bibikova et al. 1973). One of these mutants (19-8) was induced in cultures of *E. coli* B by successive exposure to methyl-methanesulfonate and N-methyl-N-nitro-nitrosoguanidine. The mutant acquired increased sensitivity to antibiotics with different mechanisms of action, as it can be seen from the data given on Table 1.

Table 1

Sensitivity of the parent culture *E. coli* B and of its mutant 19-8 to various antibiotics (minimal inhibitory concentrations, mcg/ml)

	E. coli	Mutant 19-8
Interference with nucleic acid biosynthesis		
Actinomycin D	250	25
Streptonigrin	2.5	0.02
Daunorubicin	50	25
Olivomycin	50	1.25
Interference with protein biosynthesis		
Chloramphenicol	1.2	0.62
Neomycin	10	2.5
Lincomycin	25000	6250
Kanamycin	25	6.2
Erythromycin	500	60
Interference with cell wall biosynthesis		
Ristomycin	2500	50

It is clear that this mutant is more sensitive to inhibitors of biosynthesis of nucleic acids, to inhibitors of protein biosynthesis and to inhibitors of biosynthesis of the cell wall. These observations indicate a change in the cytoplasmic membrane of the mutant, that contributes to the increased permeability of the cell to various agents.

It is of considerable interest that mutant 19-8 inherited from the parent strain the capacity to grow on synthetic nutrient media with a mineral source of nitrogen. It was therefore used in our program of screening for antimetabolites synthesized by microorganisms, as far as the latter can be detected only on synthetic media. In the rich nutrient media their action is neutralized by the metabolites present in the medium.

In a recent series of experiments 3000 cultures of actinomycetes freshly isolated from various soils were studied for antimetabolite production. Mutant 19-8 as well as the parent culture of E. coli were used as detectors. It is of considerable interest that two times more producers of antimetabolites can be detected in cultures of actinomycetes with the aid of mutant 19-8 than with the aid of the parent culture of E. coli. Some of the antimetabolites detected with the aid of the mutant cannot be detected at all with the aid of other techniques.

Mitochondrial mutant of yeast Torulopsis globosa 11-3 also represents considerable interest in the screening for new antimetabolites synthesized by actinomycetes, since it can detect products which remain unnoticed with the aid of many other tests (Gause et al. 1972). With the aid of this mutant some new antimetabolites have been isolated recently, possessing antitumor action in animal experiments.

In the screening for antitumor antibiotics in cultures of microorganisms one can also use tumor cells multiplying in test tubes for the detection of new cytostatic products. A model particularly appropriate for this work has been recently developed in our laboratories (Makukho et al. 1972). It is based on the employment of the ascites tumor cells of lymphadenoma of mice (strain NkLy) in the primary cultures. Numerous alternating passages of tumor cells through the primary culture in the test tube and through the abdominal cavity of mice produced variants of the ascites cells combining high malignancy with the capacity for rapid growth in the test tube. The rate of multiplication of these cells in the test tube was measured by the increase in the content of nucleic acids (RNA plus DNA), assayed spectrophotometrically. This screening system in vitro was found very useful for the detection of new cytostatic products. It has many of the advantages characteristic for microbiological assays.

References

Bibikova, M.V., Laiko, A.V., Selezneva, T.I. and Terechova, L.P. (1973), Antibiotiki, 18, 1074

Gause, G.F., Laiko, A.V., Kusovkova, L.I. and Selesneva, T.I. (1972), Antibiotiki, 17, 195

Hanka, L.J. (1972), Advances Applied Microbiol., 15, 147

Makukho, L.V., Ivanitskaya, L.P. and Volkova, L.Y. (1972) Antibiotiki, 17, 117

PROBLEMS RELATED TO THE DETECTION OF ACTIVITY OF ANTITUMOR ANTIBIOTICS[1]

L. J. Hanka, D. G. Martin, P. F. Wiley, and G. L. Neil

The Upjohn Company

Kalamazoo, Michigan 49001 U.S.A.

[1] Supported by Contract NO1-CM-43753 from the Division of Cancer Treatment, National Cancer Institute, National Institutes of Health, Department of Health, Education, and Welfare.

Various programs for detection of potential anticancer drugs have been developed during the last 25 years. The technology utilized in such programs commonly was based on experience in screening for antimicrobial drugs. Frequently, materials, after being tested for their antimicrobial properties, were also evaluated *in vivo* against several animal tumors. With time it became obvious that the *in vivo* systems had too many disadvantages and are not ideal as the primary screen. People began to look for *in vitro* systems - pre-screens - that would make it possible by using a simple technique to pre-select candidates for *in vivo* testing from large number of samples. Most *in vitro* pre-screens are non-specific and would detect antitumor compounds regardless of their mechanism of action. Systems based on *in vitro* inhibition of growth or metabolism of KB, HeLA or L1210 cells would fit into this category. However, it is possible to design *in vitro* pre-screens to detect only drugs with a specified biochemical effect. Thus, in our laboratories we have developed an *in vitro* system for detection of drugs with antimetabolite mode of action (1). Another good example is the system designed to detect specifically DNA-interfering drugs as that described by Dr. W. Fleck from Jena in Germany (2).

In our laboratories a program for detection of new antitumor drugs was carried out since 1954 and we have used four different types of screens in that time. Our present detection system is based on inhibition of growth of L1210 cells *in vitro* and the source of potential activities are fermentation liquors of soil microorganisms. The cultures that significantly inhibit L1210 growth *in vitro* are then tested in animal tumor systems according to protocols of the NCI. Such *in vivo* evaluation is done on clarified fermentation liquors - either in liquid form or after lyophilization.

For several years we have had some doubts whether it was proper to make final decisions on the potential producers based on *in vivo* activity of crude fermentation liquors.

During the time we were screening for antimetabolites we isolated two interesting drugs only because, for various reasons, we did not cease work on the producing microorganism when the lyophilized fermentation liquors were found to be inactive *in vivo*. The first drug was furanomycin, an antimetabolite of isoleucine. It was also isolated about the same time by Dr. Katagiri in Osaka, Japan (4). The second drug was U-42,126 an antimetabolite of histidine (5). This drug is being evaluated by the NCI at present. I have reported these findings at a symposium similar to this one at the last Congress in Athens in 1973 (6).

In the past two years we have investigated this whole area in more depth and since our findings could be of general interest I'd like to share our experience with you today.

First, we have asked ourselves the question: What percentage of the known antitumor antibiotics would be detectable by our current system if we adhered strictly to the protocol requirement of demonstrable *in vivo* activity in crude fermentation liquors. A few simple calculations are appropriate at this point and they are summarized in Table 1.

In our experience, a typical fermentation liquor of a streptomycete will produce about 20 μg/ml of pure antibiotic and will have 20 mg/ml of solids. Thus, 1 mg of lyophilized liquor contains 1 μg of pure drug.

In the routine *in vivo* testing of the whole lyophilized fermentation liquors the highest level used is - as a rule - 400 mg/kg/day of solids. Thus, a dose of 0.4 mg/kg of pure drug would be administered. As we'll see shortly this is often an inadequate amount.

The situation with drugs produced by fungi would be more favorable for detection inasmuch as the amount of solids in filtered fermentation beers tends to be smaller than in case of streptomyces. However, the weaker producers would be easily missed again by evaluating *in vivo* the whole fermentation liquors.

From the data presented in Table 2 it appears that such protocol is adequate for drugs which are *in vivo* active at low doses and which would be "detected" quite reliably: Actinomycin D, levomycin,

TABLE I

ESTIMATED CONTENTS OF A TYPICAL FERMENTATION LIQUOR

	Streptomycetes	Filamentous Fungi
Amount of solids	20 mg/ml	5 mg/ml
Average titer of pure drug	20 μg/ml	20 μg/ml
Amount of pure drug delivered in a dose of 400 mg/kg/day of solids	0.4 mg/kg	1.6 mg/kg

TABLE 2

IN VIVO ANTITUMOR EFFECT OF SOME DRUGS

Name	Approximate Optimal Dose (mg/kg/Day)[a]	Probability of Detection
A. Antibiotics		
Actidione	> 36.0[b]	−
Actinomycin D	0.1	+
Adriamycin	1.0	±
5-Azacytidine	5.0	−
Azaserine	10.0	−
Bleomycin	20.0	−
Cinerubin A	1.0	±
Daunomycin	1.0	±
Levomycin	< 0.5	+
Mithramycin	0.13	+
Mitomycin C	2.0	±
Nogalamycin	2.0	±
Porfiromycin	> 5.0	−
Streptozotocin	50.0	−
Tubercidin	1.0	±
Xanthomycin	<< 1.0	+
B. Nonantibiotics		
Ara-C	50.0	−
FUdR	150.0	−
6-Mercaptopurine	30.0	−

[a]I.P. dose, QD 1-9, L1210 or P388 leukemic mice.

[b]Effective dose must extend the mean life span by a minimum of 25% over untreated controls.

xanthomycin. All these drugs are *in vivo* active at doses under 1 mg/kg/day. It was indeed our experience in the past years that drugs like these three tend to be discovered over and over again to the point that specific techniques had to be incorporated into our screening program to eliminate these antibiotics as early as possible.

On the other hand, drugs requiring a fairly large dose to elicit a positive *in vivo* response would have been easily missed: actidione, porfiromycin, streptozotocin.

Considering these results, we felt that many cultures producing insufficient titers for demonstrable *in vivo* activity would have been discarded over the years. A program was therefore designed to explore such a possibility. From among the cultures that inhibited L1210 growth *in vitro* we selected those reported *in vivo* inactive and non-toxic at the highest level tested (usually 400 mg/kg). All such cultures were refermented using the original cultivation conditions (2-3 l. volumes) and relatively simple extraction procedures carried out before *in vivo* evaluation. Obviously not all antitumor agents will be susceptible to solvent extraction but the extracts from over 90% of these fermentation showed significant (5-fold or greater) enrichment of *in vitro* effect on growth of L1210 over crude beer solids. Alternate enrichment (resins and ultrafiltration) were attempted on those fermentations not yielding significant *in vitro* enrichment on solvent extraction. The following extraction procedure was arbitrarily selected. To date, 60 cultures have been submitted

1. Ferment *ca*. 3 l.
2. Filter
3. On aliquots (*ca*. 50 ml) of clear fermentation liquor
   a. Extract with butanol at pH 2
   b. " " " " pH 7
   c. " " " " pH 10
4. Extract mycelial pad with acetone-methanol, evaporate the organic solvents, and extract with butanol.
5. Submit residues of above extracts along with crude fermentation liquor solids for *in vitro* assay.
6. If 5-fold or greater enrichment of *in vitro* activity is achieved with solvent extracts, extract the remaining fermentation liquor at the appropriate pH giving the most *in vitro* active material.
7. Test enriched extracts *in vivo*.

to extraction procedures. Of these, 55 (92%) were susceptible to significant enrichment of *in vitro* cytotoxicity by solvent extraction and extracts were submitted for *in vivo* evaluation. *In vivo* results against P388 leukemia in mice are presently available for 42 of these 55 cultures:

2 (4.8%) had very strong *in vivo* activity (T/C > 1.80)
9 (21.4%) had strong *in vivo* activity (T/C 1.50-1.79)

7 (16.7%) had modest in vivo activity (T/C 1.36-1.49)
9 (21.4%) had weak in vivo activity (T/C 1.25-1.35)
15 (35.7%) were inactive in vivo (T/C < 1.24)

Alternate Enrichment Procedures

Ultrafiltration

1. 300 ml of clear fermentation liquor is filtered through a membrane retaining materials having molecular weights greater than 30,000.
2. The retentate and filtrate are freeze dried and submitted for in vitro assays.

Resin Extraction

1. 750 1 ml of clear fermentation liquor is stirred at 5° overnight with 50 g of XAD-2 resin.
2. The supernatant is decanted.
3. The resin is washed with 90 ml of water.
4. The resin is stirred for 2 hrs with 90 ml of methanol.
5. Decant.
6. S tir 1/2 hr with 50 ml of methanol.
7. Decant.
8. Combine the methanol extracts, filter and evaporate to dryness at below 40°. The residue is submitted for in vitro assays.

We recognize, of course, that many of these actives will eventually be shown to produce a known antitumor drug which was just present in the fermentation liquor at low concentrations (6 so far).

Furthermore, we recognize that such procedures involve a substantial amount of additional work. However, the result of our study so far indicated that this is a reasonable investment. It will detect activities that were repeatedly missed by the conventional in vivo evaluation in the past. We would like to bring our experience to the attention of our colleagues engaged in search for new antitumor drugs and who like us are using some in vitro pre-screen followed by evaluation in experimental animal tumor systems.

REFERENCES

1. Haňka, L. J. In vitro screen for antimetabolites. Proc 5th Int Congr Chemother B9/2:351-357, 1967.

2. Fleck, W. Eine neue mikrobiologische Screening Methode für die Suche nach potentiellen Carcinostatica und Virostatica mit Wirkung im Nucleinsaure-Stoffwechsel. Z. Allg. Mikrobiol., 8, 139-144, 1968.

3. Grady, J. E., W. L. Lummis and C. G. Smith. An improved tissue culture assay. III. Alternate methods for measuring cell growth. Cancer Research 20: 1114-1117, 1960.

4. Katagiri, K., Tori, K., Kimura, Y., Yoshida, T., Nagasaki, T., and Minato, H. A new antibiotic. Furanomycin, an isoleucine antagonist. J Med Chem 10: 1149-1154, 1967.

5. Haňka, L. J., D. G. Martin, and G. L. Neil. U-42,126, A new antitumor antimetabolite. Antimicrobial reversal studies and preliminary evaluation against mouse leukemia L1210 in vivo Cancer Chemotherapy Reports 57, 141-148, 1973.

6. Haňka, L. J. Results of in vitro screening for antimetabolites. Proceedings of the 8th International Congress of Chemotherapy. Vol. III: 118-122, 1974.

ATTEMPTS TO OVERCOME METHOTREXATE RESISTANCE:
THE VALUE OF DRUG RESISTANT CELL LINES

Bridget T. Hill*, L.A. Price‡, J.H. Goldie++

*Imperial Cancer Research Fund, London, U.K.

‡Institute of Cancer Research, London, U.K.

++ St. Michael's Hospital, Toronto, Canada

The potential antitumour effects of chemotherapy agents frequently are assessed in *vitro* and/or in *vivo* using experimental test systems consisting of tumour cells which show an inherent sensitivity to cytotoxic drugs (1-3). Since a major problem in cancer chemotherapy is that of drug resistance, there is a need to select agents effective against cells resistant to currently available drugs. One approach , which has received little attention, is to use drug-resistant cells in culture.

In studying methotrexate (MTX) resistance we used a range of cultured murine cells, in which resistance is associated with either (i) a reduced ability to transport MTX (MTX-resistant L5178Y cells)(4) or (ii) an elevated level of dihydrofolate reductase (MTX- resistant L1210 cells) (5). We have determined potential antitumour activity in terms of the ability of agents (i) to reduce cell viability, measured by colony-forming assays, (ii) to be transported into tumour cells, and (iii) to inhibit dihydrofolate reductase (DHFR), if the agents are classed as 'antifolates'.

This report will consider two aspects of our current work:

I - STUDIES WITH ADRIAMYCIN

Adriamycin (ADR) effectively reduces the colony-forming ability of L1210 and L5178Y cells (Table 1). Its superiority over MTX is seen in its ability to kill MTX-resistant cell lines,

TABLE 1: MOLAR DRUG CONCENTRATIONS REQUIRED TO PRODUCE A ONE LOG CELL KILL AFTER A 24HR. EXPOSURE

	L1210 cells		L5178Y cells	
	MTX	ADR	MTX	ADR
MTX-sensitive cells	$2x10^{-8}$	$6x10^{-8}$	$8x10^{-7}$	$3x10^{-8}$
MTX-resistant cells	10^{-5}	$6x10^{-8}$	$>10^{-4}$*	$7x10^{-9}$

*10^{-4}M drug results in approx. 0.5 log cell kill following a 24 exposure.

especially L5178Y cells where the cytoxicity of ADR is significantly greater against MTX-resistant cells than the parent sensitive line. In all cell lines the toxicity of ADR increases with dose and duration of exposure, indicating that the drug is a 'cycle specific' agent and confirming other earlier studies (7,8).

Transport studies with ^{3}H-ADR (donated by Pharmitalia, UK) showed that for all cell types ADR uptake is temperature dependent and is reduced in the presence of metabolic inhibitors, e.g. CN^-, F^- and DNP. These findings confirm other studies showing that ADR is actively transported into cells (9). The pattern of influx of ADR is characterised by an initial rapid association of the drug with the cells, followed by a period when uptake increases linearly with time; saturation is not reached until about 150 min. The 'steady state' levels of ADR in the various cell lines are shown in Table 2. These show that more ^{3}H-ADR is taken up by MTX-resistant L5178Y cells and that the extent of uptake parallels the degree of reduction in viability (see Table 1). Therefore, in this case, the ability of a cell to take up the drug may be correlated with the cytotoxicity of the compound. However, enhanced transport may not be taken always as a reliable guide to a drug's cell killing capacity (see below).

TABLE 2: 'STEADY-STATE' LEVELS OF ADR ACHIEVED AFTER 150 MIN. INCUBATION AT 37°C (μ moles/10^9 cells)

Cell line	Adriamycin concentration
MTX-resistant L5178Y cells	1.30
MTX-sensitive L5178Y cells	0.98
MTX-resistant L1210 cells	0.75
MTX-sensitive L1210 cells	0.75

These studies show that ADR is an effective agent in reducing viability of cells resistant to MTX by a transport defect or an elevated level of DHFR, and may therefore be a useful agent for treating neoplasms resistant to MTX, or for use in combinations with MTX against mixed cell populations.

II - STUDIES WITH DIAMINOPYRIMIDINES

Certain diaminopyrimidines possess some antitumour activity in a few experimental systems (10,11). Under certain circumstances, two of these compounds Pyrimethamine (PRM) (2,4-diamino-5-(4'-chlorophenyl)-6-ethyl-pyrimidine) and DDMP (2,4-diamino-5-(3',4'-dichlorophenyl)-6-methylpyrimidine) also have significant antitumour properties in man (12,13).

We compared the effect of a series of these compounds, including DDEP, an ethyl derivative of DDMP, against the MTX-resistant L5178Y lymphoblasts in culture. Fig. 1 shows that tested against MTX resistant cells. In constrast to MTX, PRM shows nearly equivalent activity against both MTX-sensitive and MTX-resistant cells (14,15). However, using DDMP, high level of drugs (10^{-4}M) are maintained in contact with cells for a prolonged exposure (48-72 hrs.), DDMP is more effective at reducing the viability of MTX-resistant L5178Y cells than the sensitive subline. Similar results were obtained with L1210 cells. However, in transport studies both PRM and DDMP are always taken up to a greater extend by MTX-sensitive than MTX-resistant cells. Therefore, although MTX-resistant cells have a reduced ability to take up DDMP, they are still killed as effectively or to a greater extent by exposure to the drug. This observation is in agreement with previous studies showing that the rate of influx alone is probably an inadequate criterion for evaluating a drug's possible therapeutic efficacy (16).

Further studies showed that DDMP uptake is unaffected by the presence of equimolar concentrations of other diaminopyrimidines (PRM or DDEP), or by MTX or folic acid (15,17). This implies that DDMP may enter cells by different routes from these compounds and would be in agreement with our findings that (i) MTX-resistant cells, with a transport defect of MTX, are sensitive to DDMP, and (ii) DDMP-resistant cells are sensitive to MTX. These results also suggest that combinations of DDMP and MTX may be valuable against mixed cell populations.

Of particular importance was the finding that uptake of DDMP into MTX-sensitive cell is markedly reduced by the

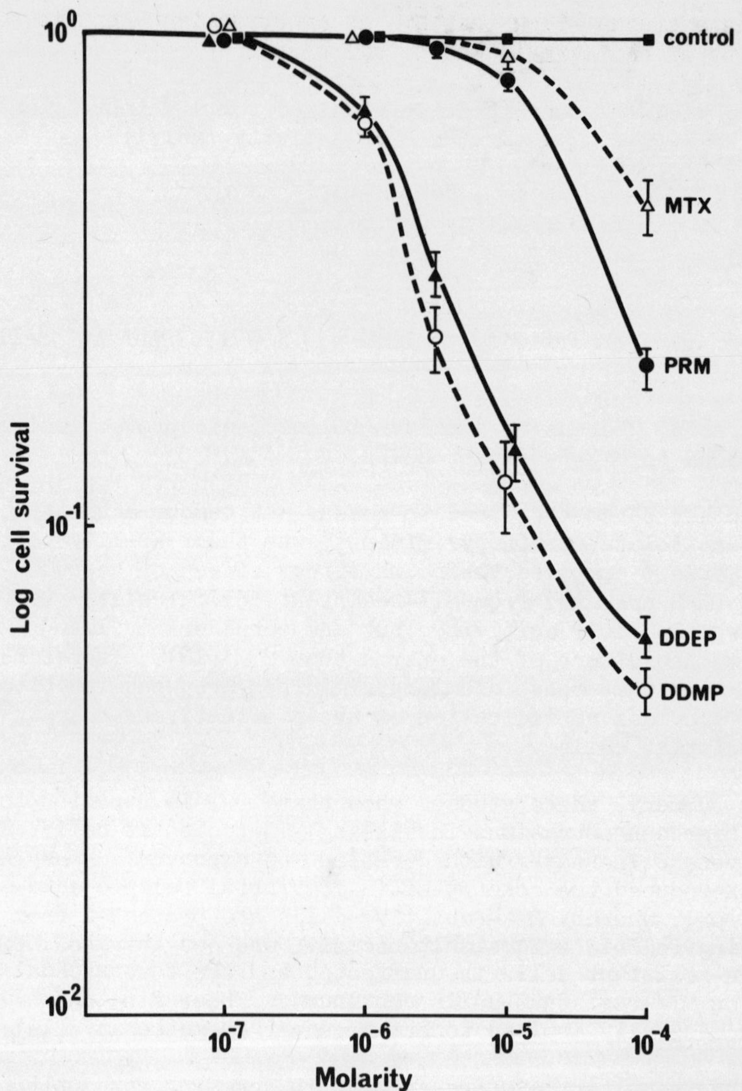

Fig. 1: A comparison of the effects on cell viability of an 18hr. exposure of MTX-resitant L5178Y cells to methotrexate and various diaminopyrimindines.

presence of equimolar folinic acid (17). In contrast DDMP transport into MTX-resistant cells is unaffected by folinic acid (15). This finding may explain our observation that, in terms of viability assays, the cytotoxic effects of DDMP on MTX-sensitive cells can be abolished by simultaneous addition of

TABLE 3: INHIBITORY EFFECTS OF 'ANTIFOLATES' ON DHFR* ACTIVITY

Drug used	Concentration required for 50% inhibition of DHFR activity (mol/l)
MTX	5.0×10^{-9}
PRM	1.8×10^{-5}
DDMP	2.4×10^{-5}

*The specific activity of DHFR was 1.9 I.U. per 10^{9} cells.

folinic acid, whereas no similar 'folinic acid protection' could be afforded to MTX-resistant cells.

Another parameter used to assess antitumour activity of these 'antifolate diaminopyrimidines' was their ability to inhibit DHFR. Table 3 compares their inhibitory effect on a crude extract DHFR prepared from MTX-resistant L5178Y cells. DDMP and PRM show comparable acitivity, but are considerably less effective inhibitors of the enzyme than MTX (18). Therefore, this finding that these diaminopyrimidines are weak inhibitors of DHFR provides no indication of their effectiveness against MTX- resistant cells.

In summary, these studies show that DDMP is superior to MTX at high concentrations in killing MTX-resistant cells: Its effectiveness increases with duration of exposure. They have also introduced the concept of 'differential folinic acid protection', whereby MTX-sensitive cells are protected from DDMP using folinic acid simultaneously, whereas entry of DDMP into MTX-resistant cells is unaffected and the tumouricidal effect on MTX-resistant cells continues. These findings have been successfully applied to human cancer chemotherapy (19).

These results therefore suggest in screeing for antitumour activity it is insufficient to assess agents on the basis of their ability (i) to reduce the viability of drug-sensitive cells, or (ii) to be readily transported into cells, or (iii) to inhibit a proposed 'target enzyme', e.g. DHFR for 'antifolates'. A series of carefully controlled experiments are needed. A valuable predictive test would appear to be their ability to reduce the viability of drug-resistant cells in culture, whilst transport studies are of particular importance in assessing competition for uptake in proposed drug combinations especially when considering mixed cell populations.

REFERENCES

1. Zubrod, C.G., Schepartz, S., Leiter, J., Endicott, K.M., Carresse, L.M. and Baker, C.G. Cancer Chemotherapy reports 50 (1966) 349.
2. Carter, S.K. Eur. J. Cancer 9 (1973) 833.
3. Dixon, G.J. Schabel, F.M., Skipper, H.E., Dulmadge, E. A. and Duncan, B. Cancer Res. (suppl) 21 (1961) 535.
4. Fischer, G.A. Biochem. Pharmacol. 11 (1960) 1233.
5. Jackson, R.C. Personal communication.
6. Chu, M.Y. and Fischer, G.A. Biochem. Pharmacol. 17, (1968) 753.
7. Hill, B.T., Goldie, J.H. and Price, L.A. Proc. Amm. Assoc. Cancer Res. 16 (1975) 44.
8. Barranco, S.C., Gerner, E.W., Burk, K.H. and Humphrey, R.M. Cancer Res. 33 (1973) 11.
9. Neol, G., Trouet, A., Zenebergh, A. and Tulkens, P. EORTC Int. Symp. Adriamycin Review (1975) 99. Brussels.
10. Burchenal, J.H. Goetchius, S.K., Stock, C.C. and Hitchings, G.H. Cancer Res. 12 (1952) 251.
11. Sugiura, K. Cancer Res. 13 (1953) 431.
12. Geils, G.F., Scott, C.W., Baugh, C.M., and Butterworth, C.E. Blood 38 (1971) 131.
13. Murphy, L.M., Ellison, R.R., Karnofsky, D.A. and Burchenal, J.H. J. Clin. Invest. 33 (1954) 1388.
14. Goldie, J.H. Furness, M.E. and Price, L.A. Eur. J. Cancer 9 (1973) 709.
15. Hill, B.T., Price, L.A. and Goldie, J.H. Eur J. Cancer (1975) in press.
16. Goldman, I.D. In 'Drug Resistance and Selectivity'. Ed. E. Mihich. (1973) 299. Academic Press.
17. Hill, B.T., Price, L.A., Harrison, S. and Goldie, J.H. Biochem Pharmacol. 24 (1975) 535.
18. Hill, B.T., Goldie, J.H. and Price, L.A. Br. J. Cancer, 28 (1973) 263.
19. Price, L.A., Goldie, J.H. and Hill, B.T. Br. Med. J. 2 (1975) 20.

IN VITRO MUTAGENESIS BY ANTI-CANCER DRUGS

Margaret Fox

Paterson Laboratories
Christie Hospital & Holt Radium Institute
Manchester M20 9BX, United Kingdom

Many of the drugs commonly used in cancer chemotherapy are known to induce chromosome damage. Some of these are listed in Table 1. Over the past few years methods have been developed which permit the assay of induced mutation in somatic mammalian cells *in vitro*[1]. A number of known mutagens have been assayed in such systems,[1] and a close correlation between lethal and mutagenic damage has been demonstrated[2-4]. A close relationship between chromosome damage and cell lethality has also been established,[3,5] and hence a relationship between lethality, chromosome aberrations and mutation induction has been proposed[6].

1 Some Anticancer Drugs Which Produce Chromosome Structural Aberrations in Human Cells

Alkylating Agents		Antimetabolites
Busulphan		Amethopterin
Cyclophosphamide		Aminopterin
Nitromin		Cytosine arabinoside
Nitrogen mustard		6-Azauridine
Trenimon		5-Fluorodeoxyuridine
TEPA		Thioguanine
ThioTEPA		6-Mercaptopurine
Hexamethylmelamine		**Alkaloids**
Hexamethylphosphoramide		Demecolcine
Imuran		Podophyllotoxin
Antibiotics		Heliotrine
Actinomycin D	Phleomycin	**Misc**
Daunomycin	Streptonigrin	Hydroxyurea
Mitomycin C	Bleomycin	Urethane

I shall discuss this idea with reference to two classes of anti-tumour agents namely the alkylating agents and antimetabolites. An immediate difference between the two classes of compound is apparent when survival curves for V79 Chinese hamster cells exposed to the two agents are compared. Fig. 1 and 2. This difference has been observed in a number of cell lines and has led to the classification of alkylating agents as "cycle specific" and antimetabolites as "phase specific" drugs[7].

Alkylating agents are known to interact with DNA of cells in all stages of the cell cycle, producing lesions which can be excised or by-passed by known cellular repair processes[5,6,8,9]. There is now increasing evidence relating the efficiency of such repair processes to cell survival, some of the possible interrelationships are illustrated Fig. 3.

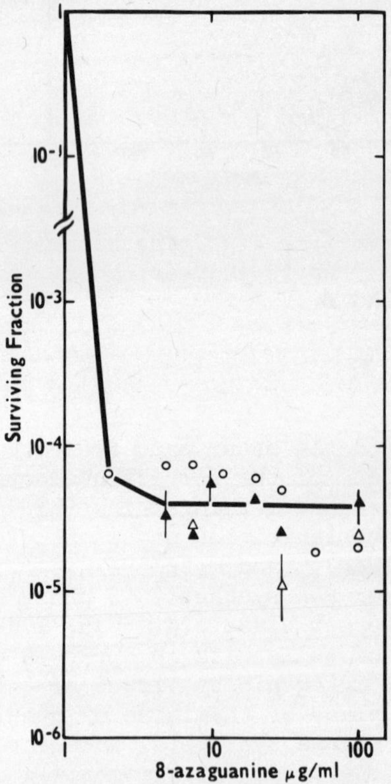

Fig. 1. Survival of V79 Chinese hamster cells after exposure to increasing concentration of 8-azaguanine *in vitro*. Drug was added to cultures 4 hrs after plating at a density of either 5×10^4 cells/dish ▲ or 1×10^5 cells/dish △ ○ 5×10^5 cells/dish.

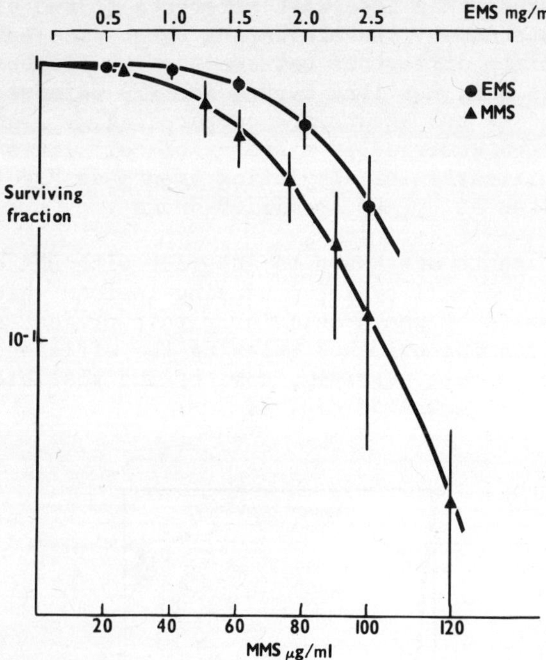

Fig. 2. Survival curves for V79 Chinese hamster cells after exposure for 3 hr to increasing concentrations of either EMS ● or MMS ▲.

Antimetabolites on the other hand are either incorporated into DNA or RNA in place of the correct nucleotide e.g. 5-iodo-2-deoxyuridine (IUdR)[10] and 6-thioguanine (6TG)[11] or interfere with DNA or RNA synthesis by inhibition of essential enzymes e.g. fluorodeoxyuridine (FUdR)[12] and methotrexate[13]. They thus kill cells undergoing DNA or RNA synthesis (S phase cells). Low doses of compounds of the former class e.g. BUdR, IUdR and 6-thioguanine, could allow survival of cells with no apparent chromosome damage but they are probably mutagenic by virtue of their known incorporation into DNA in place of thymidine or guanine[10]. High doses result in inhibition of DNA synthesis, some chromosome damage and cell lethality. The shattering of chromosomes observed after exposure of cells to high doses of FUdR a potent inhibitor of DNA synthesis will almost certainly be lethal as will the 'open' breaks observed after exposure to lower doses[14]. If sufficiently low doses are used interchanges can be produced which resemble those produced by alkylating agents[5].

I have discussed the expectation that as a result of their ability to produce chromosome breakage a large number of cytotoxic agents will also be mutagenic. How then can the mutagenicity of such compounds be measured directly, and their relative effectiveness compared?

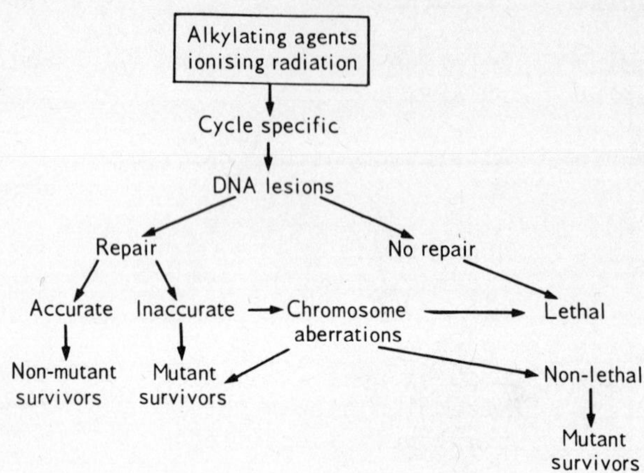

Fig. 3. Some of the possible interrelationships between DNA damage, repair, chromosome aberrations and cell lethality in mammalian cells.

A number of genetic markers are now available in mammalian cell lines[1]. These fall into two general classes examples of which are shown in Table 2. It is thus possible to select mammalian cell variants which are drug resistant; the resultant biochemical changes have also been studied. Selection of cell lines auxotrophic for certain nutritional requirements has also been reported but the biochemistry as yet is less well established.

One of the most widely used systems to date has been that of forward mutation to 8-azaguanine resistance in V79 Chinese hamster cells[1-4]. The rest of my remarks will be with reference to data obtained using this system.

There has been much controversy as to the genetic nature of drug resistant variants in mammalian cells and hence as to the validity of their use in the study of induced mutation[15]. There is now however, considerable evidence that under defined conditions 8-azaguanine resistant cells carrying mutations in the structural gene for hypoxanthine-guanine phosphoribosyl transferase (HGPRT) can be isolated[1,16,17]. Some of the main evidence in support of this conclusion is summarised in Table 3.

2 Some Markers Used in Somatic Cell Genetics

Resistance to IUdR BUdR excess TdR	Deletion or alteration of thymidine kinase	Autosomal recessive
8-azaguanine 6-thioguanine	Deletion or alteration of HGPRT	Sex-linked recessive
2-6 diamino -purine	Deletion or alteration of APRT	Autosomal recessive
Ouabain	Alteration of Na^{++}/K^{++} pump	Autosomal dominant
Auxotrophy for asparagine	Acquirement of asparagine synthetase	Autosomal recessive
glycine proline serine adenine + thymidine	Loss of specific enzymes metabolic blocks not completely identified.	Autosomal recessive
glucose fructose	Biochemistry not defined	Autosomal dominant

3 Evidence For "Point" Mutations to Drug Resistance in Mammalian Cells

1) Stable in absence of selective agent.
2) No gross chromosome change.
3) Frequency increased by mutagens e.g. EMS.
4) Low reversion frequency $\sim 1 \times 10^{-6}$.
5) Quantitative and qualitative alteration in gene product, (enzyme).

Thus, the mutagenicity of any particular compound can be assayed by measuring the increase in frequency of 8-azaguanine resistant colonies after exposure of V79 cells to a particular mutagen. In general in cultured mammalian cells, it is necessary to use doses which produce some cytotoxicity before a mutagenic effect can be demonstrated. When many diverse drugs are used, it is not possible to compare effectiveness in terms of applied dose. We therefore routinely make comparisons between different mutagens in terms of number of mutations induced by equitoxic doses. An example of such a comparison between a number of different mutagens in V79 Chinese hamster cells[2] and mouse lymphoma cells[18] is shown (Fig. 4). Data for cytosine arabinoside and 5-bromo-2-deoxyuridine plotted in the same way show a similar relationship i.e. mutation frequency increases as cytotoxicity increases[19]. FUdR however, which has been shown to break chromosomes, was apparently non mutagenic in V79 cells,[19] and 8-azaguanine was ineffective in increasing the frequency of thymidine resistant colonies in mouse lymphoma cells.

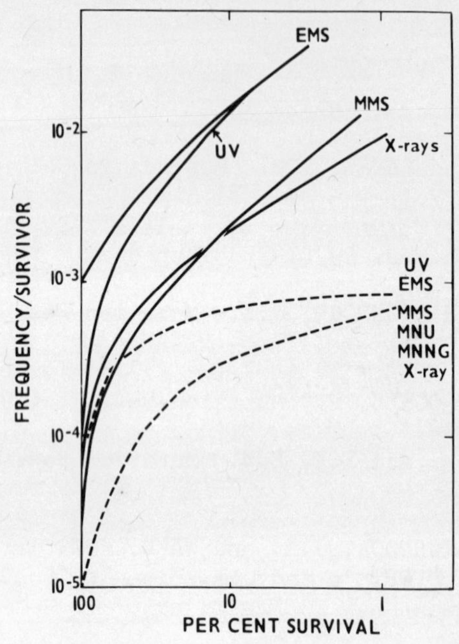

Fig. 4. Relationship between survival and frequency of $8AZ^r$ colonies or TdR^r colonies in V79 Chinese hamster cells and P388 mouse lymphoma cells respectively after exposure to a number of known mutagens. —— V79 8AZ ----- P388 TdR^r.

Thus, there is now good evidence that mammalian cells in vitro can be used to assay the mutagenic effectiveness of a variety of cytotoxic agents, and that in general a correlation exists between cell lethality, chromosome damage and mutational damage.

However, the demonstration that a particular compound produces chromosome damage does not necessarily mean that it will be mutagenic e.g. FUdR, since all chromosome damage may be lethal. Conversely, the absence of visible chromosome damage does not necessarily mean that a compound will not be mutagenic.

Thus, although on the basis of our present knowledge it is possible to make some predictions, there is an obvious need for direct evidence. From a practical point of view, it seems likely that a large proportion of the drugs at present in use in cancer chemotherapy will be mutagenic. Thus the possibility of induction of mutation in germ cells of patients of reproductive age and of new somatic mutations which may predispose treated patients to the development of new malignancies should be borne in mind. The latter may account for some of the late recurrences after apparently successful therapy of malignant disease.

REFERENCES

1) THOMPSON, L.H. and BAKER, R.M. Methods in Cell Biology VI Ch. 7 (1975) p.209-277.

2) FOX, M. Mutation Res. 29 (1975) in press.

3) ROBERTS, J.J. and STURROCK, J.E. Mutation Res. 20 (1973) 243-255.

4) DUNCAN, M. and BROOKES, P. Mutation Res. 21 (1973) 107-118.

5) SCOTT, D., FOX, M. and FOX, B.W. Mutation Res. 22 (1974) 207-221.

6) ROBERTS, J.J., STURROCK, J.E. and WARD, K.N. in Chemical Carcinogenesis. P.OPTs'o and J.A. Dipaulo (eds) Marcel Decker New York (1974).

7) BRUCE, W.R., MEEKER, B.E. and VALERIOTE, F.A. J.Nat.Canc.Inst. 37 (1966) 233-245.

8) ROBERTS, J.J., BRENT, T.P. and CRATHORN, A.R. p.5-27 in The interaction of drugs and subcellular components in animal cells. J.A. Churchill Limited London (1968).

9) FOX, M. and FOX, B.W. Mutation Res. 19 (1973) 119-128.

10) PRUSOFF, W.H. p.45-68 in The interaction of drugs and subcellular components in animal cells. J.A. Churchill Limited London (1968).

11) LePAGE, G.A. and JONES, M. Cancer Res. 21 (1961) 1590-1594.

12) HARTMAN, K.U. and HEIDEBERGER, C. J.Biol.Chem. 236 (1962) 3006-3013.

13) BERTINO, J.R. Cancer Res. 23 (1963) 1286-1306.

14) OCKEY, C.H., HSU, T.C. and RICHARDSON, L.C. J.Nat.Canc.Inst. 40 (1968) 465-475.

15) DeMARS, R. Mutation Res. 24 (1974) 335-364.

16) BEAUDET, A.L., ROUFA, D.A. and CASKEY, C.T. Proc.Nat.Acad.Sci. (US) 70 (1973) 320-324.

17) FOX, M. and BOYLE, J.M. Mutation Res. (1975) in press.

18) ANDERSON, D. and FOX, M. Mutation Res. 23 (1974) 107-122.

19) HUBERMAN, E. and HEIDEBERGER, C. Mutation Res. 14 (1972) 130-132.

IN VITRO SYSTEMS USING MICRO-ORGANISMS FOR DETECTION OF CARCINOGENIC AGENTS

R. Colin Garner

Department of Experimental Pathology and Cancer Research

University of Leeds, 171 Woodhouse Lane, Leeds. LS2 3AR

SUMMARY

A novel assay using bacteriophage lambda is described to detect activated carcinogens and mutagens. The assay may be used in *in vivo* as well as in *in vitro* studies.

It is now generally accepted that metabolic activation of chemical carcinogens is an essential step in the initiation of cancer by these substances (Miller, 1970). The reactive metabolites formed are often generated by the mixed function oxidase group of enzymes localised in the endoplasmic reticulum, although for some compounds further activating enzymes may be required. Distribution of these enzymes varies widely for compound to compound, the liver generally having highest activity as well as the highest level of detoxification enzymes. Electrophilic metabolites have been demonstrated during mixed function oxidase attack of polycyclic hydrocarbons (Sims et al., 1974), nitrosamines (Magee et al., 1975), aromatic amines (Clayson and Garner, 1975), vinyl chloride (Bartsch et al., 1975), aflatoxin (Garner, 1975) and nitrofuran (Yahagi et al., 1974) as well as for a number of other proven chemical carcinogens. All electrophilic metabolites will react with tissue nucleophiles often within the cell in which they are generated to yield covalently bound adducts (Miller and Miller, 1971). Nucleophiles attacked include RNA, DNA and protein and it is thought that one or more of these reactions initiates the cancer process.

Trapping of the metabolites by adding exogenous nucleophiles to an *in vitro* system has been used for a number of years to study the activation particularly of aromatic amines (DeBaun et al., 1968). A modification of this procedure using micro-organisms in place of added nucleophile has been suggested as a general screen for detecting metabolic activation of chemicals (Garner et al., 1972; Ames et al., 1973). Such assays could be useful as a pre-screen for chemical carcinogens and mutagens since they are rapid and cheap and could thus provide some toxicological data on the thousands of industrial and environmental chemicals for which no information is available.

Present methods of testing for production of electrophiles from compounds under study involve incubation of the chemical with bacteria or yeasts in the presence of a mixed function oxidase preparation (Fahrig, 1974). Any reactive intermediates generated will attack the micro-organisms' DNA and cause a heritable genetic alteration. Organisms used are generally nutritional auxotrophs and reversion to the wild type is assayed i.e. a back-mutational system. The disadvantage of this type of assay is that different tester strains are required to detect frame-shift, base substitution and deletion mutations. Strains deficient in repairing DNA damage are more suitable than wild type strains because of their greater sensitivity to mutagens. Compounds which have been shown to be converted to mutagens include polycyclic hydrocarbons (Ames et al., 1973), aromatic amines (Ames et al., 1972), vinyl and vinylidene chloride (Bartsch et al., 1975), and nitrofurans (Yahagi et al., 1974).

Besides the problem of needing a number of detector strain in a back-mutation assay there is the additional problem of the involvement of the bacteria themselves in any activation or detoxification process. The liver microsomal fraction can convert acetylaminofluorene to a bacterial mutagen even though some of the soluble esterification enzymes such as sulphotransferase appear to be absent. One explanation of this is that the bacteria themselves carry out the esterification step (Garner, unpublished). Similarly a bacterial reductase has been shown to convert nitroquinoline-1-oxide to a mutagen (Fukuda and Yamamoto, 1972). Membrane permeability has also been found to be important.

To get round some of these problems my group is presently investigating the use of bacteriphage lambda as a detector strain. We are using both clear plaque mutation, a forward system and phage survival as a means of detecting the production of electrophilic metabolites. Phage should have some advantages over bacteria since they have no metabolic activity. We have used lambda because it is subject to repair by bacterial enzymes, DNA repair-deficient bacterial strains can increase the sensitivity of the assay.

Incubation of lambda with 2-acetoxy-2-AAF resulted in a dose-dependent inactivation of the phage, killing resulting from reaction of the ultimate carcinogen with phage DNA. Assaying viability on a uvrA strain of E.coli showed greater inactivation than on the wild type bacteria as did the use of a λ red strain rather than a wild type phage. Phage inactivation was also demonstrated on incubation with liver mixed function oxidase enzymes and aflatoxin B_1, a carcinogen requiring metabolic activation.

Clear plaque mutation assays showed an increase in the mutation rate after reaction of the phage with either 2-acetoxy-2-AAF or 7-bromomethylbenz(a)anthracene, both direct acting carcinogens. An increase in the sensitivity of the mutagen assay was found as a result of prior irradiation of the host bacteria with UV-light before adsorption of the mutagen treated phage.

The phage assay may also be used for measuring organ specific activation of carcinogens _in vivo_. Phage can be recovered from the liver, lung, spleen, kidney and blood 24 hours after intraperitoneal injection. Work is currently in progress to see if the organotropy of carcinogens can be measured using this _in vivo_ assay (Toogood and Garner, 1975).

The _in vivo_ test described using lambda phage may give a better measure of the overall pharmaco-kinetics of metabolism than current _in vitro_ methods with their excess of co-factors and substrates. Also since phage are phagocytosed by the reticulo-endothelial system _in vivo_ and persist as viable particles for at least one week, chemical feeding studies can be carried out.

REFERENCES

Ames, B.N., Gurney, E.G., Miller, J.A. and Bartsch, H. (1972) Proc. Nat. Acad. Sci. USA, 69, 3128

Ames, B.N., Durston, W.E., Yamasaki, E. and Lee, F.D. (1973) Proc. Nat. Acad. Sci. USA, 70, 2281

Bartsch, H., Malaveille, C. and Montesano, R. (1975) Int. J. Cancer, 15, 429

Bartsch, H., Malaveille, C., Montesano and Tomatis, L. (1975) Nature, 255, 641

Clayson, D.B. and Garner, R.C. (1975) Chemical Carcinogens, Washington, D.C. American Chemical Society Monograph, in press

DeBaun, J.R., Rowley, J.Y., Miller, E.C. and Miller, J.A. (1968) Proc. Soc. Exp. Biol. Med., 129, 268

Fahrig, R. (1974) Chemical Carcinogenesis Essays p. 161, IARC, Lyon.

Fukuda, S. and Yamamoto, N. (1972) Cancer Res., 32, 135

Garner, R.C., Miller, E.C. and Miller, J.A. (1972) Cancer Res., 32, 2058

Garner, R.C. (1975) Prog. Drug. Metab. vol. 1, Wiley, in press

Magee, P.N., Montesano, R. and Preussman, R. (1975) Chemical Carcinogens, Washington, D.C., American Chemical Society Monograph, in press

Miller, J.A. (1970) Cancer Res., 30, 559

Miller, J.A. and Miller, E.C. (1971) J. Nat. Cancer Inst., 47, v.

Sims, P., Grover, P.L., Swaisland, A., Pal, K. and Hewer, A. (1974) Nature, 252, 326

Toogood, S.M. and Garner, R.C. (1975) Proc. Brit. Assoc. Cancer Res., 16th Meeting

Yahagi, T., Nagao, M., Hara, K., Matsushima, T., Sugimura, T. and Bryan, G.T. (1974) Cancer Res., 34, 2266

IN VITRO SCREENING OF CYTOTOXIC SUBSTANCES USING DIFFERENT TUMOUR CELLS

J. Fuska,*P. Vesely, ** L. Ivanickaja, A. Fuskova

Department of Microbiology and Biochemistry
Slovak Polytechnical University
Bratislava, Czechoslovakia

SUMMARY

A three-step system for the screening of potential cytostatics was devised. *In vitro* criteria used in the first two steps of the screening allow the finding of *general* cytotoxic substances and to choose from them for final evaluation *in vivo* those in which the specific effects on tumour cells were observed. The results achieved in this system are demonstrated on the PSX-1 antibiotic.

The *in vitro* screening system of potential cytostatics used in our laboratory enables *us to* evaluate the biological properties of the studied substances from different aspects. The basic scheme of the system consists of three steps (Figure 1). The first step is considered to be prescreening. Its aim is to detect and choose from a large number of the tested substances those with a cytotoxic effect. For test objects we have used the cells of the Ehrlich ascites carcinoma (EAC) as well as the leukaemia P 388 (Fuska et al. 1971). The cells of both given tumours were adapted for the growth and proliferation *in vitro* for 24 to 72 hours. The strains are passaged intermittently *in vivo* and *in vitro* and so the cells are able to induce tumours *in vivo* (Ivanickaja and Makucho, 1973).

* Institute of Experimental Biology and Genetics, Prague
** Institute of New Antibiotics, Moscow, USSR.

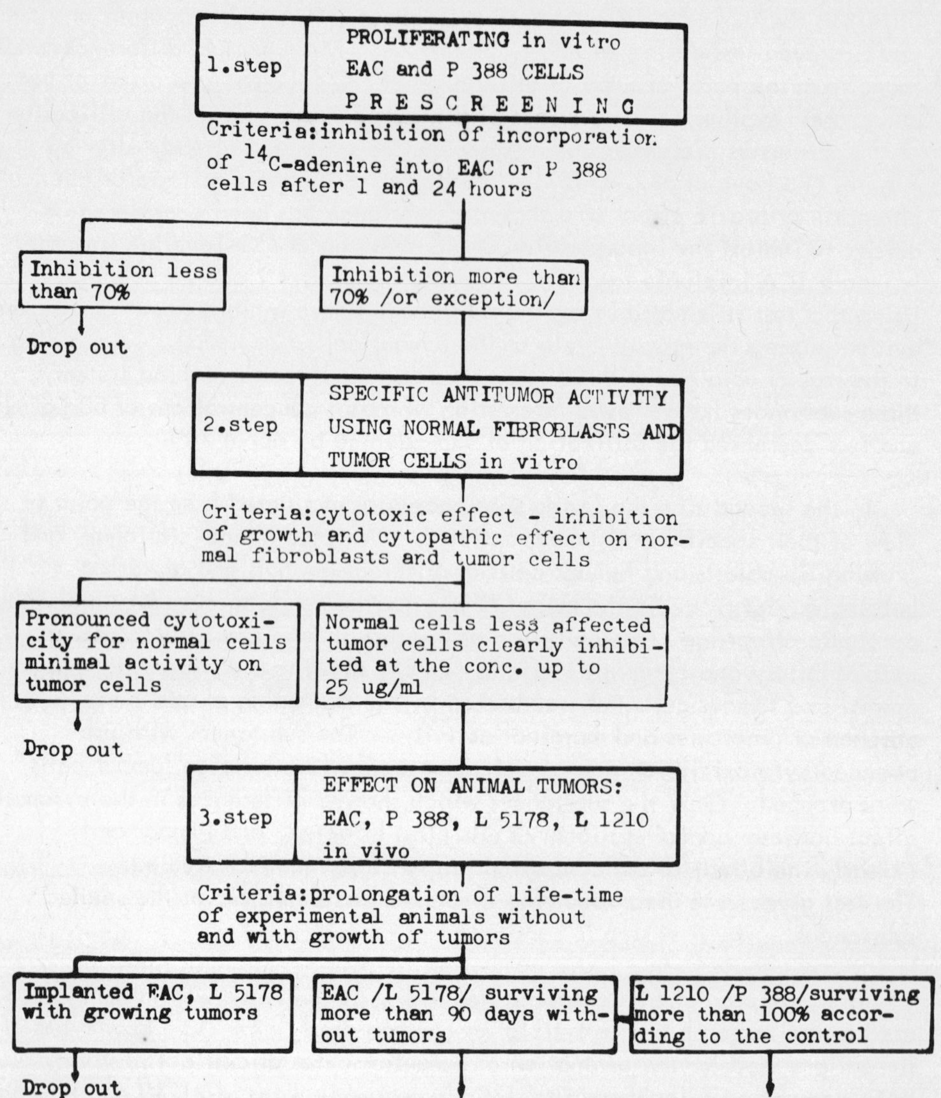

Figure 1. Screening system of the cytotoxic substances effective on tumour cells

Following the dependence of proliferation of the cells and simultaneously the synthesis of nucleic acids (NA) and protein in them upon the time it was found that the number of cells increased approximately twice, but the amount of NA in the tumour cells increased only about 80% and the content of proteins even less during 24 hours (Figure 2). More marked differences were found from the point of view of utilization of ^{14}C-labelled precursors of NA and protein synthesis. The effect of the tested substances on the utilization of the precursors present in the medium can be estimated already after 60 minutes (Fuskova et al., 1975). Therefore, as the main criteria of the potential cytotoxic effect of a screened substance has been considered its ability to inhibit the incorporation of ^{14}C-adenine or ^{14}C-1-valine into the ice-cold TCA insoluble fractions of tumour cells after 1 and 24 hours treatment. Using this test it is possible to find substances whose inhibitory action becomes evident during the growth cycle of the tumour cells (24 hours). According to the results obtained with 25 known cytostatics in our screening system, those substances have proved interesting which in concentrations of 50 μg/ml and less decreased the utilization of ^{14}C-adenine by about 70%.

In the second step the tested substances are evaluated from the point of view of their specific antitumour activity. We used normal stationary and growing fibroblasts and tumour cells of different animals and of varied aetologic origin. As the main criteria for the substances we have used the cytotoxic effect i.e. the inhibition of the growth of normal fibroblasts and cytoinhibitory and cytopathic effects (CPE), showing a different damage to normal and tumour cells, characterized by the flattening of cell body, absence of pinosomes and marginal activity. The substances with pronounced cytotoxicity on normal cells and minimal activity on tumour cells were dropped. Only the substances which showed differences in the cytopathic effect between normal stationary cells (less affected) and tumour cells (clearly inhibited) at concentrations up to 25 μg ml were studied. The test gives some idea about the cytotoxic characteristic of the studied substances.

The third step of the screening lies in the coincidence with other systems used in the research of the cytostatics (Geran et al., 1972). Four types of tumour are used for the estimation of potential cytostatic effect in vivo: EAC, lymphocytic leukaemia L 5178, lymphoid leukaemia L1210 and lymphocytic leukaemia P 388. In the first part of the experiment the prolongation of life-time of EAC and L5178-bearing mice, treated with the substance, as well as the inhibition of the growth of tumours, is evaluated. If the treated animals survive more than 90 days without tumours the substance is applied to the animal bearing L1210 and P 388 tumours. The prolongation of life-time of the treated animals (50%), compared with the control, conditioned the next studies of the substance.

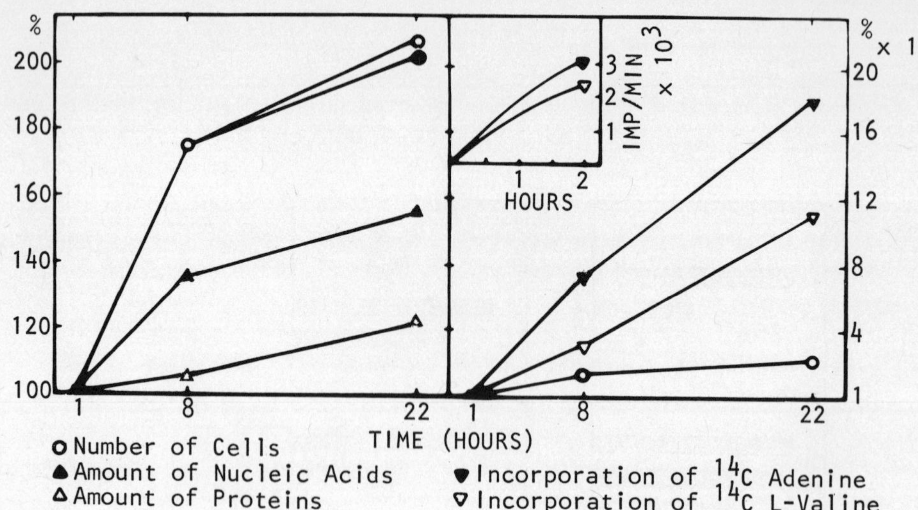

Figure 2. Utilization of ^{14}C precursors and synthesis of macromolecules by EAC cells proliferating in vitro.

Using the reported screening system, new metabolites (vermikulin, bikaverin, duclauxin, frequentin, X-80 and PSX-1) which strongly inhibited utilization of ^{14}C-adenine into tumour cells were isolated, but only the last of them passed through the criteria of the first and second, and part of the third step. This substance is used to demonstrate our screening system (Fuska et al. 1973, 1974).

An inhibitory effect of PSX-1 substance on the five tumours was compared with the known cytostatics: olivomycin, daunomycin, and streptonigrin. The results obtained show that the effect of PSX-1 (ED_{50}) is very close to that of these antibiotics (Table 1).

Table 1. Inhibition of incorporation of ^{14}C-adenine into the tumour cells caused by some antibiotics.

	ED_{50} (μg/ml)			
Tumours	PSX-1	Olivomycin	Daunomycin	Streptonigrin
EAC	2.0	0.7	0.8	6.5
P 388	6.6	4.6	4.75	56.0
L 5178	4.6	2.1	5.0	8.7
NK Ly	4.1	3.6	7.7	-
S 37	3.1	0.24	4.1	-

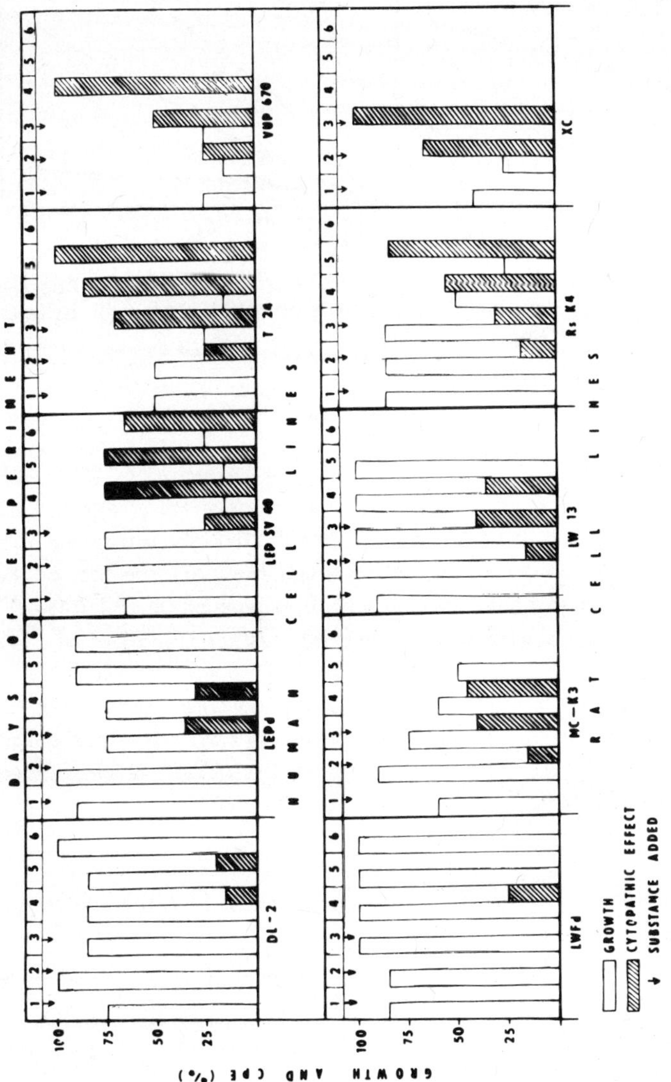

Figure 3. Cytopathic effect induced in normal and tumour cells by PSX-1 antibiotic.

Cytotoxic and cytopathic effects of PSX-1 on normal human and rat fibroblasts as well as on tumour cells were studied in the second step of the screening. The following normal fibroblasts and tumour cells were used: LWFd (normal embryonic fibroblasts), MC-K3 (sarcoma cells from tumour induced by methylcholanthrene), LW-13 (spontaneously neoplastic variant derived from LWF), RsK4 (epitheloid variant transformed by Rous sarcoma virus), XC (tumour cells obtained from Rous sarcoma induced in vivo)(Svoboda, 1960; Vesely and Weiss, 1973) and DL-2 (normal human fibroblasts), LEPd (diploid human lung embryo fibroblasts SEVAC Prague), LEP-SV 40 (LEP reinfected and transformed by SV40 virus, SEVAC Prague), T-24 (cell line from human carcinoma of the urinary bladder), VUP 670 (cells of malignant tumour melanoblastoma of choroid) (Vrba and Bucek, 1974). The substance was added within the first three days together with a fresh medium. The growth of the cells and the cytopathic effect were evaluated every day beginning 24 hours after the first application of the substance, using a light or scanning microscope, often in combination with time-lapse cinemicrography.

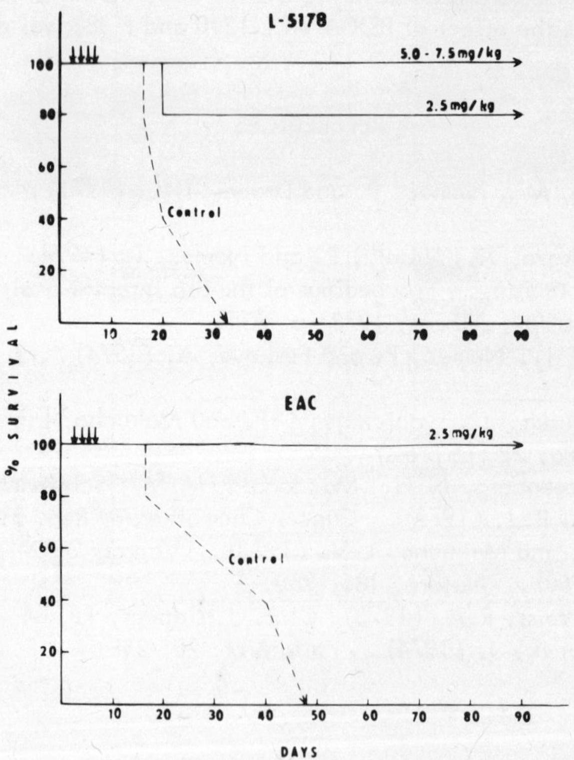

Figure 4. Life prolongation of EAC and L 5178-bearing mice treated with PSX-1 antibiotic

The graphic illustration allows immediate comparison of CPE on the cells and simultaneously of the retardation of the growth of the cells. When CPE reached more than 75% the cells were beyond repair and died. The first signs of CPE in the cells were observed within 50 hours. The substance PSX-1 in concentration of about 2.5 μg/ml showed relatively low toxicity on normal human and rat fibroblasts but caused a marked cytotoxic and CPE effects in tumour cells.

A potential cytostatic effect of PSX-1 was evaluated in vivo using gradually EAC and L 5178 tumours (Figure 4). The substance was administered in a 2.5% water solution in DMSO in the doses of 10-7.5-5.0-2.5 mg/kg/day intraperitoneally once a day for four consecutive days in a volume of 0.2 ml/mouse/day. Five mice (injected with 3.1 cells) were used for each dose in the experiment. The treatment was initiated 24 hours after the tumour cell implantation. The solution of DMSO neither influenced the surviving time nor the growth of the tumours. All animals treated with 2.5 mg/kg/day using EAC and 5.0 and 7.5 mg/kg/day using L 5178 survived for 90 days and no tumours appeared in the treated mice during this time. During these days the effect of PSX-1 on L 1210 and P 388 was evaluated.

REFERENCES

Fuska, J., Miko, M., Nemec, P. and Drobnica, Ľ. (1971). Neoplasma, 18, 631.

Fuska, J., Horáková, K., Veselý, P. and Nemec, P. (1974). Progress in Chemotherapy. Proceedings of the 8th International Congress of Chemotherapy, Athens, 1973, p. 835.

Fuska, J., Kuhr, I., Nemec, P. and Fusková, A. (1974). J. Antibiotics, 27, 123.

Fusoková, A., Fuska, J., Ivanickaja, L.P. and Makucho, L.V. (1975). Neoplasma, 22 (in press)

Geran, R.I., Greenberg, N.H., Macdonald, M.M., Schumacher, A.M. and Abot, B.J. (1972). Cancer Chemotherapy Rep. 3.

Ivanickaja, L.P. and Makucho, L.V. (1973). Voprosy onkoligii, 19, 67.

Svoboda, J. (1960). Nature, 186, 980.

Veselý, P. and Weiss, R.A. (1973). Int. J. Cancer, 11, 64.

Vrba, M. and Buček, J. (1974). Folia Biol. 20, 258.

IN VITRO METHODS FOR USE IN DRUG METABOLISM STUDIES

B.J. Phillips* and P.J. Cox

*Fellow of the Ludwig Institute for Cancer Research

Chester Beatty Research Institute, London

Cyclophosphamide is a potent and relatively specific anti-tumour alkylating agent which requires activation by liver microsomal enzymes. The drug has been under intensive study for many years and the general outline of its metabolism has been largely worked out (for a review see ref. 1). The purpose of this paper is to describe some cell culture techniques which were used as part of an extensive study of cyclophosphamide metabolism carried out at the Chester Beatty Research Institute, London. The contribution of these methods to the understanding of cyclophosphamide metabolism, and their potential usefulness in drug metabolism studies in general, will be discussed.

The basis of all the experiments described below was a cytotoxicity test, the important features of which were its technical simplicity and small scale. As described previously[2], Walker tumour cells in static suspension culture were treated with drugs for one hour, washed in fresh medium, and plated at low density in Linbro, 96-well, Microtest plates, each well containing 200µl. A number of duplicate wells was set up for each drug treatment, so that separate samples of cell suspension could be used for cell counts at 24 hr intervals. The counts were used to construct growth curves from which % inhibition of cell growth could be estimated for each treatment. ID_{50} values (drug concentration causing 50% inhibition) were obtained from dose-response curves.

This very simple and rather crude test system has given surprisingly reproducible results. Cell counting is not only probably the simplest technique for estimating cytotoxicity but is also, perhaps, the closest approximation possible, *in vitro*, to the techniques used for estimating drug response *in vivo*.

With slight modifications this test has been used for all the experiments with cyclophosphamide described below.

DEMONSTRATION OF MICROSOMAL ACTIVATION

The need for microsomal activation for cyclophosphamide to exert its cytotoxic effects has been amply demonstrated in the past[3-5]. This requirement for activation can be very simply demonstrated using the test described above. In a series of activation experiments it was found that cyclophosphamide alone had an ID_{50} of 6000μg/ml which was reduced after one hour of pre-incubation with washed liver microsomes and an NADPH generating system, to 0.5μg/ml. In fact, the method could be simplified even further by adding the microsomes and drug directly to the cell suspensions during treatment, as microsomes alone had no toxic effects. This small scale method could be adapted very simply to the routine testing of drugs for possible activation or detoxification by various enzyme systems.

CYTOTOXICITY OF KNOWN METABOLITES

The metabolites of cyclophosphamide which had been identified and which could be obtained in pure form were tested directly for cytotoxicity. Clearly, since 50% inhibition of cell growth can be obtained after the activation of only 0.5μg/ml of cyclophosphamide, the active metabolite would be expected to have an ID_{50} of the same order, while detoxification products should be much less toxic. According to the currently accepted metabolic scheme[6-8], cyclophosphamide is hydroxylated by microsomal enzymes, forming 4-hydroxycyclophosphamide which also exists as its ring-open tautomer, aldophosphamide. The latter can give rise to phosphoramide mustard probably by β-elimination of acrolein. Secondary oxidation of 4-hydroxy- and aldophosphamide by soluble enzymes may also occur, giving 4-ketocyclophosphamide and carboxyphosphamide.

The ID_{50} values for many of these compounds are given in Table 1. In agreement with the scheme given above, the presumed toxic end products, phosphoramide mustard and acrolein, were very cytotoxic, while the detoxification products, 4-keto and carboxyphosphamide were relatively non-toxic.

Although these results were satisfactory, the primary metabolites were not available for test, and an important step in the activation process could not be studied. Accordingly, a method was developed for studying the products of cyclophosphamide incubated *in vitro* with microsomes.

Table 1: Cytotoxicity of cyclophosphamide and the metabolites available in pure form

Compound	ID_{50} (μg/ml)
Cyclophosphamide	6000
Phosphoramide mustard	0.6
Acrolein	1.0
4-ketocyclophosphamide	240
Carboxyphosphamide	400

TLC PLATE CYTOTOXICITY SCANNING

$[^{32}P]$ Cyclophosphamide was incubated with washed microsomes and the metabolites were extracted, separated by TLC and identified by mass spectrometry (see ref. 6). The silica was scraped from duplicate plates, in 5mm strips, and each sample was mixed with 500μl culture medium. The silica was removed by centrifugation and the supernatant used to treat Walker cells in the standard assay system. The radioactivity of each sample was measured in order to estimate the quantity of each metabolite present. The cytotoxicity data were used to construct a scan which was compared with the corresponding radioactivity scan. When metabolites were extracted and separated as described by Connors *et al*[6], four main peaks of radioactivity were observed on scanning. Three of these corresponded exactly with peaks of toxicity observed in the cytotoxicity scan. The fourth radioactive peak was identified as cyclophosphamide itself and was non-toxic. The major products of metabolism were represented by two of the peaks of radioactivity and cytotoxicity and were identified as isomers of 4-ethoxycyclophosphamide, formed from 4-hydroxycyclophosphamide during the extraction procedure[6]. ID_{50} values for these compounds, derived from the plate scan, were 2.2μg/ml and 8.0μg/ml for the chromatographically "fast" and "slow" compounds respectively. The third cytotoxic-radioactive peak, which was chromatographically immobile, contained phosphoramide mustard.

The results of these plate scanning experiments demonstrated the cytotoxic activity of a derivative of the major product of cyclophosphamide activation and also the absence of an alternative candidate for the role of primary metabolite.

The usefulness of the method for this work was due to its small scale, which allowed microgram quantities of metabolites to be tested. The scanning technique has the potential advantage, should it find application in the study of other drugs, of being able to detect cytotoxicity on any part of a TLC plate, regardless of the presence of absence of labels.

DEACTIVATION

From the metabolic scheme outlined above, the primary metabolites, 4-hydroxycyclophosphamide and its tautomer aldophosphamide can be enzymatically converted to 4-ketocyclophosphamide and carboxyphosphamide respectively. Both of these compounds have relatively low cytotoxicities (see above). This secondary oxidation would prevent the chemical breakdown of the aldophosphamide to release the highly cytotoxic compounds, acrolein and phosphoramide mustard. The selective action of cyclophosphamide *in vivo*, compared with other alkylating agents, has been attributed to the balance between chemical breakdown and secondary oxidation of aldophosphamide[6]. Thus the capacity of various tissues to deactivate cyclophosphamide should be inversely related to their sensitivity to the activated drug.

This deactivation capacity was tested for a number of tissues. A series of concentrations of cyclophosphamide were activated by microsomal incubation, as described previously. Rat tissue supernatants were prepared by homogenization and sonication followed by centrifugation and adjusted to approximately equal protein concentration[9]. A similar concentration of bovine serum albumin was used as a control in addition to a buffer control. Two volumes of buffer, protein solution, or tissue supernatant were added to one volume of activated cyclophosphamide and incubated at 37° for 1 hr followed by centrifugation for 1 hr at 37° to remove microsomes, and the supernatant used to treat Walker cells as in the normal assay. Percentage growth inhibition was plotted against final concentration of cyclophosphamide, and ID_{50} values were obtained for activated cyclophosphamide treated with the various solutions and supernatants. The ratios between the ID_{50} value after supernatant incubation and after incubation with buffer (i.e. Dose Reduction Factors (DRF)) give an indication of the capacity of the tissues for deactivation. Table 2 shows ID_{50} values and DRF's for the tissues tested.

The observed DRF's correspond well with the known sensitivities of tissues to cyclophosphamide. BSA deactivated to a certain extent, presumably non-enzymatically, and spleen had little more deactivating ability than BSA. Tumour and gut mucosa, both sensitive to cyclophosphamide *in vivo* gave much less deactivation than the resistant tissues, liver and kidney.

In a similar way, DRF's were obtained for phosphoramide mustard incubated with BSA, spleen and liver (Table 3). The value obtained for liver suggests that deactivation of cyclophosphamide cannot be due to an effect on phosphoramide mustard and is therefore probably due to the secondary oxidations mentioned above.

The value of tissue culture in deactivation experiments also depends largely on the small scale of the test. Only small amounts of tissue supernatants, and therefore very few animals, were needed even though large numbers of drug concentrations and supernatants were used. In addition, the results were obtained after only 3 days, compared with up to several weeks for bioassay test systems (see ref. 9) where cells incubated *in vitro* are reimplanted *in vivo*, and high % cell kills result in long delays before tumours appear. Another advantage of the tissue culture method was that accurate estimations of growth inhibition were obtained in the range 10-90% inhibition. Sensitivity in this range was essential for distinguishing the lesser deactivation capacities of BSA, and spleen, tumour and gut supernatants. Bioassay systems are normally accurate only at high cell kills above 90%.

Table 2: Cytotoxicity of activated cyclophosphamide after incubation with tissue supernatants

	ID_{50} (μg/ml)	DRF
Buffer alone	0.6	1.0
BSA	0.8	1.4
Spleen	0.7	1.3
Walker tumour	1.6	2.9
Gut mucosa	4.1	7.3
Kidney	9.5	17
Liver	27	49

Tissue culture tests have been in widespread use for many years and their value is now accepted. Their potential in many fields, however, has yet to be fully realised. It is hoped that the experiments described above, while they only relate to cyclophosphamide metabolism may demonstrate some ways in which cell culture can be useful in drug metabolism studies.

Table 3: Cytotoxicity of phosphoramide mustard after incubation with tissue supernatants.

	ID_{50} (μg/ml)	DRF
Buffer alone	3.8	1.0
BSA	3.6	0.95
Spleen	4.9	1.3
Liver	10.5	2.7

REFERENCES

1. Montgomery, J.A. and Struck, R.F. Progr.Drug Res., 17: 320, 1973.
2. Phillips, B.J. Biochem.Pharmacol., 23: 131, 1974.
3. Foley, G.E., Friedman, O.M. and Drolet, B.P. Cancer Res., 21: 57, 1961.
4. Brock, N. and Hohorst, H.J. Arzneimittel-Forsch., 13: 1021, 1963.
5. Connors, T.A., Grover, P.L. and McLoughlin, A.M. Biochem. Pharmacol., 19: 1533, 1970.
6. Colvin, M., Padgett, C.A. and Fenselau, C. Cancer Res., 33: 915, 1973.
7. Connors, T.A., Cox, P.J., Farmer, P.B., Foster, A.B. and Jarman, M. Biochem.Pharmacol., 23: 115, 1974.
8. Struck, R.F. Cancer Res., 34: 2933, 1974.
9. Cox, P.J., Phillips, B.J. and Thomas, P. Cancer Res. in press.

SOME PROBLEMS IN THE USE OF SHORT TERM CULTURES OF HUMAN TUMOURS FOR IN VITRO SCREENING OF CYTOTOXIC DRUGS

P.P. Dendy

Department of Medical Physics
University of Aberdeen
Aberdeen, Scotland

INTRODUCTION

A number of papers in this volume have already been devoted to *in vitro* screening tests. They have illustrated the diversity of studies that can be made including (a) mechanisms of cancer induction (b) causes of cancer spread and metastasis, (c) screening for new drugs (d) studies on the mechanism of acquired drug resistance and (c) methods of killing resistant cells.

There has also been increasing interest recently in the possibility of developing *in vitro* screening tests to make the best use of existing drugs for each patient (Dendy in press). It has been suggested that the tumour cells from each patient will only respond to certain drugs and that these must be selected by sensitivity tests carried out on an individualised basis (Oncobiogram Tanneberger & Bacigalupo, 1970). To obtain this information, experimentation is necessary on human tumour biopsy material which has only been in culture for a very short time. Evaluation of the responses of cells to drugs under these conditions presents special problems, some of which are considered in this paper.

HOW SHOULD DRUG SENSITIVITY BE EVALUATED IN SHORT TERM CULTURE?

The standard accepted criterion for cell viability is reproductive integrity. However, present technical skills with short term cultures do not yet give high enough plating efficiencies for this technique to be reliable. In any event, the time delay between starting the culture and getting an answer might be unacceptably long if the information were required by the clinician.

On the other hand it is well known that the study of a single biochemical parameter shortly after treatment with a cell killing agent frequently does not give a true measure of cell survival. An obvious example is the response of sensitive and resistant strains of bacteria to radiation. Although survival studies show that the strain E coli B_{S-1} is 3-4 times more sensitive to radiation than the strain E coli B/r, the immediate effect of radiation on incorporation of a 1 min. pulse of ^{3}H thymidine into DNA is exactly the same for both strains (Cramp & Elgat 1972).

For many drugs we now know enough about biochemical modes of action to anticipate these problems. For example methotrexate inhibits the enzyme dihydrofolate reductase preventing reduction of folic acid to tetrahydrofolic acid. This in turn limits the conversion of deoxyuridylic acid to thymidylic acid, thereby blocking endogenous DNA synthesis. The incorporation of an exogenous source of the end product of thymidylate synthesis (e.g. ^{3}H thymidine (^{3}HTdR) into DNA will not necessarily be affected. This probably explains our own observation that although ^{125}iododeoxyuridine (^{125}IUdR) incorporation into cells in culture is inhibited by low doses of methotrexate, above 150 μgm/ml ^{125}IUdR incorporation increases again.

Other problems are not resolved so easily. Certain drugs, for example cyclophosphamide, have little or no cytotoxic action but are converted in vivo to highly toxic products (see previous paper by Phillips). If these drugs are to be used in vitro we must be able to imitate the in vivo biochemical conversions. Other drugs are known to disturb the cell cycle and Wells (personal communication) has recently suggested that vinblastine may be self-protecting in terms of its principle mode of action. Damage to DNA at higher doses most probably results in the cells spending an extended period in S phase, thus decreasing the number of cells at risk during a limited period of exposure to this drug. Some groups (Knock et al 1974), Dickson & Suzanger (in press) have overcome many biochemical problems fairly successfully by a multiparameter approach, studying several of the following:- incorporation of isotopically labelled thymidine, uridine and leucine; respiration, anaerabic glycolosis and succinic dehydrogenase inhibition in the same specimen.

Freshney et al (1975) have used HeLa cells to search for optimum times of drug treatment and recovery prior to assay. Their assay end point is the drug concentration (in μM) which reduces incorporation of ^{3}H leucine to 50% (I D 50). Results show that when the interval between drug treatment and assay is varied, as one might expect the ID 50 changes, but also that the <u>way</u> the ID 50 changes is very different for different drugs. Recent work with both HeLa cells and human glioma cells suggests that prolonged exposure to drug followed by prolonged recovery may be necessary to get a stable minimum ID 50 but other methods of analysis may also be possible. Most workers have

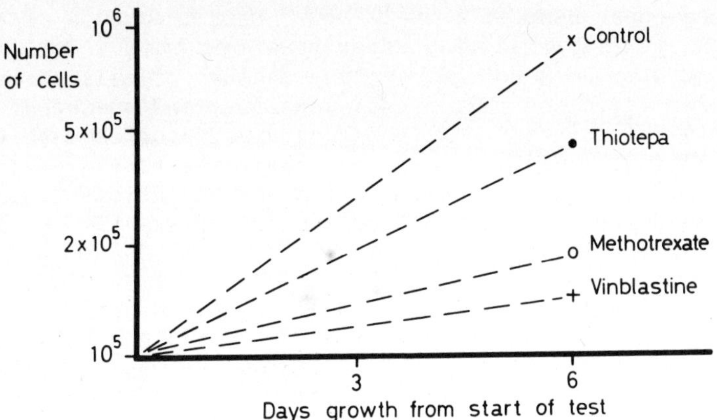

Fig. 1: Increase in cell numbers during 6 days growth for a culture from a solid biopsy of carcinoma of the stomach after one passage in vitro. Thiotepa 0.6 µg/ml, Methotrexate 0.1 µg/ml, Vinblastine 0.03 µg/ml (adapted from Wells et al. 1975).

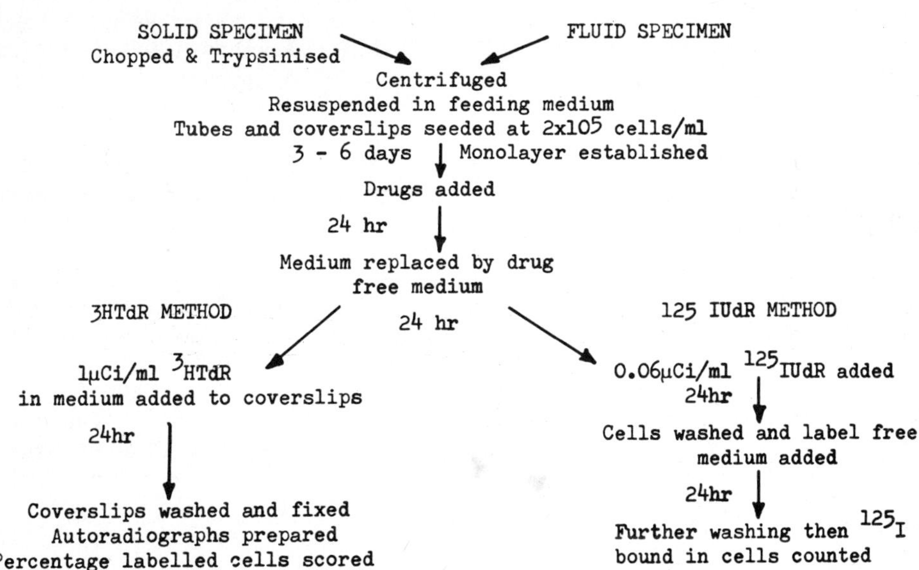

Fig. 2: Summary of two test procedures which measure the ability of cells to proceed through the DNA synthetic phase of the cell cycle after drug treatment.

therefore allowed at least a couple of days between treatment and assay. Several who grow monolayer cultures have studied the effect of different drugs by counting the number of cells present at different times after treatment (Berry et al 1975, Holmes & Little 1974, Lickiss et al 1974). Perhaps within the context of cancer management this is a more relevent parameter than reproductive integrity. I am grateful for permission to adapt results recently reported by Berry, Wells and Laing (1975) to illustrate a six day growth test (fig. 1.) A feature of the results, well illustrated here is that the increase in cell numbers over 6 days for the controls is quite low. (If the population doubled daily like HeLa cells the factor would be 64). This suggests either 1) the cell cycle time is long, 2) the percentage of cells cycling is low, 3) there are many cells lost from the glass surface, or 4) a combination of all three.

In experiments where the number of cells present at the end of a test is counted, it is important to distinguish between a true growth test where the increase in cell numbers due to cell division is compared for drug treated and untreated cells, and tests in which the major drug effect is to cause cell loss, usually by loss of attachment in the first instance. If the number of cells remaining after fixation is scored, "Drug A" which causes total mitotic inhibition and loss of cellular attachment is apparently more cytotoxic than "Drug B" which also causes total mitotic inhibition but no loss of cellular attachment. I think such a conclusion must be examined very carefully.

Our own tests are of intermediate duration. They are summarised in Fig. 2 and are designed to challenge the cells to proceed through the DNA synthetic phase after drug treatment and a suitable period of recovery. The cells studied are those which are still capable of cycling and we have shown by independent work that these cells have abnormal DNA values and are presumably malignant (Wright & Dendy in press).

^{3}HTdR labelling, autoradiography and microscopic examination is valuable because it permits examination of single cells. Thus the size and nature of the cells can be examined, anomalous labelling patterns noted and if a mexed cell population has grown, different cell types may be distinguishable. Table 1 shows good correlation between the thymidine labelling index and morphological appearance after treatment with triaziquone. For routine use the ^{125}IUdR method is preferable because it is quicker. 90% of our test reports are available by 12 days after receipt of a specimen.

HOW SHOULD DRUG CONCENTRATIONS BE CHOSEN FOR IN VITRO TESTS?

For drugs already being used to treat patients it now seems possible to interpolate from the *in vivo* dose, converting a therapeutic dose in mgm/kgm body weight to μgm/ml. For example if a daily dose of 10 mg methotrexate is uniformly distributed to the plasma of a 50 kg man containing 5 litres of blood, the equivalent concentration is about 4 μgm/ml medium. Exact methods of calculation differ from one group to another but Table 2 shows that there is general agreement on the in vitro doses that should be used for this work. Note also that when more than one dose is used, a factor of 10 is chosen.

Tumour Type	Control labelling index after 24 h ^{3}HTdR%	Labelled cells per 1000 after drug treatment / Labelled cells per 1000 in controls %	Morphological damage
Ovary	35	110	none
Melanoma	12	75	none
Breast	47	11	some
Ovary	37	6	some
Ovary	46	0	severe

TABLE 1 : Correlation of ^{3}HTdR results with morphological damage

Cultures from 5 different human tumour biopsies were treated with 10^{-2} μgm/ml triaziquone for 24 h and subsequently with ^{3}HTdR in accordance with the schedule in Fig. 2. Results show good correlation between reduction in the percentage of cells labelled with ^{3}HTdR and morphological damage.

	Drug concentration μgm/ml			
	5-FU	Vin B	Thiotepa	MTX
Dickson	25	2.5	6	4
Volm	15	-	-	1
Wheeler	15&1.5	0.1&0.01	1&0.1	-
Holmes	20	0.2	0.4	1
Lickiss	150-1.5	1.0-0.01	3-0.03	50-0.5
Berry	20&2	0.3&0.03	0.6&0.06	0.1&0.01

TABLE 2: Drug concentrations used in recent work on human tumour cells in short term culture.

Drug concentrations used by various workers in recent studies on human tumour biopsies. For a list of references see end of paper.

The use of at least two drug concentrations is highly desirable as the hypothetical dose reponse curves in Fig. 3. show. The curves can be expected to be approximately sigmoid with an overall shift to the left showing increased sensitivity, so if only one drug concentration is used and it is too high (conc. A) a quite appreciable difference in sensitivity may not be detected. With the limited material available, more detailed dose response curves will rarely be possible unless micro methods of culture can be developed. Experimental results on four different specimens treated with 5-fluorouracil are shown in Fig. 4. There is a factor of 30 between the drug concentrations required to cause 40% inhibition of ^{125}IUdR incorporation, and for one specimen, growth was actually stimulated by low doses of 5-fluorouracil.

When a large number of specimens from different patients have been tested against the same drug under the same experimental conditions, a histogram like Fig. 5. taken from our work can be drawn. There is a wide range of sensitivities for specimens from different patients. To check that this was not caused by uncontrolled variables in the experimental system, we tested cultures of human embryonic skin and muscle cells 7 times over a period of 7 weeks at a range of concentrations from 4×10^4 - 2×10^5 cells/ml. The results are superimposed as crosses on Fig. 5. They support the view that the *in vitro* test is showing real differences in the drug sensitivity of cells from different tumours. Now it is established that 5-fluorouracil is clinically useful against some tumours, so the whole rationale behind an in vitro predictive test depends on being able to say that patients whose values fall well to the left on the histogram (sensitive cells) will derive benefit from 5-fluorouracil therapy, while those whose values fall well to the right will not.

For new drugs, the clinical value of which has not yet been clearly established, it is more difficult to decide the level of in vitro response that will justify use of the drug clinically.

CLINICAL SITUATION

The requirements of the clinician are rarely compatible with those of the scientist. The scientist will study a few carefully selected specimens, often chosen because they provide a well behaved laboratory system. He will study in detail growth requirements, parameters of the cell cycle and the effects of one or at the most two drugs. A wide range of drug concentrations will be used and the cells may be tested in rapidly growing and overcrowded (plateau) phases. There is no particular urgency to produce an answer.

Although these studies are essential and in the long term will improve the value of predictive tests, they are often no use to the clinician who would like a quick answer to the effects of as many different drugs as possible on as many different specimens as possible.

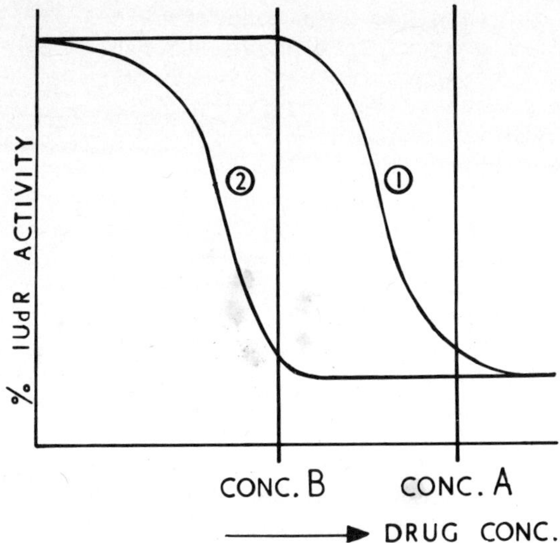

FIGURE 3: Hypothetical curves showing response, measured by ^{125}IUdR uptake, of sensitive and resistant specimens of different drug concentrations.

This information may seem very superficial to the scientist who may feel that time spent obtaining it is wasted. However the ultimate purpose is to improve the treatment of patients and I believe very strongly that within the limitations of ethical considerations we must be continually putting our data to the clinical test.

A retrospective survey of the work done in Cambridge from 1968-71 has already been made (Wheeler et al 1974). Patients were selected on well defined physical criteria and the essential details are:-

(a) At the time of test all patients had at least 100 ml free fluid (pleural or ascitic)
(b) Malignancy was confirmed by independent histology.
(c) The tissue culture test was successful.
(d) The patients received a course of chemotherapy.
(e) The patients survived at least 3 months.

For group A treatment followed the test closely. For group B treatment did not follow the test predictions. Results showed that at one year 22/32 patients in group A but only 9/31 in group B were alive, figures which are significantly in favour of group A ($p = 0.004$). This suggests that the tissue culture test does indicate the drugs that will bring the tumour under control most effectively. Because of the poor selectivity of existing drugs

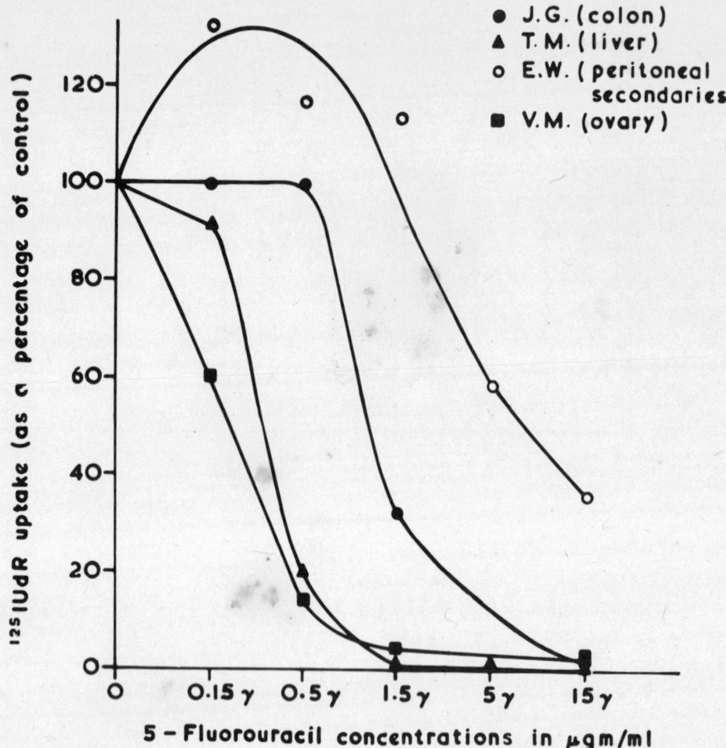

FIGURE 4 : Inhibition of incorporation of ^{125}IUdR into four human tumour biopsies in short term culture by a 24 h exposure to various concentrations of 5-fluorouracil.

for tumour cells this control cannot be maintained, probably due to the development of resistant cells, and the test will not influence cure rates for disseminated solid tumours until better drugs are available. Some improvement is evident and many patients may have been spared the unpleasant side effects of drugs to which their tumour cells were resistant so it is important to decide if and/or how clinical trials of this type should be planned in the future.

CONCLUSION

There are many difficulties associated with the use of human tumour biopsy specimens for experimental work. Certain culture procedures may select only one cell type from the biopsy population, other methods may not take account of the heterogeneity from one part of the tumour to another. The proportion of cells in cycle may change and cell cycle parameters, particularly the duration

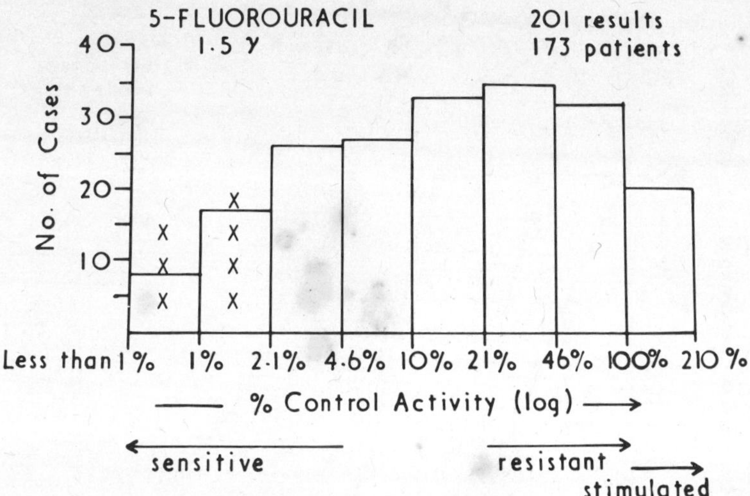

Figure 5: Histogram showing the effect of 1.5 μg/ml 5-fluorouracil on cultures prepared from 201 human tumour biopsies. x axis, ^{125}IUdR uptake as a percentage of control; y axis, number of cultures. The crosses show results for cultures of human embryonic skin and muscle cells tested in the same way on various occasions.

of S-phase may be different in culture. No detailed studies have yet been made of the effects of overcrowding on cells in short term culture. Above all, consistent reproducible results are hampered by the limited supply of material.

When the effects of drugs in this system are investigated, consideration must be given to the optimum duration of drug treatment, drug stability, and host tissue drug sensitivity as well as the factors discussed in this paper. However, it is generally accepted that loss of remission and failure to cure with chemotherapy is due to drug resistance at the cellular level. With some improvements, existing methods should be capable of indicating unsuitable drugs for a particular patient because of exceptional cellular resistance. Much more work may be required before optimum therapy can be selected in this way.

REFERENCES

1. Berry, R.J., Laing, A.H., & Wells, J. Fresh explant culture of human tumours in vitro and the assessment of sensitivity to cytotoxic chemotherapy. Br. J. Cancer (1975) 31, 218.

2. Cramp, W.A. & Elgat, M. The effects of ionizing radiations on thymidine uptake into Escherichia Coli B/r and BS-1. Rad. Res. (1972) 51, 121.

3. Dendy, P.P. (editor) Human Tumours in Short term culture - techniques and clinical applications (Acad. Press to be published 1975).

4. Dickson, J.A. & Suzanger, M. In Vitro sensitivity testing of human tumour slices to chemotherapeutic agents - its place in cancer therapy in "Human tumo tumours in short term culture - techniques and clinical application". Ed. Dendy P.P. Acad. Press (in press).

5. Freshney, R.I., Paul, J. & Kane, I.M. Assays of anti-cancer drugs in tissue culture; conditions affecting their ability to incorporate 3H leucine after drug treatment. Br. J. Cancer (1975) 31, 89.

6. Holmes, H.L. & Little, J.M. Tissue culture micotest for predicting response of human cancer to chemotherapy. Lancet Oct 26 (1974) p. 985.

7. Knock, F.E., Galt, R.M., Oester, Y.T. & Sylvester R. In Vitro estimate of sensitivity of individual human tumours to antitumour agents. Oncology (1974) 30, 1.

8. Lickiss, J.N., Cane K.A. & Baikie, A.G. In vitro drug selection in antineoplastic chemotherapy. Europ. J. Cancer (1974) 10, 809.

9. Tanneberger, S. & Bacigalupo, G. Eininge Erfahrungen mit der individuellen zytostatischen Behandlung maligner Tumoren nach prätherapeutischer Zytostatika. Sensibilitäts - Prüfung in vitro (Onkobiogramm) Arch. Geschwulstforsch (1970) 35, 44.

10. Volm., Kaufmann, M., Wayss, K., Goerttler, Kl. & Mattern, J. Gezielte Tumour - Chemotherapie durch Onkobiogramme (Aimed tumour chemotherapy using oncobiogram) Dtsch med. Wschr. (1974) 99, 38.

11. Wheeler, T.K., Dendy, P.P., Dawson, Anne. Assessment of an in vitro screening test of cytotoxic agents in the treatment of advanced malignant disease. Oncology (1974) 30, 362.

12. Wright, J.E.M. & Dendy, P.P. Identification of abnormal cells in short term monolayer cultures of human tumour specimens Acta Cytologica (in press).

COMBINATION OF CORYNEBACTERIUM PARVUM AND CYTOSTATIC DRUGS IN DISSEMINATED HUMAN CANCERS

Lucien ISRAEL and Alain DEPIERRE

Centre Hospitalier Universitaire Lariboisière

2, rue Ambroise Paré. PARIS. FRANCE

It is now known that C. parvum is a very potent experimental immunopotentiator that can increase macrophage production, increase phagocytosis and activation of macrophages, and activate the alternate pathway of complement. It also induces lymphocyte trapping and increases antibody production against both T-cell dependent and T-cell independent antigens, whereas it decreases GVH reactions and, in certain conditions, PHA transformation. C. parvum has also been shown to increase the production of colony stimulating factor. These properties explain why C. parvum has shown potent antitumor activity in a variety of animal systems, including T-cell deprived mice and has shown also synergism with cytostatic agents when applied to disseminated tumors.

We will summarize here our clinical findings and the concepts that can be derived from our studies - which started in 1967 and include at the time of this congress (July 1975) more than 600 patients, treated with Pasteur C. parvum until 1972 and with Merieux C. parvum since 1973.

I - SURVIVAL OF PATIENTS RECEIVING C. PARVUM AND CHEMOTHERAPY AS COMPARED TO CHEMOTHERAPY ALONE

Four randomized studies have been completed thus far and their results published (1) (2) (3). In all of these studies patients with disseminated cancers (miscellaneous in the first trial, then separately oat cell bronchial carcinomas, epidermoid bronchial carcinomas and breast cancers) were allocated at random to one group receiving a combination chemotherapy every two weeks and a group receiving the same chemotherapy plus C. parvum weekly, 4 mg per subcutaneous route. Our protocols call for a discontinuation of chemotherapy under 4000 white cells per cubic millimeter and a resumption after these counts were again reached.

The results of the four studies were unequivocal. The survival was generally twice as long for patients receiving C. parvum as it was for those treated by chemotherapy alone (p ranging from 0.05 to 0.0001 according to the study considered and at various time intervals). It must be noted that the response rates to chemotherapy were only slightly increased. The main difference was in terms of duration of response - which was very significantly increased in patients receiving C. parvum and accounted for the global difference seen between the two arms, where responders and non responders were mixed.

It must be noted also that these results were similar in the four studies, with no evidence of a difference with respect respect to cell type or site of cancer.

II - THE ROLE OF IMMUNE COMPETENCE AT START OF THERAPY

When these studies were initiated, the only test performed before therapy started was a PPD skin test, which showed a variable proportion, according to study, of responders. It is noteworthy that in all these studies, patients with a positive pretherapeutic test had a much longer survival than those with a negative skin test ($p < 0.01$). It was seen that negative controls had the worst prognosis, that positive controls did slightly better than negative patients receiving C. parvum and that positive patients receiving C. parvum were by far the best group in terms of survival.

III - C. PARVUM, TOLERANCE TO CHEMOTHERAPY AND RESISTANCE AGAINST INFECTIONS

All our studies showed that patients on C. parvum had significantly less periods of leukopaenia, a finding that is in accordance with the role of C. parvum on bone marrow colony formation. Less than half the interruptions of cytostatic agents, were seen in patients receiving C. parvum (which was continued during leucopoenia) and the delay of recovery was shortened.

Concomitantly infections - microbial or viral - were much less frequent in these patients as they were in patients receiving chemotherapy alone and their general condition was certainly better, although this is a very subjective parameter.

One of the consequences of these phenomena was that patients on C. parvum could receive more chemotherapy during the course of the disease than controls. As we have already seen, this did not result in increased response rates - which is not a surprise since we have shown that responses, whenever they are registered, are seen after two or at most three courses of chemotherapy - but this resulted in maintenance of occuring responses for a much longer period of time. It is difficult to separate this role of C. parvum from its autonomous role as an antitumor immunopotentiator, under the conditions of these trials, and it may well be that the protection of patients against some deleterious effects of chemotherapy is of a major importance in our results.

IV - C. PARVUM AND IMMUNE PARAMETERS

The in vitro immune parameters that we have investigated included T and B cell rosettes, PHA and Con A stimulation, total complement and C_3 levels, and immunoglobulin levels. None, except C_3 were found to be modified by the use of C. parvum. In many, but not all patients, levels of C_3 were significantly lowered, which might be explained by the activation of the alternate pathway, as seen in animals.

The skin tests applied at 2 month intervals during the treatment showed a variety of changes that led us to distinguish two types of non specific immunodeficiency in these patients : the first is due to the use of chemotherapeutic agents and is mainly a quantitative one. It can be counteracted and even reversed by the use of C. parvum, which is consistent with the fact that patients on C. parvum experience less leukopaenia than controls. The second is due to the progression of the tumor and is mainly qualitative. With or without chemotherapy, patients whose tumor progress show a progressive loss of immune competence. This cannot be counteracted by C. parvum, and neither - in our experience - by other immunopotentiators. In this respect it appears that, under the special conditions of the studies reported here, the main role of C. parvum was to protect the immune competence of the host, in responders to chemotherapy, presumably by increasing the production of immune competent cells.

V - CONCLUSION

We have restricted ourselves here to the role of C. parvum in conjunction with chemotherapy - a situation that has been also explored experimentally by Fisher, by Pearson and by Chirigos among others. It is clear from our results that :

1. Non specific immuno stimulation and chemotherapy given together are not detrimental to the host but on the contrary they are synergistic. It may be that under some experimental conditions pretreatment with one agent may induce adverse effects, but in patients with cancers already disseminated the reverse is true. C. parvum and cytostatic agents act in a synergistic way. Chemotherapy, given in greater quantities, kills more tumor cells and immunotherapy protects the host against leukopaenia infections and loss of immune competence, allowing thus the patients to receive more cytostatic drugs.

2. Non specific immuno stimulation has a role to play in disseminated disease - at least when combined with chemotherapy - a concept which is also gaining momentum from our studies with C. parvum IV daily as a single agent (4).

But it must be stated that the best dose, the best route, and the best timing with respect to chemotherapy are not yet known. It will be the task of large cooperative studies - to provide answers to these crucial questions.

REFERENCES

1. ISRAEL L. et HALPERN B. : Le corynebacterium dans les cancers avancés. - N. Presse Méd. 1972, 1, 19-23.

2. ISRAEL L. : A randomized study of chemotherapy versus chemotherapy and immune therapy with corynebacterium parvum in advanced breast cancer. - in : Conferences, Symposium, Workshops of the XIth International Cancer Congress. Vol. I. 222-223. 1974. Florence. Ambrosiana Milano Ed.

3. ISRAEL L. : Non specific immuno-stimulation in bronchogenic cancer. - Scand. J. Resp. Dis. Suppl. 89, 95-105,1974.

4. ISRAEL L., EDELSTEIN R., DEPIERRE A. and DIMITROV N. : Brief communication : Daily intravenous infusions of corynebacterium parvum in twenty patients with disseminated cancer : A preliminary report of clinical and biologic findings. - Journal of the National Cancer Institute, 1975, (in press).

RADIOTHERAPY AND CHEMOTHERAPY IN ACUTE LEUKAEMIA RELATED TO FATAL INFECTION DURING REMISSION

I.C.M. MacLENNAN on behalf of the British Medical Research Council's Working Party* on Leukaemia in Childhood

Nuffield Department of Clinical Medicine
Radcliffe Infirmary, OXFORD OX2 6HE. England

There has been steady improvement in the survival of patients with acute lymphoblastic leukaemia over the past twenty years. This has mainly been due to the use of multiple drug maintenance chemotherapy given over a prolonged period and effective prevention of central nervous system (CNS) relapse. Pinkel and his group in Memphis made the break-through in prophylaxis against CNS leukaemia by the introduction of cranio-spinal irradiation(Pinkel et al, 1971). Subsequently, the British Medical Research Council carried out a trial of CNS irradiation (UKALL I) and confirmed the Memphis observations (MRC Leukaemia Committee Report, 1973). In this trial only one out of 75 patients who received CNS prophylaxis relapsed from CNS leukaemia while 26 out of 80 patients in the control group developed this complication. There was, however, a price to pay for this prophylactic treatment in that five of the CNS irradiation group died in complete remission while no remission deaths occurred in the non-irradiated group.

The most striking haematological difference between the two groups was seen in lymphocyte count(Campbell et al, 1973). The

---

*The Members of the Working Party are as follows: Professor J.M. Hutchinson(Chairman), Professor R.M.Hardisty(Secretary), Dr.K.D. Bagshawe,Dr.J.M.Bridges, Professor Neville Butler, Dr.J.M.Chessells Dr.P.F.Deasy, Sir Richard Doll, Dr.P.M.Emerson, Dr.H.W.Everley Jones, Dr.D.I.K.Evans, Dr.D.M.J.Gairdner, Dr.D.A.G.Galton, Dr.R.J. Guyer, Dr.C.B.Howarth, Dr.E.M.Innes, Dr.P.Morris Jones, Dr.H.E.M. Kay, Dr.T.J.McElwain, Dr.I.C.M.MacLennan, Dr.J.Martin, Professor I.C.S.Normand, Mr.P.G. Smith, Dr.J.Stuart, Dr.E.W.Thompson, Dr. M.L.N. Willoughby.

irradiation group consistently had in the region of 800 fewer peripheral blood lymphocytes per cubic millimetre than the control group. It is interesting that the fluctuations in lymphocyte count with chemotherapy seen in both groups was quantitively similar. This would appear to indicate that the lymphocytes lost, in the long term, after irradiation are different from those temporarily lost as the result of Methotrexate and 6 Mercaptopurine therapy. We have analysed the nature of lymphocytes lost in these two groups of patients (Campbell et al, 1973). This analysis showed that the difference between the irradiated and non-irradiated groups was mainly attributable to loss of PHA responsive cells following irradiation. On the other hand, the chemotherapy reduced K cell numbers but also affected some PHA responsive lymphocytes.

It would be tempting to conclude that the deaths in remission in the irradiated groups in UKALL I were attributable to lymphopenia. However, analysis of individual deaths showed that four out of the five deaths were likely to have been caused by pyogenic infection. Three of these cases had observed associated profound neutropenia at the time of death while no haematological data were available in the fourth case. When the degree of neutropenia was assessed in the irradiated and non-irradiated groups by plotting the proportion of patients with counts below 1000/μl more neutropenia was seen in 16 out of the 18 weeks after methotrexate courses in the patients who had had CNS irradiation. This difference was highly significant (MRC Working Party Report 1975a).

The importance of drug timing in relation to immunosuppression and myelosuppression is well demonstrated by comparing neutrophil and lymphocyte counts in the UKALL I trial, which we have been discussing, with those in the second UKALL trial, UKALL II. UKALL II maintenance chemotherapy was similar to that in use in UKALL I in that twelve week cycles of maintenance chemotherapy were given in both trials. Both protocols contained three five day courses of methotrexate and a reinduction period of prednisolone and vincristine. Again in both trials the rest of the course was given up to treatment with 6 Mercaptopurine. The main difference in the maintenance was that in UKALL I the methotrexate courses were given at the beginning of the cycle and were spaced by nine day gaps whereas in UKALL II the three methotrexate courses were evenly distributed throughout the cycle. In UKALL I the 6MP was given for four weeks after the courses of methotrexate, whereas in UKALL II it was spaced between the courses of methotrexate. Also in UKALL II the maximum period without treatment was only two days as opposed to nine days in UKALL I. The neutropenia of UKALL I was largely avoided in UKALL II. On the other hand the more continuous therapy of UKALL II was associated with prolonged lymphopenia(MRC Working Party Report, 1975b). It may be that the wider spacing of methotrexate courses interspersed with 6MP in UKALL II meant that the next course of methotrexate was given during a time of recovery of the myeloid progenitors when an accelerated growth phase was occurring. Vogler and his colleagues (1973) analysed methotrexate toxicity to the myeloid system in mice and showed that a second course of methotrexate given soon after the first and during the period of maximum myeloid recovery was considerably more myelotoxic than one given when the bone marrow had returned to quiescence. Analysis of deaths in UKALL II have again shown some correlation with the haematological findings. In this trial only one out of the eight remission deaths was associated with pyogenic infection and neutropenia. Four were clearly associated with viral infection and profound lymphopenia. Two further cases may have been associated with viral infections and the eighth death occurred during prednisolone therapy and was caused by perforation of the stomach. Although the number of remission deaths in these two trials are fortunately too small to allow certain correlations to be made between neutropenia, lymphopenia and the type of death which occurred there is a strong suggestion that the major toxic complication of UKALL I chemotherapy was neutropenia with associated pyogenic infection whereas in UKALL II lymphopenia was far more serious and this was associated with viral infection. These data then indicate that relatively minor alterations in the timing of drug therapy in the maintenance period for acute leukaemia can markedly alter the extent and type of toxic side effects.

In the UKALL III trial a further example has occurred which shows that small changes in chemotherapy schedules can make profound differences to the incidence and type of remission deaths. In this trial induction therapy was similar to that in UKALL II. The main differences in the schedules occurred in the three weeks immediately after CNS irradiation, where in UKALL III weekly doses of methotrexate were given with continuous 6MP. At the equivalent time in UKALL II reinduction with prednisolone and vincristine was given. In UKALL III, eight remission deaths occurred in the immediate post-irradiation period. It seems very likely that these were attributable to the methotrexate and 6MP given in the three weeks following irradiation as no remission deaths occurred at this stage in UKALL II, when a similar number of patients were at risk. This conclusion is confirmed by the fact that since finding that these early remission deaths were occurring, the UKALL III post-irradiation schedule was altered to give prednisolone and vincristine in place of the methotrexate and 6MP. No further deaths at this period have occurred although the maintenance schedule of UKALL III continues to be continuous 6MP and weekly methotrexate starting three weeks after irradiation. Analysis of deaths occurring after the induction of remission and during the first year of remission in UKALL III before the modification described above, has shown that more patients died in complete remission than succumbed to leukaemia following relapse. This was not the case in UKALL I and UKALL II where the majority of deaths in the first year were following relapse. However, if one divides the patients with acute lymphoblastic leukaemia into good and poor prognostic groups on the basis of presenting white cell count and age, then the patients with the more favourable prognosis are very much more likely to die in complete remission than those with a poor prognosis. Sixty three per cent of the patients in UKALL I and UKALL II presented with white cell counts below 20,000/μl and were under the age of 13. In this good prognosis group 26 deaths occurred in patients who had achieved remission before 85 weeks. Nearly 40% of these were in complete remission. On the other hand in the poor prognosis group of 57 deaths in patients who had achieved remission only one occurred during remission. These data indicate that intensification of the treatment schedules in the good prognosis group must be made with great caution as the danger of causing more deaths from the treatment than from the disease is considerable. On the other hand in patients with known poor prognosis there is considerable justification for attempting more aggressive chemotherapy.

In conclusion it seems to us that careful analysis of simple haematological parameters offers a powerful tool which has often been overlooked for the analysis of cancer therapy. The data shown here clearly indicate that it is dangerous to generalise about the immunosuppressive and myelosuppressive action of a single drug out of the context of the whole treatment, for the same combination of drugs given with different timing can have markedly different effects. On the other hand, these data indicate that there is a considerable chance that careful manipulation of drug schedules can reduce toxic complications without losing anti-leukaemic effect.

REFERENCES

CAMPBELL, A.C. et al (1973). British Medical Journal 2, 385.

MEDICAL RESEARCH COUNCIL(1973). British Medical Journal 2, 381.

MEDICAL RESEARCH COUNCIL WORKING PARTY REPORT (1975a) British Medical Journal (In Press).

MEDICAL RESEARCH COUNCIL WORKING PARTY REPORT (1975b) Submitted.

PINKEL, D. et al (1971). Cancer 27. 247.

VOGLER, W.R. et al (1973). Cancer Research 33, 1628.

THE TARGET CELL OF IMMUNOSUPPRESSIVE AGENTS

Jean Francois Bach

Hopital Necker

161 rue de Serves, Paris

The four classes of immunosuppressive agents which are most widely used clinically are thiopurines (6-mercaptopurine, azathioprine), alkylating agents (cyclophosphamide, chlorambucil), corticosteroids and antilymphocyte serum. Their effects differ very much from one another and these differences in activity are probably related to differences in target cells.

Thiopurines seem to act preferentially on T-cells at least at the relatively low doses given to man. The main arguments in favour of such a selective action on T-cells are (1) their particular action on T-cell mediated immune responses such as the mixed lymphocyte reaction, cell-mediated lympholysis, organ graft rejection and delayed hypersensitivity reactions with much less effect, if any, on humoral antibody formation; (2) the selective inhibition of T-rosette forming cells by azathioprine and the loss of azathioprine sensitivity after thymectomy; (3) the favourable action on T-cell mediated experimental allergic disease such as experimental allergic encephalomyelitis or thyroiditis contrasting with the absence of clear effect on the autoimmune disease of NZB mice which associates T-cell functions depression and B cell hyperactivity, and lastly (4) the preferential promotion of T-cell dependent viral infections and relatively little promotion of B-cell dependent bacterial infections.

Alkylating agents act on B cells rather than on T-cells at least at high dosage. This is mainly suggested by (1) the decrease in the percentage of theta bearing cells (T-cells) in mice given one single injection of 300 mg/kg cyclophosphamide; (2) the atrophy of the bursa of Fabricius of chicks given cyclophosphamide in ovo; (3) their remarkable action on antibody production contrasting with the modest effect on delayed hypersensitivity reactions; and (4) the suppressive effect of cyclophosphamide on the autoimmune disease of NZB mice. However chronic treatment with cyclophosphamide may alter T-cell mediated immune reactions and PHA responsiveness is, (for example), depressed in cyclophosphamide treated patients. The point remains however that alkylating agents act both on B- and T-cells and eventually according to the schedules of administration employed, better on B-cells than on T-cells.

Corticosteroids have complex effects on mononuclear cells. Paradoxically, they have little action on T-cells although they induce thymus lysis in the mouse. The only well documented action on T-cells is on Cytotoxic cells at the effector phase of cell-mediated immune reactions. This action may have some importance in transplantation and tumour immunity. The corticosteroid effects on B-cells are not great either, except perhaps at the level of the progenitor of antibody-forming cells. The main action of steroids on immune responses might well be on phagocytes: they depress significantly monocyte production and alter some *in vitro* and *in vivo* phagocyte function including their susceptibility to T-cell mediators such as MIF or MAF.

Antilymphocyte sera are not widely used clinically any more. They are however the most potent depressor of T-cell function in the mouse, prolonging, for example, nearly indefinitely skin allograft survival. Their selective action on T-cells is assessed by the decrease in the number of theta positive cells and the depletion of thymus dependent areas of lymph nodes and spleen induced by short-term treatments. It is corroborated by the synergistic effects of ALS and adult thymectomy.

REFERENCES

All references will be found in: Bach J.F. (1975). The mode of action of immunosuppressive agents. North Holland-American Elsevier, Vol. 41. Amsterdam, New York, 379P.

IMMUNOLOGICAL ASPECTS OF ANTI-CANCER DRUGS

D.A.L.Davies

Searle Research Laboratories

Lane End Road, High Wycombe, Bucks, England

Drugs used in various combinations, have had considerable influence in cancer therapy but, unless improved products appear, they are not likely, alone to be capable of controlling the disease. Immunological methods have, so far, made little impact on cancer therapy although tumour specific antigens provide a difference between normal and neoplastic cells which should be taken advantage of. Encouragement of active immunity in cancer suffers from the disadvantage of being imposed upon an immunologically depressed state, normally encountered in cancer and increased by the use of drugs which are frequently immunosuppressive in themselves. We are using passive immunity, for example animals are immunised against human tumours and the sera absorbed to remove anti-human and to leave anti-tumour antibodies. These we use to attach drugs to "home" to the tumour site. Various claims have been made for such an effect, but no therapeutic agent has emerged. Following work in mouse models, such drugged antibodies now exist and will be discussed elsewhere at this meeting. In the meantime we also have a synergism between drugs and antibodies which will be illustrated by mouse data. These systems are being tested clinically with encouraging results.

List of Contributors

Adams, G.E.
Anderson, T.

Bach, J.F.
Bachur, N.R.
Brock, N.
Bull, J.

Calliauw, L.
Cleare, M.J.
Cox, P.J.

Davies, D.A.L.
Dendy, P.P.
Denekamp, J.
Depierre, A.
Double, J.A.
Dowsett, M.

Easty, D.M.
Easty, G.C.

Foster, J.L.
Fowler, J.F.
Fox, M.
Frei, E. III
Fuska, J.
Fuskova, A.

Garfield, J.
Garner, R.C.
Gause, G.F.
Goldie, J.H.
Goldin, A.
Gregoriadis, G.

Hanka, L.J.
Hansen, H.S.
Hellmann, K.
Hill, B.T.

Israel, L.
Ivanickaja, L.

Jaspan, T.
Jordan, V.C.

Levin, V.A.
Loo, T.L.

MacLennan, I.C.M.
Martin, D.G.
McMenamin, M.G.
Mihich, E.
Moertel, C.G.

Neil, G.L.
Neville, A.M.
Norpoth, K.

Phillips, B.J.
Povlsen, C.O.
Powles, T.J.
Price, L.A.

Ryall, R.D.H.
Rygard, J.

Sadee, W.
Schein, P.S.
Schmahl, D.

Schmidt, C.G.
Schutt, A.J.
Scott, D.
Sykes, J.A.C.

Tattersall, W.H.N.
Tisdale, M.J.

Umezawa, H.

Venditti, J.M.
Vesely, P.

Walker, M.D.
Wiley, P.F.
Willson, R.L.
Wilson, C.B.
Wolpert-Defilippes, M.K.